AGING MEDICINE

Robert J. Pignolo, MD, PhD; Mary Ann Forciea, MD;
Jerry C. Johnson, MD, Series Editors

For further volumes:
http://www.springer.com/series/7622

David R. Thomas • Gregory A. Compton
Editors

Pressure Ulcers
in the Aging Population

A Guide for Clinicians

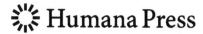 Humana Press

Editors
David R. Thomas, MD
Division of Geriatric Medicine
Saint Louis University
Saint Louis, MO, USA

Gregory A. Compton, MD, CMD
Geriatric Medicine and Palliative Care
Wound Care Consultant
Hospice Care of South Carolina
Johns Island, SC, USA

ISBN 978-1-4939-6316-4   ISBN 978-1-62703-700-6 (eBook)
DOI 10.1007/978-1-62703-700-6
Springer New York Heidelberg Dordrecht London

Humana Press is a brand of Springer
Springer is part of Springer Science+Business Media (www.springer.com)

Drs. Thomas and Compton would like to dedicate this book to their ever-patient wives, Janice and Bonnie, respectively, who support them in their lifelong learning and pursuit of excellence in geriatric care. Many a long days were spent in putting this project together.

Preface

The Pressure ulcer volume is a welcome addition to the Springer Aging Medicine Series. It is written for the nursing and medical generalist, student, or practitioner. It is a collection of scholarly review articles written by respected active wound care clinicians and teachers. One additional aim is to be a reference for medical and surgical trainees caring for older adults in all settings.

The subjects range from basic biology of skin and the cellular response of injured tissue to wound assessment, prevention, and treatment. The role of nutrition and bacterial colonization augments the sections on specific medical and surgical treatment. A chapter is devoted to palliation and skin as an organ failure. Legal issues are addressed in an afterword.

Much has been learned about the causes, prevention, and treatment of pressure ulcers since the publication of *Pressure Ulcers in America: Prevalence, Incidence and Implications for the Future by the NPUAP* in 2001. In 1989 the prevalence of pressure ulcers in all groups in all settings varied from 3 % to as high as 25 %. More recent data from larger, multisite studies show a gradual downward trend in prevalence from 2004 to 2009. It is too early to say, based on the data, that the trend is significant. Overall the current prevalence rate of 12–16 % did not meet the Healthy People 2010 Objective 1–16 to reduce the prevalence of pressure ulcers in nursing homes by 50 %.

One explanation for not significantly reducing pressure ulcer prevalence over the last decade is case-mix. The elderly experience the vast majority of the pressure ulcers in the USA. Prevalence numbers are more difficult to impact than incidence rates because of ongoing technical advancements in treatment that is based on better understanding of the mechanisms of healing and its impediments. The pressure ulcer patient is sicker and living longer. The typical elderly inpatient or nursing home resident is older and has multiple comorbidities, hence the emphasis of this treatise on the aging population.

To the extent that consensus exists, best practices are identified in this volume. Several of the contributors have spent their careers teaching and advancing excellence in geriatric wound care.

The book's scope is purposely narrow, pressure ulcers in the elderly, so to provide in-depth coverage of the subject. It covers the entire range of care from prevention and assessment to surgical care. It exposes the reader to newer concepts such as deep tissue injury and differentiating heavy bacterial wound colonization from infection. The editors' intention is to provide focused knowledge to allow the generalist to be more involved in the care of pressure ulcer patients. Pressure ulcers are one of the major geriatric syndromes that all primary providers need to address. The training of most generalists involves little or no wound care exposure. This volume is designed to bridge that gap.

Saint Louis, MO, USA   David R. Thomas
Johns Island, SC, USA   Gregory A. Compton

Contents

Contributors

Barbara M. Bates-Jensen RN, PhD Associate Professor, School of Nursing & David Geffen School of Medicine, University of California, Los Angeles, USA

Dan Berlowitz MD, MPH Bedford VA Hospital, Bedford, MA, USA

Janet Cheng RN, MSN, MPH School of Nursing, University of California, Los Angeles, USA

Gregory A. Compton MD, CMD Geriatric Medicine and Palliative Care, Wound Care Consultant, Hospice Care of South Carolina, Johns Island, SC, USA

Kim W. House MD, CMD Department of Medicine, Atlanta VA Medical Center/ Emory University, Decatur, GA, USA

Theodore M. Johnson MD, MPH Department of Medicine, Atlanta VA Medical Center/Emory University, Decatur, GA, USA

Dean P. Kane MD, FACS Baltimore, MD, USA

Jan Kottner Department of Dermatology and Allergy, Clinical Research Center for Hair and Skin Science, Charité-Universitätsmedizin Berlin, Berlin, Germany

Diane L. Krasner PhD, RN, CWCN, CWS, MAPWCA, FAAN Wound and Skin Care Consultant, York, PA, USA

Kathrin Raeder Department of Nursing Science, Charité Universitätsmedizin Berlin, Berlin, Germany

R. Gary Sibbald BSc, MD, FRCPC (Med, Derm), MACP, FAAD, Med, MAPWCA Dermatology Clinic, Ontario, Canada

David R. Thomas MD, FACP, AGSF, GSAF Division of Geriatric Medicine, Saint Louis University Health Sciences Center, Saint Louis, MO, USA

Kevin Y. Woo PhD, RN, FAPWCA School of Nursing, Queen's University, Kingston, ON, Canada

West Park Health Center, Toronto, ON, Canada

Chapter 1
The Biology of Wound Healing

Gregory A. Compton and David R. Thomas

Abstract The skin is the largest organ in the human body. It receives 5–10 % of the cardiac output. Pressure ulcers, rare in the general patient population, are a common chronic skin disorder in the neurologically impaired and the frail elderly. Recognition and treatment initially falls to the generalist nurse and physician. Dermatologists are usually not involved in pressure ulcer care. At times nurse specialists and surgeons are called as consultants.

A basic knowledge of skin anatomy and wound healing physiology is imperative to optimal treatment of chronic wounds. The skin is more than a passive barrier that heals itself. Wound healing is a complex highly orchestrated interaction of cells and cellular mediators operating in the extracellular matrix.

This chapter outlines normal skin anatomy and function as a foundation to build an understanding of normal and impaired wound healing physiology. The concepts outlined can be applied to healing in all acute and chronic wounds. Special emphasis is placed on age-related skin changes and wound healing. Abnormalities of and delays in healing in older patients with chronic wounds are covered. The chapter is an introduction to many of the concepts covered in the volume.

Keywords Pressure Ulcer • Skin • Skin anatomy • Wounds • Wound healing

G.A. Compton, M.D., C.M.D. (✉)
Geriatric Medicine and Palliative Care, Wound Care Consultant, Hospice Care of South Carolina, 2948 Seabrook Island Road, Johns Island, SC 29455, USA
e-mail: gacompton@comcast.net

D.R. Thomas, M.D., F.A.C.P., A.G.S.F., G.S.A.F.
Division of Geriatric Medicine, Saint Louis University, 1402 South Grand Blvd. M238, Saint Louis, MO 63104, USA

D.R. Thomas and G.A. Compton (eds.), *Pressure Ulcers in the Aging Population:*
A Guide for Clinicians, Aging Medicine 1, DOI 10.1007/978-1-62703-700-6_1,
© Springer Science+Business Media New York 2014

Basic Skin Anatomy

The Epidermis

The outermost layer of the skin is the epidermis. The epidermis is composed primarily of cells and is between 50 and 150 μm thick. The layer contains three cell types: keratinocytes, melanocytes, and Langerhans cells (sentinel dendritic cells). The most abundant epidermal cell type is the keratinocyte (approximately 90 % of cells). The keratinocyte begins as a stem cell attached to the basement membrane. Keratinocytes are roughly divided into four layers: basal (stratum germinativum), spinous (stratum spinosum), granular (stratum granulosum), and cornified (stratum corneum) keratinocytes [1].

Basal keratinocytes differentiate and migrate to the surface to become the stratum corneum over 2 weeks. They reside in the stratum corneum for another 2 weeks before sloughing off. The surface-differentiated keratinocytes act as a semipermeable membrane and a physical barrier [2]. The melanocytes protect the skin from UV radiation and the Langerhans cells have an important immunologic role.

Multiple factors control keratinocyte proliferation, differentiation, and apoptosis-like cornification, including growth factors, neuropeptides, adrenergic and cholinergic signaling, calcium, and cell–cell and cell–matrix interactions [1].

The Dermis

The dermis is the highly vascularized skin layer below the epidermis that provides structure and nutritional support. The dermis varies in thickness from 0.3 mm on the eyelid to 3.0 mm on the back. It contains three types of connective tissue: collagen, elastic tissue, and reticular fibers. The relatively few cells within the dermis are interspersed in an extracellular matrix that is composed mainly of collagen, approximately 72 % of the dry weight. There are currently 21 recognized "types" of cutaneous collagen. Type I and type III collagen are the most abundant in adult dermis [3]. The enzyme collagenase degrades exposed native and denatured collagen by peptide bond cleavage at physiological pH [4]. Both topical and natural collagenase solubilize denatured collagen fiber that anchor the eschar plug to the wound base.

The dermis has two layers: the thin upper layer is referred to as the papillary dermis is composed of thin, irregularly arrayed collagen fibers. The thicker lower layer, the reticular dermis, extends from the base of the papillary layer to the subcutaneous tissue and is composed of thick collagen fibers that are roughly parallel to skin surface. The dermis also normally contains histiocytes, macrophages [5] that collect hemosiderin, melanin, and debris caused by inflammation. Mast cells, located around blood vessels, release histamine also reside in the dermis.

Dermal collagen fibers and elastic fibers are embedded in a "ground substance" formed by large proteoglycans of approximately 100–2,500 kDa that account for up to 0.2 % of the dry weight of the dermis [1, 6]. Proteoglycans influence dermal volume and compressibility through their capacity to bind water. They also influence dermal cell activity by binding growth factors, such as basic fibroblast growth factor (bFGF) and vascular endothelial growth factor (VEGF).

The basement membrane (BM) separates the dermis and epidermis. Also referred to as the dermal–epidermal junction, it is the boundary between the epidermis and the dermis and functions to join the epidermis to the dermis. It is an acellular collection of attachment molecules. It can be subdivided into three layers by electron microscopy: hemidesmosome-anchoring filament (including the lamina lucida), basement membrane (lamina densa), and anchoring fibril layers [7]. The BM is composed mainly of basal keratinocyte products, with a minor contribution from dermal fibroblasts. In addition to connecting the epidermis and dermis, it functions to protect against mechanical shear, to orientate cell growth, and to serve as a semipermeable barrier [8]. The dermis is attached to the sublamina densa region by anchoring fibrils and anchoring plaques that adhere to dermal fibers and collagen.

The BM is a dynamic structure that is constantly remodeled [9]. It is bidirectionally penetrated by Langerhans cells under normal conditions. Lymphocytes cross the BM in inflammatory and neoplastic disease. Metalloproteases (MMPs) expressed by immune or malignant cells are responsible for the abnormal cell penetration. The MMPs are thought to play a role in thinning of the epidermal BM in aged and photoaged skin.

Dermal macrophages are bone marrow-derived phagocytic cells that differentiate from blood monocytes after entering peripheral tissues [5]. The functions of macrophages in skin are numerous and include processing and presentation of antigen, wound healing activities, and microbe and tumor killing.

The sensations of pain, itch, and temperature are received by unmyelinated nerve endings in the papillary dermis. Low intensity stimulation due to dermal inflammation causes itching, whereas high intensity stimulation of dermal receptors created by inflammation causes pain. Therefore scratching converts the intolerable sensation of itching to the more tolerable sensation of pain and temporarily eliminates pruritus.

The skin connects to the central nervous system and has a wide array of efferent and afferent fibers in the dermis [10]. Control is exerted over the sweat glands, blood vessels, and the pilosebaceous system. Afferent fibers also control vascular tone.

The autonomic system innervates the skin. Adrenergic fibers control blood vessels through vasoconstriction and motor fibers to hair erector muscles. Autonomic fibers to eccrine sweat glands are cholinergic. The sebaceous glands are under endocrine control and are not innervated by autonomic fibers.

Functions of Skin

The skin is one of the three barrier organs in humans. The other two, the lung and the gastrointestinal tract are internal. Intact skin is protective. It prevents loss of fluids, electrolytes, and proteins [11]. Wound exudate can result in loss of visceral proteins.

Skin plays a role in calcium metabolism. Vitamin D_3 is produced in the epidermis. UV radiation acts on 7-hydrocholesterol, which is hydroxylated in the liver and kidney to the active form of vitamin D 1,25 dihydrocholecalciferol.

The skin has two distinct circulatory systems, the vascular system that is "two-way" and the lymphatic that is one-way out. The arteriolar blood flow supplies nutrients and delivers leukocytes. The dermal vascular bed also has a thermoregulatory function. The movement of cellular elements from the blood into the tissues is directed by a complex sequence of cellular signaling. Lymphatic capillaries are blind ended and lead out of the dermis and drain into regional lymph nodes. Interstitial fluid and cells exit through these channels [12].

The skin has an important immunological function [13]. Initial recognition of "non-self" antigens occurs when sentinel dendritic cells in the epidermis and dermis become activated. These cells, upon activation, engulf and process particles then migrate via the lymphatic channels to lymph nodes. In the node helper T cells enable B-lymphocytes to produce antibodies. The helper and cytotoxic T cells recirculate to the skin to fight infection. Keratinocytes and vascular endothelial cells produce a wide range of interacting regulatory molecules now generally known as cytokines. These proteins exert influence on healing and other skin function. Further research will be needed to better understand the role of these agents.

Trauma and physical injury to skin is common. Breaks in skin from blunt and sharp impact, UV solar penetration, and thermal injury all evoke the skin's repair mechanism. The skins healing system evokes a complex orchestrated interaction of cells and cellular mediators operating in the extracellular matrix. It is a continuous process that starts with some form of trauma and ends with remodeling that continues long after epithelization.

Failure of the repair system results in delayed wound healing. There is no well-accepted time line to delineate an acute, orderly healing wound from a chronic or delayed wound. Wound depth, size, and host factors will influence the time to heal [14].

The Wound Healing Society has defined the term chronic wound. A committee developed definition, and after holding public hearings, published the "Definitions and Guidelines for Assessment of Wounds and Evaluation of Healing" in 1994 [15, 16]. This publication defined a chronic wound as one that has failed to proceed through an orderly and timely reparative process to produce anatomic and functional integrity or that has proceeded through the repair process without establishing a sustained anatomic and functional result. Simply stated, wounds may be classified as those that can repair themselves or can be repaired in an orderly and timely process (acute wounds) and those that do not (chronic wounds) [17] (see Box 1.1).

Phases of Acute Wound Healing

Acute wound healing is an orderly sequence of overlapping cellular events leading to tissue repair of the skin. Healing can be divided into four sequential phases. Some texts lump the first two (coagulation and inflammation) into one phase. The phases are mediated by a complex array of cellular mediators (see Table 1.1).

> **Box 1.1 Pathologic Processes in Chronic Wounds**
>
> The biochemistry of the wound base is what allows an acute wound to heal in a reasonable amount of time or prevents a chronic wound from healing. Chronic wounds have a more pathologic process that includes some or all of the following:
>
> - A prolonged inflammatory phase.
> - Cellular senescence (older less viable cells). Defined as a change in the cell's ability to proliferate.
> - Deficiency of growth factor receptor sites.
> - No initial bleeding event to trigger cascade.
> - Higher level of proteases.

Table 1.1   Cytokine families affecting wound healing

Cytokine	Major effects
Epidermal growth factor family	
Epidermal growth factor	Cell mobility and proliferation
Transforming growth factor α	Cell mobility and proliferation
Heparin-binding epidermal growth factor	Cell mobility and proliferation
Fibroblast growth factor family	
Basic fibroblast growth factor	Angiogenesis and fibroblast proliferation
Acidic fibroblast growth factor	Angiogenesis and fibroblast proliferation
Keratinocyte growth factor	Epidermal cell motility and proliferation
Transforming growth factor β family	
Transforming growth factor β1 and β2	Epidermal cell motility, chemotaxsis of macrophages and fibroblasts, extracelluar matrix synthesis and remodeling
Transforming growth factor β3	Anti-scarring effects
Other	
Platelet-derived growth factor	Fibroblast proliferation and chemotaxis, macrophage chemoattraction and activation
Vascular endothelial growth factor	Angiogenesis and vascular proliferation
Tumor necrosis factor α	Expression of growth factors
Interleukin-1	Expression of growth factors
Insulin-like growth factor 1	Re-epithelialization and granulation formation
Colony-stimulating factor 1	Macrophage activation and granulation formation

From Thomas DR. Age Related Changes in Wound Healing. Drugs & Aging 2001;18(8):607–620 [51]. With permission

The Coagulation Phase

The first response of the integument to wounding is coagulation. It has a both a cellular and a vascular response. The first cells on the scene are platelets.

They initiate hemostasis, adhere to damaged vessel walls, and release growth factors[1] such as PDGF. Platelets also release transforming growth factor beta 1 and 2 (TGF-beta-1, TGF-2). These factors initiate the next phase in the healing cascade, inflammation. Wounding also causes local vasodilatation, leakage of extravascular fluid, and lymphatic obstruction, which manifest as local redness, induration, and swelling. The inflammatory phase typically lasts 24–48 h. A prolonged inflammatory phase is one of the reasons wounds do not progress and become chronic.

Hemostasis has two parts, formation of the fibrin plug and initiation of the coagulation cascade. Wounding also damages blood vessels and exposes collagen. Platelets are activated at the wound site by thrombin and exposed collagen fibrils. The proline and hydroproline in collagen activate platelets. Activated platelets degranulate releasing serotonin, ADP, fibrinogen, and other mediators. Other platelets are induced to form an unstable platelet plug to stop bleeding. Endothelial cells also produce prostacyclin that inhibits platelet aggregation.

PDGF, TGF-beta1, and TGF-2 are chemotatic and mitogenic and attract fibroblasts, macrophages, and neutrophils [18]. Activated platelets also play an early role in angiogenesis.

The Inflammatory Phase

In a very short time after injury, disrupted blood vessels are covered with marginating neutrophils and monocytes. These cells release chemical mediators of inflammation (histamine, serotonin, kinins, and prostaglandins) and migrate through the vessel wall to phagocytize bacteria and matrix proteins. Monocytes arrive on the scene immediately after neutrophils, attracted by factors produced by the coagulation cascade. Once migrated into the tissues, monocytes are transformed into macrophages. Continued monocyte recruitment occurs through monocyte-specific chemoattractants such as thrombin and TGF-beta1. The inflammatory phase resolves with apoptosis of the inflammatory cells. A number of anti-inflammatory cytokines have been identified but their exact role and interaction is poorly understood [19].

Macrophages are essential components to wound healing, but neutrophils are not critical [20]. The macrophage is the most important cell in the regulation of the inflammatory phase. They produce a sizable array of cytokines that induce cell migration, proliferation, and matrix production. Along with other leukocytes they kill microorganisms, scavenge tissue debris, and ultimately eliminate remaining neutrophils [21]. This is one of the mechanisms by which they control the inflammatory response.

---

[1] Growth factors, cytokines, and hormones share many similarities and act as biochemical messengers and have roles in stem cell-related growth and regulation. The terms growth factor and cytokine and often used interchangeably. Some cytokines and hormones are growth factors and the distinction between them is arbitrary and is relate to the timing of their discovery rather than a difference in function. See Box 1.2.

> **Box 1.2   Cytokines Are Glycoprotein Mediators That Have the Following Properties**
>
> - Signal between cells and coordinate the immune response
> - Delivered by cells either to the systemic circulation or to the local environment
> - Bind to high affinity surface receptors
> - Produced by immune and nonimmune cells (fibroblasts, endothelial cells)

> **Box 1.3   Actions of Growth Factors and Cytokines**
>
> Autocrine mode—action on cell of origin.
> Paracrine mode—action on neighboring cells.
> Exocrine mode—action on distant cells.

The process of macrophage phagocytosis and cellular destruction is accomplished by release of active oxygen intermediates and proteases. This process induces early angiogenesis and early formation of granulation tissue. Macrophages tolerate tissue hypoxia well. Hypoxic macrophages produce a growth factor that promotes neovascularization. If macrophages are removed from a wound bed, autolysis and angiogenesis cease.

The inflammatory phase is influenced by a number of chemical mediators. These include histamine, serotonin, kinins, and prostaglandins. Their precise role as agonists and inhibitors of inflammation is not well understood [22].

Most cellular and local signs of inflammation are absent with 2 weeks. Granulocytes disappear and mononuclear cells predominate. If a wound has excessive necrotic tissue, is heavily colonized with pathogens, or contains material that cannot be phagocytized during the acute inflammatory phase, mononuclear cells persist and inhibit the cellular activity of the proliferative phase.

The Proliferative Phase

The proliferative phase follows as inflammation subsides. Growth factors produced by inflammatory cells and migrating epidermal and dermal cells induce and maintain proliferation of fibroblasts and keratinocytes [22] that form the granulation tissue that fills the defect (also see Box 1.3). This new tissue requires adequate blood supply.

The proliferative phase is characterized by neovascularization. New blood vessels develop by forming de novo networks in the wound space that re-couple with existing vessels. New capillary buds form and endothelial cells undergo a phenotypic alteration and migrate into the wound bed. The migration depends on the presence of chemotactic factors, an extracellular matrix and the absence of adjacent endothelial cells [23]. Migration of endothelial cells causes them to divide and proliferate. Growth factors released by macrophages, low oxygen tension, and lactic acid stimulate angiogenesis. Tissue hypoxia also stimulates TGF-beta and collagen synthesis. Chronic hypoxia can cause excess fibrosis seen in some chronic wounds. New blood vessels are a critical for transporting oxygen and nutrients into the wound bed. They are a conduit for cell migration and bioactive substances.

A clinical sign of healthy wound healing is the presence of granulation tissue. Wound voids are filled with extracellular matrix (ECM) and fibroblasts into which new blood supply is continuously growing. The key cell in the production of the dermal matrix is the fibroblast. Fibroblasts migrate into the wound bed within 48 h of wounding. They perform several functions including production of fibers and the amorphous ground substance; they also undergo phenotypic transformation to myofibroblasts to provide dermal structure. Myofibroblasts also participate in wound contraction during healing.

The dermal connective tissue is composed of cells, fibers, and an amorphous viscous gel known as ground substance. Fibroblasts secrete the ECM, which is comprised of the ground substance and the extracellular fibers (principally collagen). The dermal ground substance provides flexibility and integrity to the dermis. It holds tissue fluids and allows diffusion of nutrients and waste products.

Collagen is the principle protein of the dermis. It comprises 70 % of its dry weight and provides structure and strength. Collagen fibers themselves are not elastic and have a high tensile strength. They are arrayed in a loose interlacing network that permits skin stretch. Elastin is the other major structural protein fiber in the dermis. It is a long thin retractile fiber that makes up 2 % of the dermis. It allows for skin recovery after deformation.

Type I collagen predominates in adult dermis and other connective tissue (90 % type I). In addition to dermis it is found in tendons, fascia, and bone. Upon wounding, the initial collagen produced by fibroblasts is gel-like similar to type III collagen. As wounds remodel there is gradual turnover from type III to type I collagen.

The epidermis reacts almost immediately to injury. Within 12 h they flatten and lose their desmosomal cell–cell attachments and begin to migrate. In partial thickness wounds, epidermal stem cells can originate in adnexal structures as well as the wound free edge. Migrating free keratinocytes can cover a small partial thickness (i.e., stage II pressure ulcer) in a week, under ideal conditions. This process requires loss of tight binding between cells. Neither BM nor the underlying dermis is required for keratinocyte migration. There is a provisional matrix of fibrin, fibronectin, and type V collagen. Fibronectin appears to be a critical component in keratinocyte migration [24]. The provisional matrix allows the advancing keratinocyte edge to dissect under superficial eschar and debris covering a wound bed. The process requires a moist wound environment. This accounts for the success of occlusive wound dressings that promote moist (but not wet) wound beds.

The basal keratinocyte secrets collagenase-1 that degrades fibrillar collagen that allows for ongoing keratinocyte migration. Once the wound is fully re-epithelialized, the keratinocytes bind to alpha2 and beta1 integrin and production of collagenase-1 stops. Once a single layer of epidermal cells covers the wound, the migrating cells bind and proliferate to re-form an intact normal epidermis. Approximately 7–10 days after the single layer of epidermal cells forms, the BM zone returns and cell adhesion returns. In the early days of re-epithelization the new skin is very fragile.

The Remodeling Phase

Remodeling is the final phase of wound healing. Dermal remodeling is occurring over approximately 1 year after the skin barrier has been restored. In 1 month the tensile strength is 40 % of preinjury strength. At 1 year it is 80 %, but never returns to 100 % [18]. The principal activity occurring during the remodeling phase is lysis of type III collagen and its replacement with type I collagen.

Structural Changes in Aging Skin

As the skin ages, or with chronic disease, some of the protective properties are lost or diminished. There is a reduction in sebum production and the skin becomes drier and less elastic. Dryness leads to small cracks in the skin, which will support bacterial invasion. Combined with a chronic disease such as vascular disorders or diabetes, reduction in blood flow to the skin will occur, directly impacting wound healing.

Aging skin is more susceptible to damage due to thinning and increased friability. Other issues are a decrease in the inflammatory response, cell senescence, decrease in cytokines and growth factor production, and a reduction in cell receptor sites.

A number of structural and functional changes in aging skin are known to occur. These include (1) decrease in dermal thickness, (2) a decline in collagen content, and (3) a loss of elastin. Changes in the skin with aging are difficult to discern from the effects of exposure to solar ultraviolet radiation. The effect of solar exposure on skin is cumulative. Older individuals show more changes in skin structure. It is difficult to distinguish the effects of photoaging and chronological aging in human skin. In 90 individuals, aged 18–94 years, changes in thickness of sun-exposed regions were compared to the nonexposed skin of the buttocks. A progressive, age-related decrease in thickness was found in sun-exposed regions (dorsal forearm, forehead), but not in moderately exposed regions (ventral forearm, ankle). In the buttocks an increase in thickness was observed [25]. It appears that photoaging causes a decrease in skin thickness in the upper dermis, but chronological age is associated with an increase in thickness in the lower dermis. No general relationship between overall skin thickness and age was observed [25].

In the absence of solar damage (photoaging), the thickness of the stratum corneum is largely unchanged over time [26]. Whether a slight overall thinning of the epidermis occurs with aging is controversial. No difference in epidermal or dermal thickness was noted in a study of wound healing comparing young and old volunteers [27].

The dermis becomes less cellular and less vascular with age. There is flattening of the dermal interface and dermal rete pegs are less deep [28, 29]. These changes predispose to epidermal–dermal shear-type injuries. These are often referred to as "skin tears" and are common in the frail elderly and occur with minimal force. Melanocytes decrease by 8–20 % per decade, beginning at age 30, in both sun-exposed and nonexposed skin [30]. An overall thickening of subdermal collagen fibers occurs with aging and paradoxically makes the skin becomes more lax. The elastic fiber network in the papillary dermis slowly disappears with aging, causing wrinkles.

The distribution of subcutaneous fat changes significantly with age. Subcutaneous tissue atrophies on the face, hands, and shins with aging, while subcutaneous fat increases in the abdomen of men and thighs in women. There is minimal reduction in capillary blood flow between older and younger subjects [31]. In vitro fibroblast migration declines with age [32].

The accumulation of solar injury appears to account for a major part of observed skin structural change over time. In nonexposed skin, there seems to be little overall effect of chronological aging, other than a decline in elastin content that contributes to a decrease in skin elasticity with aging. A decrease in responsiveness to growth factors appears to occur with aging. The impact of these changes on human wound healing is not clear.

Changes in Wound Healing with Age

Progress in understanding the effect of cytokines on wound healing has provided a mechanism to study age-related effects on wound healing. Wound healing is usually measured in one of three ways (1) determination of force needed to break a healed or healing wound (tensile strength), (2) a measure of some product of the healing process in the wound bed, or (3) the rate of closure of an open wound. Each method produces its own set of difficulties.

Most of the research on wound healing has been done in animal models. The models are useful for measuring response to pharmacological products and for measuring toxicities of topical wound products. But no animal model is considered ideal for analysis of chronic wounds or extensive burns. Pig models have been particularly useful for graft donor site evaluation because of the similarity of cutaneous architecture to human skin. Angiogenesis has been studied in a chick chorioallantoic membrane or rabbit corneas. Tensile strength has been tested in the rat.

Each model has some advantages and limitations. The translation of animal data to human healing may introduce error. Some animal models have been extremely useful in directing clinical research.

Tensile Strength

Tensile strength has been measured in a number of animal models, but in few human studies. The dehiscence of surgical wounds has been observed to be higher in elderly persons, which formed the basis for the first reports on impaired healing in elderly persons. A dehiscence occurred in 0.9 % of surgical wounds in patients aged 30–39, in 2.5 % in patients aged 50–59, and in 5.5 % in patients over age 80, suggesting that tensile strength declines with age [33]. However, adjustment for comorbidity or other potential confounders was not done.

A single study [34] found that less force was needed to disrupt wounds in older subjects. Surprisingly, the visual quality of scarring and microscopic evaluation of the healing wound have been shown to be superior in older subjects [35]. A trial of experimental forearm wounding demonstrated that persons more than 80 years of age had a 6 % decrease in tensile strength compared to persons less than 70 years of age [36].

Measurement of Wound Healing

The accumulation of hydroxyproline in polytetrafloroethylene (PTFE) implanted tubes has been frequently used as a proxy measure wound healing, but the ideal wound healing product to measure is controversial. Subcutaneous insertion of PTEE tubes was developed by Goodson and Hunt in 1982 [37] and has been used extensively in wounding models. In surgical patients, collagen deposition is frequently decreased [38]. The accumulation of wound healing products is also confounded by several factors. For example, nutritional state greatly influences hydroxyproline accumulation. In 66 adult surgical patients, the hydroxyproline content of subcutaneously implanted Goretex tubes was higher in the 36 normally nourished patients than the 21 patients with mild or severe protein energy malnutrition [39]. Thus, nutritional status, which may be more compromised in elderly persons with comorbid conditions, must be adjusted for in wound healing studies using this method.

Collagen deposition appears to be similar in both young and old wounded subjects. In nine experimentally wounded, healthy volunteers whose mean age was 34 years, no difference in hydroxyproline accumulation in PTFE tubes was seen compared to 15 healthy volunteers whose mean age was 72 years [40]. Age has no effect on collagen synthesis 2 weeks after wounding [26, 40].

Rate of Wound Closure

The rate of wound closure is probably more associated with a meaningful clinical outcome than measures of wound healing product studies mentioned above. Complete wound healing requires longer observation than frequently used partial closure endpoints. The rate of epithelialization appears to differ with age. Complete epithelialization of partial thickness wounds occurred 1.9 days faster in nine young healthy volunteers (mean age 34 years) compared to 15 old healthy volunteers (mean age 72 years) [36]. In 12 subjects with skin-graft-donor sites treated with silver sulfadiazine with or without epidermal growth factor, time-to-complete-healing was accelerated by 1.5 days (95 % confidence limits 0.3–2.5 days) [41].

A difference in in vitro growth of epidermal cells has been shown among newborn, young, or old adults. Although there was large interdonor variability, growth of keratinocytes obtained from upper arm biopsies of young (22–27 years) and old (60–82 years) adult donors significantly decreased with age. Cell yields at 7 days showed an eightfold increase for young adults but only a fourfold increase for old adults [42].

Cultured neonatal keratinocytes release factors that stimulate the growth of other keratinocytes, whereas adult keratinocytes fail to do so. Epidermal growth factor failed to stimulate growth for either adult age group [42]. Keratinocytes of older individuals grow more slowly in culture with a reduced culture life span and mitogen responsiveness [43]. Although adult cells may be initially slower to culture, once grown the production growth factor is the same as neonatal cells [40].

Fibroblasts have a major role in the synthesis and remodeling of the extracellular matrix during wound repair. An impaired biosynthetic or functional response of these cells to stimulation by growth factors might contribute to the delayed wound healing reputed in aging. Cultures of dermal fibroblasts from young and elderly individuals exposed to transforming growth factor-beta 1 (TGF-beta 1) demonstrated a 1.6- to a 5.5-fold increase in the levels of secreted type I collagen and extracellular matrix proteins and exhibited a 2.0- to a 6.2-fold increase in the amounts of the corresponding mRNAs. The dose response to TGF-beta 1 was as vigorous in biosynthetic and contractile properties in cells from aged donors as in cells from a young donor [44].

Inflammatory Response

The response of cultured fibroblasts to cytokines or growth factors does not appear to change with age. In 28 fibroblast cell lines derived from persons aged 3 days to 84 years, mitogenesis and synthesis of collagen in response to epidermal growth factor, tumor necrosis factor-α, PDGF, and transforming growth factor-β did not vary with the age of the cell donor [45].

At least five cell adhesion molecules (CAM) have been identified on the surface of endothelial cells in the presence of inflammatory cytokines. The expression of specific CAM modulates the inflammatory response early in the inflammatory phase. Differences in CAM expression occur with aging. When cutaneous punch biopsies were taken from 138 healthy subjects, aged 19–96 years, and compared to repeated biopsies at fixed time points from day 1 up to 3 months post-wounding, a marked early increase in the neutrophil response occurred in the aged with a less pronounced peak in the wounds of young subjects. Monocyte/macrophage and lymphocyte appearance was delayed in the aged, peaking at day 84, compared to day 7 for monocytes and day 21 for lymphocytes in the young. An increased number of mature macrophages were observed in the aged. Intracellular CAM-1 and vascular CAM-1 expression exhibited an age-related delay in appearance and a reduction in staining intensity [46]. The effect of this altered CAM profile in the early inflammatory response of aged humans on clinical wound healing is not known.

Matrix metalloproteinases (MMPs) have been implicated in arthritis, Alzheimer's disease, and wound healing. These proteins (such as collagenases, stromelysins, and gelatinases) degrade the extracellular matrix of the wound, leading to remodeling. This proteolysis is an essential component of wound healing but, if uncontrolled, it may lead to degradation of the wound matrix and a delay in wound repair. Examination of a punch biopsy in 132 healthy humans aged between 19 and 96 years showed an age-related increase in MMP-2 and MMP-9 immunostaining. Aging seems to be associated with the upregulation of the MMPs associated with chronic wound healing. This may predispose to tissue breakdown disorders because of MMP-2 upregulation in normal skin [47].

Specific tissue inhibitors of matrix metalloproteinases (TIMP-1 and TIMP-2) modify the activity of MMPs, thereby acting to prevent an accelerated breakdown of connective tissue. TIMP-1 and TIMP-2 proteins are upregulated from 24 h postwounding, with a decrease in staining intensity by day 7 for TIMP-2 and by day 14 for TIMP-1. In biopsied tissue, steady-state mRNA levels for both TIMPs were significantly greater in normal young skin than in aged skin. In the young, a significant increase in mRNA expression for TIMP-1 and TIMP-2 by day 3 post-wounding has been observed, which decreased by day 14 and returned to basal levels at day 21. In the wounds of the aged subjects, no increase was observed for TIMP-1 and -2 at all time points. These results suggest that intrinsic cutaneous aging is associated with reduced levels of TIMP mRNA both in normal skin and during acute wound repair. The lower levels could lead to a dermal tissue breakdown in normal skin, retarded wound healing, and the predisposition of the elderly to chronic wound healing states [48].

Clinical observations have suggested that older persons have less wound tensile strength than younger persons. However, adjustment for factors other than chronological age was not done in early studies. Other studies have suggested that microscopic structure of wounds in older persons is better than younger persons. There does not appear to be a decrease in wound tensile strength in advanced age in the single reported study in humans. The accumulation of collagen in wounds does not appear to differ with aging. Clinically there does not appear to be a large difference in surgical wound healing between younger and healthy older persons undergoing elective surgery. The rate of epithelialization does appear to be different in older persons, but the magnitude of the delay may not be clinically important. The response to epidermal growth factor or TGF-beta 1 and wound contractility does not appear to be different with aging. Most age-related effects on the inflammatory process are modest. Little in vivo evaluation of aging and the inflammatory response has been done [45].

Box 1.4 Medications That Impair Wound Healing

Corticosteroids
Antiplatelet/nonsteroidal anti-inflammatory drugs
Antibiotics
Cytotoxic medications
Nicotine
Anticoagulants
Immunosuppressives
Anti-RA medications
Vasoconstrictors

The overall clinical experience with growth factors and other mediators to accelerate wound healing has been discouraging. This is not surprising, considering that wound repair is the result of a complex set of interactions among soluble cytokines, formed blood elements, extracellular matrix, and cells. Among these factors, only recombinant platelet-derived growth factor has been approved by the US Food and Drug Administration for the treatment of diabetic ulcers. Some concern has been raised for association with malignancy [49].

Summary

Evidence for age-related effects on wound healing has been derived for the most part from empirical observations without adjustment for confounders other than age. Changes in the structure of the skin have been observed with aging, but the effects in skin unexposed to solar radiation appear modest. Age-related changes in function of the skin include a decrease in elastic fibers and a slowing of re-epithelialization [28]. Regular sunscreen use slows skin aging in exposed areas, but oral beta-carotene and other topical agents are not effective [50]. The clinical impact of age-related changes in acute wound healing seems to be small. Poor healing in chronic wounds, largely seen in the older population, is more often related to comorbid conditions and medications (see Box 1.4) rather than age alone.

References

1. Chu DH, Haake AR, Holbrook K, et al. The structure and development of skin. In: Freedberg IM, Eisen AZ, Wolff K, et al., editors. Fitzpatrick's dermatology in general medicine. 6th ed. New York, NY: McGraw-Hill; 2003. p. 58–88.
2. Madison KC. Barrier function of the skin: "la raison d'etre" of the epidermis. J Invest Dermatol. 2003;121:210–6.

3. Uitto J, Pulkkinen L, Chu ML. Collagen. In: Freedberg IM, Eisen AZ, Wolff K, et al., editors. Fitzpatrick's dermatology in general medicine. 6th ed. New York, NY: McGraw-Hill; 2003. p. 165–79.
4. Brett DW. A historical review of topical enzymatic debridement. New York, NY: The McMahon Publishing Group; 2003. p. 33–4.
5. Lu KQ, McCormick TS, Gilliam AC, et al. Monocytes and macrophages in human skin. In: Bos JD, editor. Skin immune system. 3rd ed. Boca Raton: CRC Press LLC; 2004. p. 183–209.
6. Gallo RL, Towbridge JM. Proteogylcans and glycosaminoglycans of skin. In: Freedberg IM, Eisen AZ, Wolff K, et al., editors. Fitzpatrick's dermatology in general medicine. 6th ed. New York, NY: McGraw-Hill; 2003. p. 210–6.
7. Burgeson RE, Christiano AM. The dermal-epidermal junction. Curr Opin Cell Biol. 1997;9:651–8.
8. Ghohestani RF, Li K, Rousselle P, Uitto J. Molecular organization of the cutaneous basement membrane zone. Clin Dermatol. 2001;19:551–62.
9. Burgeson RE. Basement membranes. In: Freedberg IM, Eisen AZ, Wolff K, et al., editors. Fitzpatrick's dermatology in general medicine. 5th ed. New York, NY: McGraw-Hill; 1999. p. 271.
10. Oaklander AL, Siegel SM. Cutaneous innervation: form and function. J Am Acad Dermatol. 2005;53:1027–37.
11. Ponec M, Gibbs S, Pilgram G, et al. Barrier function in reconstructed epidermis and its resemblance to native human skin. Skin Pharmacol Appl Skin Physiol. 2001;14:63–71.
12. Cueni LN, Detmar M. New insights into the molecular control of the lymphatic vascular system and its role in disease. J Invest Dermatol. 2006;126:2167–77.
13. Janeway Jr CA. How the immune system works to protect the host from infection: a personal view. Proc Natl Acad Sci USA. 2001;98:7461–8.
14. Mustoe TA, O'Shaughnessy K, Kloeters O. Chronic wound pathogenesis and current treatment strategies: a unifying hypothesis. Plast Reconstr Surg. 2006;117:35–41.
15. Lazarus GS, Cooper DM, Knighton DR, Margolis DJ, Pecoraro RE, Rodeheaver G, Robson MC. Definitions and guidelines for the assessment of wounds and evaluation of healing. Arch Dermatol. 1994;130:489–93.
16. Wound Healing Society. Guidelines for the best care of chronic wounds. Wound Repair Regen. 2006;14:647–710.
17. Menke NB, Ward KR, Witten TM, Bonchev DG, Diegelmann RF. Impaired wound healing. Clin Dermatol. 2007;25:19–25.
18. Eming SA, Krieg T, Davidson JM. Inflammation in wound repair: molecular and cellular mechanisms. J Invest Dermatol. 2007;127:514–25.
19. Singer AJ, Clark RA. Cutaneous wound healing. N Engl J Med. 1999;341:738–46.
20. Simpson DM, Ross R. The neurophilic leukocyte in wound repair. A study with antineutrophilic serum. J Clin Invest. 1972;51:2009–23.
21. Doughty D, Sparks-Defriese B. Wound-healing physiology. In: Bryant RA, Nix DP, editors. Acute & chronic wounds: current management concepts. 3rd ed. St. Louis, MO: Mosby/Elsevier; 2007. p. 56–81.
22. Falanga V. Growth factors and wound healing. J Dermatol Surg Oncol. 1993;19:711–4.
23. Folkman J. Angiogenesis: initiation and control. Ann N Y Acad Sci. 1982;401:21–7.
24. Grove GL. Age-related differences in healing of superficial skin wounds in humans. Arch Dermatol Res. 1982;272:381–5.
25. Gniadecka M, Jemee GB. Quantitative evaluation of chronological ageing and phtoageing in vivo: studies on skin echogenicity and thickness. Br J Dermatol. 1998;139(5):815–21.
26. Holt DR, Kirk SJ, Regan MC, et al. Effect of age on wound healing in healthy human beings. Surgery. 1992;112:293–8.
27. Lavker RM. Structural alternations in exposed and unexposed aged skin. J Invest Dermatol. 1979;73:59–66.
28. Kurban R, Bhawan J. Histological changes in skin associated with aging. J Dermatol Surg Oncol. 1990;16:908–14.

29. Montagna W, Carlisle K. Structural changes in aging human skin. J Invest Dermatol. 1979;73:47–53.
30. Gilchrest BA, Blog FB, Szbo G. Effects of aging and chronic sun exposure on melaoncytes in human skin. J Invest Dermatol. 1979;73:141–3.
31. Kelly RI, Pearse R, Bull RH, et al. The effects of aging on the cutaneous microvasculature. J Am Acad Dermatol. 1995;33:749–56.
32. Pienta KJ, Coppey DS. Characterization of the subtypes of cell motility in ageing human skin fibroblasts. Mech Ageing Dev. 1990;56:99–105.
33. Mendoza Jr CB, Postlethwait RW, Johnson WD. Incidence of wound disruption following operation. Arch Surg. 1970;101:396–8.
34. Sandblom PH, Peterson P, Muren A. Determination of the tensile strength of the healing wound as a clinical test. Acta Chir Scand. 1953;105:252–7.
35. Horan MA, Ashcroft GS. Ageing, defense mechanisms and the immune system. Age Aging. 1997;26:15S–9.
36. Lindstedt E, Sandblom P. Wound healing in man: tensile strength of healing wounds in some patient groups. Ann Surg. 1975;181:842–6.
37. Goodson III WH, Hunt TK. Development of a new miniature method for the study of wound healing in human subjects. J Surg Res. 1982;33:394–401.
38. Jorgensen LN, Kallehave F, Karlsmark T, et al. Reduced collagen accumulation after major surgery. Br J Surg. 1996;83:1591–4.
39. Haydock DA, Hill GL. Impaired wound healing in surgical patients with varying degrees of malnutrition. JPEN J Parenter Enteral Nutr. 1986;10:550–4.
40. Compton C, Tong Y, Trockman N, et al. Transforming growth factor and gene expression in cultured human keratinocytes is unaffected by cellular ageing. Arch Dermatol. 1995; 132:683–90.
41. Brown GL, Nanney LB, Griffen J, et al. Enhancement of wound healing by topical treatment with epidermal growth factor. N Engl J Med. 1989;321:76–9.
42. Stanulis-Praeger BM, Gilchrest BA. Growth factor responsiveness declines during adulthood for human skin-derived cells. Mech Ageing Dev. 1986;35:185–98.
43. Phillips T, Gilchrist BA. Cultured allogenic keratinocyte grafts in the management of wound healing: prognostic factors. J Dermatol Surg Oncol. 1989;15:1169–76.
44. Reed MJ, Vernon RB, Abrass IB, et al. TGF-beta 1 induces the expression of type 1 collagen and SPARC, and enhances contraction of collagen gels, by fibroblasts from young and aged donors. J Cell Physiol. 1994;158:169–79.
45. Freedland M, Karmiol S, Rodriguez J, et al. Fibroblast responses to cytokines are maintained during aging. Ann Plast Surg. 1995;35:290–6.
46. Ashcroft GS, Horan MA, Ferguson MW. Aging alters the inflammatory and endothelial cell adhesion molecule profiles during human cutaneous wound healing. Lab Invest. 1998;78:47–58.
47. Ashcroft GS, Horan MA, Herrick SE, et al. Age-related differences in the temporal and spatial regulation of matrix metalloproteinases (MMPs) in normal skin and acute cutaneous wounds of healthy humans. Cell Tissue Res. 1997;290:581–91.
48. Ashcroft GS, Herrick SE, Tarnuzzer RW, et al. Human ageing impairs injury-induced in vivo expression of tissue inhibitor of matrix metalloproteinases (TIMP)-1 and −2 proteins and mRNA. J Pathol. 1997;183:169–76.
49. Prescribing information, Ortho-McNeil, Division of Ortho-McNeil-Janssen Pharmaceuticals, Inc. Raritan, NJ. Becaplermin Concentrate provided by: Novartis NPC 2010 Cessna Dr., Vacaville, CA, US License No. 1244. Revised May 2011.
50. Hughes MCB, Williams GM, Baker P, Green AC. Sunscreen and prevention of skin aging. Ann Intern Med. 2013;158:781–90.
51. Thomas DR. Age related changes in wound healing. Drugs Aging. 2001;18(8):607–20.

Useful General References for More Detail on the Anatomy, Function and Biology of the Skin

52. Adkinson NF. Middleton's allergy: principles and practice. 7th ed. Philadelphia, PA: Mosby Elsevier; 2008.
53. Freedberg IM, Eisen AZ, Wolff K, et al., editors. Fitzpatrick's dermatology in general medicine. 6th ed. New York, NY: McGraw-Hill; 2003.

Useful General References for More Detail on the Cytokines and Growth Factors

54. Kaushansky K. Lineage-specific hematopoietic growth factors. N Engl J Med. 2006;354(19):2034.
55. McInnes IB. Cytokines. In: Harris E, Budd R, Firestein G, et al., editors. Kelley's textbook of rheumatology. 7th ed. London: Elsevier; 2004.

Chapter 2
Incidence and Prevalence of Pressure Ulcers

Dan Berlowitz

Abstract Understanding pressure ulcer epidemiology is central to understanding disease burden and to efforts to improve pressure ulcer care. A variety of measures are commonly used, including incidence, prevalence, and facility acquired rates. Each of these measures has specific strengths and limitations when used in assessing pressure ulcer rates. Pressure ulcer rates are highly dependent on the data source and rates calculated from one source can never be compared to rates from a different source. Estimates of pressure ulcer rates from different settings vary considerably but indicate that pressure ulcers are among the most common conditions seen in hospitalized individuals.

Keywords Pressure ulcer • Epidemiology • Incidence • Prevalence • Outcome assessment

Epidemiology involves understanding the frequency and distribution of disease in a well-defined population. For many clinicians, their knowledge of pressure ulcer epidemiology is limited to being aware that pressure ulcers are among the most common conditions encountered in clinical practice and that regardless of specialty, they are likely to see many patients with pressure ulcers or at risk for developing an ulcer. This underscores the need for nearly all clinicians to understand the basics of prevention and treatment. However, for those clinicians with special expertise in wound care, additional knowledge on pressure ulcer epidemiology is often required. Pressure ulcers are more than a condition affecting the individual patient; they provide information on the burden of disease in a group of patients and on the quality of the care being provided to those patients. Pressure ulcer information can help

D. Berlowitz, M.D., M.P.H. (✉)
Bedford VA Hospital, 200 Springs Road, Bedford, MA 01730, USA
e-mail: dan.berlowitz@va.gov

D.R. Thomas and G.A. Compton (eds.), *Pressure Ulcers in the Aging Population: A Guide for Clinicians*, Aging Medicine 1, DOI 10.1007/978-1-62703-700-6_2,
© Springer Science+Business Media New York 2014

address the question of how good is the care that we are providing and how do we compare to others. This information is typically provided through measurements of pressure ulcer rates, especially incidence and prevalence.

While incidence and prevalence are widely used, the interpretation of these rates is not always straightforward and there are a number of important considerations when analyzing these data. In addressing these considerations, this chapter will specifically describe the different measures that are available and their strengths and limitations. Next, we will examine the interpretation of these rates particularly when incidence and prevalence are used in describing performance of individual facilities or units. Finally, this chapter will conclude with a description of what is presently known about pressure ulcer prevalence and incidence in the key settings of hospitals and nursing homes.

Defining What You Measure

Any consideration of pressure ulcer epidemiology must include a clear definition of what is considered a pressure ulcer. While standardized definitions of pressure ulcers do exist, many epidemiological studies fail to provide the specific definition used or they use different definitions. This complicates comparisons of different studies. For example, in defining incidence and prevalence, some studies consider all pressure ulcers while others only include stage 2 and higher ulcers. Moreover, the definition of a pressure ulcer, and how it is interpreted, has changed in a number of ways over time. First, there is a much greater appreciation of moisture-associated dermatitis as a distinct entity from pressure ulcers. Many sacral and gluteal lesions that previously might have been considered a pressure ulcer are now more appropriately classified as moisture-associated dermatitis. Second, in 2007 the National Pressure Ulcer Advisory Panel (NPUAP) added deep tissue injury as a distinct stage of pressure ulcers [1]. This raises the possibility that lesions that previously were not counted are now recognized as a pressure ulcer. Finally, the important role of medical devices as a cause of pressure ulcers, particularly those in atypical locations, is now better recognized. These pressure ulcers are more likely to be counted in more recent studies. The net effect of all these changes on epidemiological studies is uncertain.

Measures of Pressure Ulcer Rates

Efforts to describe the frequency of pressure ulcers have typically relied on incidence or prevalence rates [2, 3]. Both of these are measures of disease frequency and provide a perspective of the scope of the pressure ulcer problem in a given setting and at a specific time. Yet both incidence and prevalence rates have limitations. To address some of these limitations, recent efforts to describe pressure ulcer rates have relied on a "hybrid" approach known as the facility acquired or nosocomial rate. These approaches are described below.

Prevalence is a measure of the number of cases of pressure ulcers at a specific time, providing a description of the total burden of the disease. By providing insights into the magnitude of the pressure ulcer problem, it allows for the planning for health resource needs. The cases used in calculating prevalence may have recently developed or they may have been present for months or years. Prevalence may be described two ways. Point prevalence describes the situation at a specific point in time such as a specific date (first of the month) or an event (date of discharge). Period prevalence, in contrast, describes the cases over a prolonged time period such as the entire hospitalization. The main advantage of prevalence rates is their ease of calculation. However, since the cases may have developed elsewhere, prevalence rates provide fewer insights into the quality of care being delivered.

Incidence describes the number of new pressure ulcers in people without an ulcer at baseline. Since it only captures new cases, it provides the most direct measure of quality of care as well as allowing the identification of causative factors for pressure ulcer development. Calculation of incidence, though, is more complicated as it requires several assessments of pressure ulcer status, first to determine that there is no ulcer at baseline and subsequently to determine whether or not an ulcer has developed. Time plays a critical role when describing incidence as longer periods of follow-up will result in more pressure ulcers and a higher incidence rate. Consequently, it is often preferable to describe incidence over a defined time span such as 1 or 2 weeks rather than over an event such as an entire hospitalization that may sometimes last for a month or longer. An alternate approach is to describe incidence density which describes number of new pressure ulcers per 1,000 days of care rather than per patient. Central to this calculation is the assumption that pressure ulcer risk is stable over time so that the chance of developing a pressure ulcer on day 1 is the same as on day 30. This is most likely to be true in long-term care settings where people tend to be stable on admission rather than acute hospitals where people are generally sickest on admission and then improve.

Prevalence rates have the advantage of ease of calculation while incidence rates provide a better indication of quality of care. The facility acquired rate attempts to combine these advantages through a two-step process. First, prevalence is determined. Then, among those patients with a prevalent pressure ulcer, a further review is undertaken to determine whether the pressure ulcer was present on admission. Those present on admission are not counted in determining the rate.

Data Sources for Calculating Pressure Ulcer Rates

There are four main sources of data that could be used in calculating pressure ulcer rates; direct examination of patients, use of medical records, administrative databases, and patient survey. Each of these data sources has distinct advantages and limitations. Moreover, the pressure ulcer rate that is calculated will vary considerably depending on the source so that rates calculated from one data source should never be compared to another.

Direct examination of the skin, performed as part of a comprehensive skin assessment, provides the most accurate information regarding pressure ulcer status. When performed by an appropriately trained assessor, results should be reliable and valid, and even stage 1 ulcers will be detected. By performing assessments at regular intervals, nearly all pressure ulcers will be detected and this approach may be considered the "gold standard." However, direct examination of the skin is labor-intensive and expensive. The examinations are also intrusive so that informed consent will be required when performed as part of a research study. Consequently, pressure ulcer studies involving direct examination tend to be small and involve only a few sites.

Accurate data on pressure ulcer status may also be obtained from medical record reviews. Available data relies on detection of the pressure ulcer by a clinician, entry of this data into the medical record, and collection of the data during the medical record abstraction. The complexity of this process indicates the many ways in which information may be missed. In particular, stage 1 pressure ulcers will often not be detected. This suggests that pressure ulcer rates calculated from medical record abstraction may be lower than that obtained from direct examination of patients [4]. While chart abstractions are often labor-intensive, it involves less effort than examining patients.

Administrative databases, because of their widespread availability and ease of use, have frequently been utilized in epidemiological studies of pressure ulcers. Because they often have been developed for reimbursement purposes, they typically will provide information on thousands, or even millions of patients. There are two main types of databases. First are databases, such as hospital discharge abstracts, that provide a summary description of pressure ulcer status during an entire episode of care. Typically, this relies on an ICD-9 code for pressure ulcer listed among the discharge diagnoses. Until recently, though, databases based on discharge diagnoses did not contain information on pressure ulcer stage and whether the ulcer was present on admission. This would limit the ability to differentiate incident from prevalent ulcers. Second are databases such as the nursing home Minimum Data Set (MDS) or homecare Outcome and Assessment Information Set (OASIS) that capture pressure ulcer status on a specific date [5]. As assessments are repeated at periodic intervals, by examining serial entries for a patient, changes in pressure ulcer status over time can be determined allowing the identification of incident ulcers. However, rates cannot be determined for patients discharged prior to a second assessment. This may introduce bias in calculating rates as both healthier patients discharged home and sicker patients who die may be missed [6]. Databases often may miss information on pressure ulcer status due to incomplete entry. While this is particularly true for stage 1 ulcers, discharge diagnoses may miss even larger pressure ulcers [7]. As a result, rates calculated using administrative data tend to be lower than rates based on direct examination.

Finally, patients (or surrogates) may self-report their pressure ulcer status [8]. This approach has rarely been used in epidemiological studies due to its many limitations including difficulties in data collection, patients' unawareness of pressure ulcer status, and failure to recollect past events. Rates collected by patient self-report would be expected to be very low.

Understanding Differences in Pressure Ulcer Rates

Pressure ulcer rates are often measured in order to compare the relative performance of different providers or to examine changes in performance over time. The assumption is that a lower rate is indicative of better quality of care. Whenever comparing rates, the first question must be whether the same method was used in calculating the different rates. Very simply, pressure ulcer rates calculated with different methods are not comparable. However, even when the same methods are used, two other factors must be considered before assuming that differences in pressure ulcer rates reflect differences in quality of care.

Individual patients differ in their risk of pressure ulcer development. A mobile, incontinent patient will be at lower risk than one who is comatose. Some providers are likely to have more of these high-risk patients than others, and these providers would then be expected to have a higher rate of pressure ulcers even when providing similar quality of care as a provider with many low-risk patients. These differences in case mix are important to account for when considering differences in pressure ulcer rates [9]. Case mix of providers may also change over time, such as in response to changes in reimbursement policies. Thus, even for a single provider, case mix may need to be considered when evaluating changes in pressure ulcer rates over time [10]. A variety of approaches to case mix adjustment are available including a simple stratification into high- and low-risk groups as done by the Centers for Medicare and Medicaid Services (CMS) or the development of detailed statistical models [5]. Without such adjustments, it will always be uncertain whether higher rates are due to worse quality of care or care of a "sicker" population.

Pressure ulcer rates may also differ among providers due to random variation [11]. When we measure pressure ulcer rates, we try to infer the "true" rate indicative of quality based upon observations in a finite sample of patients. However, when this sample is relatively small, we may be uncertain as to what is the true rate. In a 50 bed nursing home, one additional pressure ulcer will raise the rate by 2 % and we would not be surprised if a 10 % rate in one time period is followed by a 6 % or 14 % rate in a subsequent period. In contrast, with 1,000 patients, we would be surprised if there was much variation in the pressure ulcer rate over time due to chance. Estimates of provider performance based on relatively few observations should be viewed with caution.

Pressure Ulcer Rates in Specific Settings

Pressure ulcer rates have been examined in many studies and in a variety of clinical settings. The National Pressure Ulcer Advisory Panel (NPUAP) has recently reviewed this literature for the years 2000 through 2011 [12] and contrasted results with an earlier data synthesis [13]. While results of this literature are readily summarized, it must be recognized that due to the multitude of methods employed, it remains difficult to provide an accurate assessment of pressure ulcer incidence and prevalence. Results from three settings are described below.

Critical Care

Reflecting the high frequency of serious medical conditions that predispose to pressure ulcer development, reported rates in critical care units are often high. As one example, an old randomized clinical trial performed in an intensive care unit described an incidence rate of over 50 % in patients placed on a standard bed [14]. Most of these incident pressure ulcers were stage 1. More recently, the NPUAP review for the years 2000–2011 performed by Cuddigan identified 23 studies on pressure ulcer rates with 6 being from the USA [15]. Although rates generally were not as high as seen in some of the earlier studies, pressure ulcers remain a significant problem. A study performed in a neurological intensive care unit reported a 12.4 % incidence rate for stage 2 or greater pressure ulcers [16]. The most comprehensive data comes from the International Pressure Ulcer Prevalence surveys which has been collecting data using a standardized methodology for over 20 years and typically includes over 90,000 acute care patients in each of its surveys. In 2009, facility acquired rates for critical care units ranged from 8.8 % in cardiac care to 10.3 % in surgical intensive care units [17]. Around one in three of these ulcers were stage 3 or deeper. Prevalence rates in various types of intensive care units were in the range of 15–20 %. These results illustrate that significant opportunities exist for improving pressure ulcer preventive practices in critical care.

General Acute Care

As with critical care, pressure ulcer rates from general acute care settings tend to vary considerably depending on the data source and methods used. In the NPUAP review performed by Goldberg, 42 studies were identified of which 18 were from the USA [18]. Highest rates are generally seen in smaller studies of high-risk patients. For example, following hip fracture, pressure ulcers developed in 14.6 % of the patients during the initial hospital stay and increased to 36.1 % by day 32 following surgery [19]. The hospital rate translated into 48 incident ulcers per 1,000 days of care. Databases based on hospital discharge diagnoses can examine pressure ulcers among millions of patients and have reported, for example, that in 2006 there were 503,300 hospital stays with a pressure ulcer diagnosis [20]; the actual prevalence rate, though, was not calculated in this analysis. More accurate data is available from some of the large surveys that have been performed using standard data collection protocols. In the previously described International Pressure Ulcer Prevalence survey, prevalence rates in 2009 on various acute care medical and surgical units were in the 8–14 % range with the facility acquired rate in the range of 3–5 % [17]. Another large study that has collected data over several years at multiple sites reported a prevalence rate of 16.0 % among nearly 32,000 patients in 2004 [21]. The incidence rate in this study was described as 7 %. Results had shown little change compared to preceding years, again illustrating the tremendous opportunities for improvement.

Nursing Homes

Pressure ulcers are also very common among nursing home residents. An early study using a forerunner of the Minimum Data Set examined nearly 20,000 residents of 51 nursing homes and found that 11.3 % possessed a stage 2 or deeper pressure ulcer on admission and among those ulcer-free residents remaining in the nursing home for 1 year, 13.2 % developed a new pressure ulcer [22]. The NPUAP review by Pieper identified 34 distinct studies published between 2000 and 2011 of which 20 were from the USA [23]. Further complicating an analysis of this literature is the fact that prevalence studies have looked at pressure ulcers on admission to the nursing home, at some point during the stay, or when nursing home residents are admitted for an acute hospital stay. Each of these approaches conveys different information. Prevalence rates in most studies have been in the 8–12 % range, although both higher and lower rates have been noted depending on the methodology employed. Incidence rates have varied so much that it is difficult to make any firm conclusions. It will be interesting to determine whether the enhanced pressure ulcer data collected as part of the new Minimum Data Set Version 3.0 will allow for better assessments of pressure ulcer rates.

Conclusions

Clinicians will encounter data on pressure ulcer rates in a variety of settings. There rates may be calculated from different data sources and there are many options in subsequently presenting these pressure ulcer rates. It is very clear that there is no preferred approach to calculating pressure ulcer rates that should be used in every situation. Rather the selected approach will depend on many factors. The wound care specialist should understand the strengths and limitations of whichever approach is selected.

References

1. National Pressure Ulcer Advisory Panel. NPUAP pressure ulcer stages/categories [Internet]. 2007 [cited 2012 Sept 9]. Available from: http://www.npuap.org/wp-content/uploads/2012/01/NPUAP-Pressure-Ulcer-Stages-Categories.pdf
2. Baharestani MM, Black JM, Carville K, Clark M, Cuddigan JE, Dealey C, DeFloor T, Harding KG, Lahmann NA, Lubbers MJ, Lyder CH, Ohura T, Orsted HL, Reger SI, Romanelli M, Sanada H. Dilemmas in measuring and using pressure ulcer prevalence and incidence: an international perspective. Int Wound J. 2009;6:97–104.
3. DeFloor T, Clark M, Witherow A, Colin D, Lindholm C, Schoonhoven L, Moore Z. EPUAP statement on prevalence and incidence monitoring of pressure ulcer occurrence 2005. EPUAP Rev. 2005;6:74–80.
4. Gunningberg L, Ehrenberg A. Accuracy and quality in the nursing documentation of pressure ulcers: a comparison of record content and patient examination. J Wound Ostomy Continence Nurs. 2004;31:328–35.

5. Berlowitz D, Intrator O. Risk adjustment for long-term care. In: Iezzoni LI, editor. Risk adjustment for measuring health care outcomes. Chicago, IL: Health Administration; 2012.
6. Berlowitz DR, Brandeis GH, Brand HK, Halpern J, Ash AS, Moskowitz MA. Evaluating pressure ulcer occurrence in long-term care: pitfalls in interpreting administrative data. J Clin Epidemiol. 1996;49:289–92.
7. Goode PS, Allman RM, Bartolucci AA, Burst N. Accuracy of pressure ulcer diagnosis by discharge diagnosis coding [Abstract]. Clin Res. 1993;41(2):200A.
8. Guralnik JM, Harris TB, White LR, Cornoni-Huntley JC. Occurrence and predictors of pressure sores in the National Health and Nutrition Examination survey follow-up. J Am Geriatr Soc. 1988;36:807–12.
9. Berlowitz DR, Ash AS, Brandeis GH, Brand HK, Halpern J, Moskowitz MA. Rating long-term care facilities on pressure ulcer development: importance of case-mix adjustment. Ann Intern Med. 1996;124:557–63.
10. Berlowitz DR, Bezerra HQ, Brandeis GH, Kader B, Anderson JJ. Are we improving the quality of nursing home care: the case of pressure ulcers. J Am Geriatr Soc. 2000;48:59–62.
11. Berlowitz DR, Anderson J, Ash AS, Brandeis G, Brand HK, Moskowitz MA. Reducing random variation in reported rates of pressure ulcer development. Med Care. 1998;36:818–25.
12. Pieper B, National Pressure Ulcer Advisory Panel, editors. Pressure ulcers: prevalence, incidence, and implications for the future. Washington, DC: NPUAP; 2012.
13. Cuddigan J, Ayello E, Sessman C, National Pressure Ulcer Advisory Panel, editors. Pressure ulcers in America: prevalence, incidence, and implications for the future. Reston VA: NPUAP; 2001.
14. Inman KJ, Sibbald WJ, Rutledge FS, Clark BJ. Clinical utility and cost-effectiveness of an air suspension bed in the prevention of pressure ulcers. JAMA. 1993;269:1139–43.
15. Cuddigan J. Critical care. In: Pieper B, National Pressure Ulcer Advisory Panel, editors. Pressure ulcers: prevalence, incidence, and implications for the future. Washington, DC: NPUAP; 2012.
16. Fife C, Otto G, Capsuto EG, Brandt K, Lyssy K, Murphy K, Short C. Incidence of pressure ulcers in a neurologic intensive care unit. Crit Care Med. 2001;29:283–90.
17. VanGilder C, Amlung S, Harrison P, Meyer S. Results of the 2008–2009 International Pressure Ulcer Prevalence™ Survey and a 3-year, acute care, unit-specific analysis. Ostomy Wound Manage. 2009;55(11):39–45.
18. Goldberg M. General acute care. In: Pieper B, National Pressure Ulcer Advisory Panel, editors. Pressure ulcers: prevalence, incidence, and implications for the future. Washington, DC: NPUAP; 2012.
19. Baumgarten M, Margolis DJ, Orwig DL, Shardell MD, Hawkes WG, Langenberg P, Palmer MH, Jones PS, McArdle PF, Sterling R, Kinosian BP, Rich SE, Sowinski J, Magaziner J. Pressure ulcers in elderly patients with hip fractures across the continuum of care. J Am Geriatr Soc. 2009;57:863–70.
20. Russo CA, Steiner C, Spector W. Hospitalizations related to pressure ulcers among adults 18 years and older. Rockville, MD: Agency for Healthcare Research and Quality; 2006. 2008 Dec. HCUP Statistical Brief #64.
21. Whittington KT, Briones R. National Prevalence and Incidence Study: 6-year sequential acute care data. Adv Skin Wound Care. 2004;17:490–4.
22. Brandeis GH, Morris JN, Nash DJ, Lipsitz LA. The epidemiology and natural history of pressure ulcers in elderly nursing home residents. JAMA. 1990;264:2905–9.
23. Pieper B, Pieper B. Long term care/nursing homes: incidence and prevalence data. In: Pieper B, National Pressure Ulcer Advisory Panel, editors. Pressure ulcers: prevalence, incidence, and implications for the future. Washington, DC: NPUAP; 2012.

Chapter 3
Prevention of Pressure Ulcers

Kim W. House and Theodore M. Johnson

Abstract Pressure ulcers (PU) cause significant morbidity in the frail elderly and neurologically impaired individuals. The cost of care may exceed $70,000 and treatment in the USA is estimated at $1.1 billion annually. New products and support surfaces are continually entering the marketplace. There has been heightened awareness of the problem and many evidence-based guidelines have been disseminated over the last decade. In spite of this there has been not been a dramatic decline in PU incidence worldwide.

Experts agree that not all PUs are avoidable. There are occasions when an ulcer develops in the face of good care. This chapter outlines the best practices for risk assessment and prevention. The tools and practices discussed can be applied to all care settings with the goal to reduce the incidence and, thereby, the prevalence of PUs.

Keywords Pressure ulcer • Prevention • Staging • Aging • Support surface • Skin assesment • Braden scale

Introduction

Pressure Ulcers (PU) are defined as "localized injury to the skin and/or underlying tissue usually over a bony prominence as a result of pressure, or pressure in combination with shear and/or friction" [1]. Pressure ulcers occur when soft tissue is compressed between a bony prominence and an external surface for a prolonged

K.W. House, M.D., C.M.D. (✉)
Department of Medicine, Atlanta VA Medical Center/Emory University,
1670 Clairmont Road, Decatur, GA 30075, USA
e-mail: Kim.house@va.gov

T.M. Johnson, M.D., M.P.H.
Department of Medicine, Atlanta VA Medical Center/Emory University,
1670 Clairmont Road, Decatur, GA 30033, USA
e-mail: Ted.Johnson@va.gov

D.R. Thomas and G.A. Compton (eds.), *Pressure Ulcers in the Aging Population:*
A Guide for Clinicians, Aging Medicine 1, DOI 10.1007/978-1-62703-700-6_3,
© Springer Science+Business Media New York 2014

time [1]. Compression causes diminished blood supply, which in turn leads to decreased oxygen and nutrient delivery to the affected tissues. These decreases cause the affected tissue to become ischemic and potentially necrotic [2].

Reports of PU incidence vary widely, from 0.4 to 38 % in acute care, from 2.2 to 23.9 % in long-term care, and from 0 to 17 % in home care, according to a report from the NPUAP [3]. Prevalence rates show the same variability: 10–18 % in acute care, 2.3–28 % in long-term care, and 0–29 % in home care [3]. The National Pressure Ulcer Advisory Panel has provided a mechanism for grading the stage of a pressure ulcer. The system has six stages: suspected deep-tissue injury, Stage I, Stage II, Stage III, Stage IV, and stageable. Because pressure ulcers are costly, take a substantial time to heal, and are a significant cause of morbidity and mortality, it is important to discuss prevention of pressure ulcers.

The Centers for Medicare and Medicaid ruling on the Inpatient Prospective Payment System states that hospitals are no longer reimbursed for care related to Stage III and Stage IV pressure ulcers that develop during a hospital admission [4].

Skin Assessment

On admission to an acute care, long-term care, or on first contact in the outpatient setting, an admission assessment should be completed that includes both a skin assessment to identify and describe any breakdown present on admission and a risk assessment to identify any patient at risk for breakdown. The skin assessment is a key component to prevention of pressure ulcers. The medical provider (MD, NP, PA) may delegate the skin assessment to other staff; however if there is inappropriate supervision, they may be at risk of litigation [5]. National Institute for Health and Clinical Excellence Pressure ulcer Guidelines [6] suggests that patients should be assessed in the hospital or emergency room within 6 h of their first episode of care, and on first contact in the outpatient setting. Assessment findings should be documented and reviewed at least weekly. A reassessment should be carried out whenever there is a change in the patient's physical and/or mental state, whether it is improving or deteriorating [6]. For Stage I pressure ulcers, the definition requires non-blanchable erythema [7]. The absence of blanching implies that the blood supply is not intact [7]. There has been a suspicion that Stage I presure ulcers are unrecognized and underreported in patients with darker skin. In these patients, the area of discolouration may be observed as being slightly darker than the surrounding skin. The blanch test will not show the pallor usually seen in lighter skin because of the presence of melanin. Therefore, other key indicators should be used alongside this test in patients with darker skin [8]. An increase or decrease in skin temperature can be indicative of pressure damage. An increase in temperature at the area can indicate inflammation or infection with cool skin indicating poor perfusion and ischemia [7]. Skin areas should be palpated for edema, which occurs in the tissues as the skin layers become separated and interstitial fluid accumulates between them [7]. Depending on staff expertise, classification/staging may be done by staff or staff describing the wound and utilizing a specific wound team or physician to classify and stage a wound. A certain level of expertise may be required to differentiate between a pressure ulcer and moisture-associated skin damage.

Pressure Ulcer Risk Assessment Scales

Pancorbo-Hildago et al. conducted a systematic review of 33 studies regarding PU risk assessment scales currently available for use. They found that the use of these scales has not changed the incidence of PUs, but they are still better risk predictors than nurses' clinical judgment [9]. Pressure ulcer risk assessment tools currently used worldwide are the Norton Scale, published in England in 1962, the Waterlow Scale, published in England in 1984, and the Braden tool, published in the USA in 1987 [10]. The most widely used and tested of all risk assessment tools is the Braden Scale for Predicting Pressure Sore Risk developed by Barbara Braden and Nancy Bergstrom [11]. The Braden Scale is an instrument that has undergone repeated testing (with varying reports of inter-rater reliability) and consists of six subscales/subscores used by healthcare providers to assess risk factors that are associated with PU development [12]. The Braden tool, like its predecessors, was developed and initially tested for validity among elderly populations in nursing home settings [11].

Braden Scale

The Braden scale is an overall numeric rating comprised of six subscales: sensory perception, mobility, activity, moisture, nutrition, and friction and shear. The six subscales are rated from 1 to 4 except the friction and shear subscale, which is rated from 1 to 3. Each numerical rating has a definition of patient characteristics to evaluate when assigning a score. A total of 6–23 points is possible, with lower numbers representing increased risk. The original critical cutoff point for defining high risk is 16 [11]. Other investigators have suggested setting 18 as the cutoff score to increase specificity and reduce the risk of false-positive screens for older patients and African-American and Latino patients [13, 14]. Certain Braden subscale definitions (such as patient's dietary intake or frequency of skin being moist) are more difficult for nurses to objectively measure or appropriately quantify than other Braden subscale factors such as activity level [10].

Gosnell Scale

The Gosnell Scale consists of five parameters—mental status, continence, mobility, activity, and nutrition with varying points (1–3 for nutrition; 1–4 for continence, mobility, and activity, and 1–5 for mental status). The scoring for each parameter is clarified by brief descriptive statements. The Gosnell Scale documents additional variables, including body vital signs, skin appearance, diet, 24-h fluid balance, medication, and interventions; however, these variables are not given weight in the final score. Possible Scores for the Gosnell Scale range from 5 to 20, with higher scores representing increased risk [15].

Norton Scale

The first pressure ulcer risk assessment scale was the Norton scale. It consists of five parameters: physical condition, mental state, activity, mobility, and incontinence. Each parameter is rated on a scale from 1 to 4, with a 1-, 2-, 3-word descriptor for each rating. The sum of the ratings for all five parameters yields a score ranging from 5 to 20, with lower scores indicating an increased risk. A score of 14 or lower indicates a risk for pressure ulcer formation [16].

Waterlow Scale

The Waterlow scale is based on the Norton Scale but is considered to be more comprehensive. The Waterlow Scale consists of eight items: build/weight for height, visual assessment of the skin in the area at risk, sex and age, continence, mobility, appetite, medication, and special risk factors. The highest and lowest scores of each item vary. The scores of mobility range from 0 to 5; scores for appetite range from 0 to 3. Patients scoring 10–14 are identified as being at risk for pressure ulcer formation. A score of 16 or below is the usual cutoff point for at-risk patients in clinical studies again with lower scores indicating a higher risk for pressure ulcer development [17].

Ramstadius Tool

The Ramstadius tool is the only assessment tool with just two questions. One question relates to skin integrity and the other to mobility. If both questions are answered "yes" the patient is considered at high risk for pressure ulcer development. However, the Ramstadius tool is not widely used and requires validation for its use as a predictive tool in a nursing home population [18].

Special Populations

SCI Patients

Salzberg et al. mailed a questionnaire to almost 2,300 members of the Eastern Paralyzed Veterans Association that sought to measure 45 potential risk factors for pressure ulcers. The survey had a 42 % response rate. There were seven risk factors that were independent predictors of pressure ulcer development: level of activity, level of mobility, complete spinal cord injury, urine incontinence or moisture, autonomic dysreflexia, pulmonary disease, and renal disease. In addition two other variables added to the predictive value, being prone to infection that causes breathing problems and paralysis caused by trauma as opposed to disease. Using these nine risk factors, the authors developed a new pressure ulcer risk assessment scale specifically for persons with paralysis who are living in a community setting. It appears to be more accurate than other scales in this population [19].

Pressure ulcer risk assessment scales, including the Braden Scale, tend to over-predict risk; as noted, this may be due to an inherent weakness in the tool itself or may reflect the effectiveness of currently used prevention protocols. Bolton in 2007 reviewed the MEDLINE electronic data base from January 1966 through March 2007 for the key term "pressure ulcer risk assessment" combined with the search terms (1) controlled study, (2) validity, (3) positive predictive value, (4) sensitivity, (5) negative predictive value, and (6) specificity. The majority of ICU patients in this review were found to be at risk for PU development based on the Braden Scale Score but did not develop a PU; it is unknown whether this represents true over-prediction or is the result of preventive care. In the first scenario, over-prediction may be the result of an intrinsic weakness of the scale and results in the unnecessary implementation of prevention protocols, which could impact healthcare costs. In this case, the refinement or development of a scale that better measures PU risk in the population would be warranted. In the second scenario, the apparent over-prediction may reflect the successful implementation of PU-prevention protocols; identification of the patient as being "at risk" triggered preventive care that actually prevented PU occurrence. Clinically, the second scenario validates the benefits of a comprehensive PU-prevention program. Since withholding PU-prevention strategies would be unethical, it is impossible to conduct a study to definitively determine whether the apparent over-prediction is true over-prediction or the result of effective care. In clinical practice, the consequences of under-prediction would far outweigh the costs of over-prediction (see Table 3.1).

Care Settings: Because pressure ulcer prevention differs so significantly by setting and by the patients seen in such settings, we have broken down further discussion of prevention by setting of care.

Table 3.1 Key points from Bolton review (2007) on pressure ulcer assessment tools [20]

1. The Braden and then Norton and Waterlow PU risk assessment scales have been found valid for the prediction of PU risk in a variety of healthcare settings and in multiple countries (level of evidence 1)
2. The Braden and Norton Scales have demonstrated inter-rater reliability when administered by RN's and LPNs (level of evidence 2)
3. A validated PURAS (Pressure ulcer risk assessment scale) should be administered by a professional nurse. Limited evidence suggests that the predictive validity of the Norton scale may be increased if it is administered by a nurse who has provided direct care of the patient undergoing risk assessment (level of evidence 2)
4. A cut point that differentiates clinically significant risk for PU development should be used for each scale. This value may vary based on setting (level of evidence 2)
5. A PURAS should be administered to all patients with 1 or more risk factors for pressure ulceration when admitted to a hospital's surgical, intensive care, orthopedic, cardiovascular, medical or step-down units, home care, hospice, or an extended care facility (level of evidence 2)
6. Administration of a PURAS is not indicated for patients without risk factors who undergo a brief period of immobility owing to surgery (level of evidence 2)
7. Pressure ulcer risk assessment should be performed on home care patients upon admission, and then weekly or biweekly until discharge (level of evidence 2) [20]

Acute Care

The acute care setting is an important site for pressure ulcer prevention because patients are acutely ill, often have limited mobility with resultant difficulty in relieving pressure, and may be nutritionally compromised. Fogerty conducted a large case–control study that reviewed admission and discharge data from over six million subjects (Nationwide Inpatient Sample) within acute hospital settings to identify risk factors and demographic differences between those who developed PU Pus and those who did not. Using multivariate logistic regression (LR) analysis examining the 45 most common diagnoses identified in persons with pressure ulcers, they reported the odds ratios (ORs) for the most significant risk factors associated with developing pressure ulcers. Analysis was also conducted stratifying the sample by age, race, and gender. Age over 75 years was the strongest PU risk factor identified with an OR of 12.63. Other strong risk factors identified by Fogerty included more than 28 medical diagnoses with an OR > 2. Age 59–75 years was a strong risk factor (OR 5.99), as was African-American race (OR 5.71). Other significant findings identified in the study highlight some of the strongest risk factors that are non-modifiable (age, paralysis, and race) while others are potentially modifiable (infection and nutritional deficiencies). A majority of the strongest risk factors identified are not accounted for in the Braden tool [21].

Cowan sought to determine if a PU predictive model could be identified specific to acute care to enhance the Braden scale which is currently utilized within facilities caring for US veterans. They investigated diagnosis of gangrene, anemia, diabetes, malnutrition, osteomyelitis, pneumonia/pneumonitis, septicemia, candidaisis, bacterial skin infection, device/implant/graft complications, urinary tract infection,

Table 3.2 Comparison of pressure ulcer risk assessment scales

Predictive power	Sensitivity (%)	Specificity (%)	PPV (%)	NPV (%)	Accuracy (%)
Norton	49	100	100	52	66
Braden	53	100	100	58	71
Gosnell	85	83	59	95	83
Waterlow	63	82.5	61	84	77

Table created from data in [23]

PPV postive predictive value, *NPV* negative predictive value

paralysis, senility, respiratory failure, acute renal failure, cerebrovascular accident, or CHF during hospitalization, patient's age, race, smoking status, history of previous PU, surgery, hours in surgery, length of hospitalization, and ICU days. Retrospective chart review and logistic regression analysis were used to examine Braden scores and other risk factors in 100 acutely ill veterans with PUs and 113 without PUs. Cowan found that malnutrition, pneumonia/pneumonitis, candidiasis, and surgery have stronger predictive value (sensitivity 83 %, specificity 72 %, area under receiver opering characteristic curve (ROC) 0.82) for predicting pressure ulcers in acutely ill veterans. The Braden scale total scores alone had sensitivity of 65 %, specificity 70 %, and an area under the ROC curve 0.70 (with 0.5 equivalent to chance, and 1.0 as perfect discrimination). Combining the four medical factors and two Braden sub-scores (activity and friction) demonstrated better overall model performance (sensitivity 80 %, specificity 76 %, and area under the ROC curve of 0.88) [22].

Jalali conducted a prospective clinical design study in which 230 subjects free of pressure ulceration on admission were assessed using the Braden, Gosnell, Norton, and Waterlow scales within 48 h of admission. Subjects' skin condition was assessed once every 24 h for a minimum of 14 days to identify any skin breakdown. As this study was conducted in Iran, the results may not be widely applicable to acute care settings elsewhere [23] (see Table 3.2).

Webster performed a single blind randomized control trial in Australia to assess the effectiveness of two-pressure ulcer screening tools against clinical judgement in preventing pressure ulcers. 1,231 patients were allocated to either a Waterlow or Ramstadius screening tool or to a clinical judgment group. There were 5.8 % of the patients who had an existing pressure ulcer on admission. Incidence of hospital-acquired pressure ulcers was similar between groups, clinical judgment (6.8 %), Waterlow (7.5 %), or Ramstadius (5.4 %) $P=0.44$. Significant associations with pressure injury in regression included requiring a dietetic referral, being admitted from a location other than home, and age over 65 years [24].

Surgical: Acute Care

Pressure ulcers can develop in a short time (as quickly as 3 days for postoperative patients) [25]. Patients undergoing surgical prodedures who are immobile for long periods and are unable to change positions are at greater risk than patients who are mobile. Because of sedation, anesthesia, and paralysis, surgical patients cannot meaningfully sense the numbness or pain that prolonged pressure causes and subsequently are unable to change position to relieve the pressure. The incidence of pressure ulcers among surgical patients can be as high as 45 % and the risk increases among older adults [26]. Bales performed a quasi-experimental clinical trial to test the efficacy of using intravenous bags as compared to a commercially available heel suspension foam boot. The target population was individuals admitted to the hospital for a hip or knee replacement between the ages of 55 and 70 years old. No patients using a foam boot (0/15) showed signs or symptoms of pressure, but 6/15 using an IV bag to "float" the heel had blanchable erythema and warmth present upon assessment [27].

Tschannen examined the relationship between patient characteristics (age, sex, BMI, history of diabetes, and [28] Braden Scale Score at admission) and care characteristics (total operating room time, multiple surgeries, and vasopressor use) and the development of pressure ulcers. The cohort study reviewed data from 3,225 surgical patients from November 2008 to August 2009. 12 % of the patients ($N=383$) had at least 1 pressure ulcer devlop during their hospitalization. According to logistic regression analysis, scores on the Braden Scale at admission ($P<0.001$), low body mass index ($P<0.001$), number of vasopressors ($P=0.03$), multiple surgeries during the admission ($P<0.001$), total surgery time ($P<0.001$), and risk for mortality ($P<0.001$) were significant predictors of pressure ulcers [29]. Schoonhoven found that total operating room time was significantly associated with the occurrence of pressure ulcers. For every 30 min the surgery went beyond 4 h, and the risk for a pressure ulcer increased by approximately 33 %. Further surgeries may result in more episodes of increased pressure on the capillaries when a patient is immobile because of sedation. This increase may in part be rleated to the amount of time a patient is completely immobile and unable to relieve pressure on bony prominences [30]. Pressure ulcers that are first noticed in postoperative units such as the Surgical Intensive Care Unit may be a result of unrelieved pressure in the operating room. Patient's recovery from the surgical operation would be lengthed with increased cost and morbidity due to an acquired pressure ulcer.

Long-Term Care

The long-term care setting is an appropriate site for discussion of prevention because the nursing home population is at increased risk for pressure ulcer development. The long-term care patient may have physical limitations that result in dependance on staff for bed mobility and pressure relief, cognitive limitations that make compliance with positioning difficult, malnutrition for various reasons, and a problem list of medical diagnosis such as vascular disease and diabetes that predispose them to the development of pressure ulcers. Ba'Pham used a validated Markov model to compare current prevention practices with four quality improvement strategies (1) pressure redistribution mattresses for all residents (bed); (2) oral nutritional supplements for high-risk residents with recent weight loss (vitamin); (3) skin emollients for high-risk residents with dry skin (lotion); and (4) foam cleansing for high-risk residents requiring incontinence care (continence). Primary outcomes included lifetime risk of stages II–IV pressure ulcers, QALYs, and lifetime costs. The NNT for each strategy was 45 (bed), 33 (vitamin), 158 (lotion), and 63 (continence), respectively, by number. Strategy 1 (bed) and 4 (continence) minimally improved QALYs and reduced the mean lifetime cost by $115 and $179 per resident. The cost per QALY gained was $78,000 for strategy 3 (lotion) and $7.8 million for strategy 2 (vitamin). If decision makers are willing to pay $50,000 for 1 QALY gained, the probability that improving prevention is cost-effective is 94 % (continence), 82 % (bed), 43 %(lotion), and 1 %(vitamin) [31].

Home Care

Home Care is an understudied area for pressure ulcer prevention and it is important to discuss because development of pressure ulcers in the home can result in costs associated with home health nursing for treatment, an increase in hospitalizations due to complications from pressure ulcers, and increased risk of nursing home placment for treatment and further prevention. Although numerous studies have examined risk factors for pressure ulcer development among hospitalized and long-term care patients, only one study and its secondary analysis have examined risk factors for pressure ulcer development in home health care. Risk factors for pressure ulcers differed from those found in long-term care studies, including oxygen use, having an adult child as the primary caregiver, and skin damage. The complete model with risk factors for higher PU development, using Cox regression analysis using time until incident ulceration, included male sex, needing assistance with dressing, being wheelchair bound, bowel/bladder incontinence, anemia, and recent fracture [32, 33].

Home healthcare agencies must collect OASIS data, which are nationally standardized and have established validity and reliability for payment of services provided to Medicare and Medicaid patients in the USA [34]. Researchers have attempted to utilize the OASIS data as a predictive model for the development of pressure ulcers. Bergquist-Beringer measured OASIS data on 3,323 females (61.6 %) and 2,072 males (38.4 %) ranging in age from 60 to 103 years. The cumulative incidence of pressure ulcers for the population was 1.3 % ($N=71$). Multiple logistic regression analyses revealed that bowel incontinence, needing assistance with grooming, dependence in ability to dress the lower body, dependence in toileting, inability to transfer, being chairfast or bedfast, and the presence of a pressure ulcer on admission were positively associated seating surfaces to patients only if they have a wheelchair. CMS also added process measures to their data collection in Outcome and Assessment Information Set (OASIS)-C. There are three that relate to pressure ulcers (1) whether or not a pressure ulcer risk assessment was conducted, (2) whether or not a pressure ulcer prevention plan was present in the plan of care, and (3) whether or not a pressure ulcer prevention intervention was evident in the short-term episode of care. This indicates the degree to which CMS is serious about pursuing a decline in the number of pressure ulcers occurring across all settings. These indicators are reported to the federal government and published on the CMS Web Site comparing a home care agency's outcomes in these areas to national and regional benchmarks since 2000 [35].

Hill-Brown in 2011 carried out a quality improvement project to provide pressure reduction cushions for veterans at high risk for pressure ulcers that did not have a wheelchair cushion. Pressure ulcers were reduced in this population of approximately 1,200 patients from around 23 pressure ulcers per year to 2 pressure ulcers per year following cushion distribution [36].

Patient Specific Risk Factors

Advanced Age

Increasing age has been found to be significantly associated with pressure ulcer development. While an important risk factor, age is essentially non-modifiable. The skin of older patients is drier, fragile, and easily injured [37]. The epidermis thins and cell turnover slows, with cell loss occurring more rapidly than cell replacement. Protective function of the epidermis is compromised. Temperature control is lessened with the loss of sweat glands and collagen renewal deteriorates with age. Emollients are helpful for dry skin [38].

Nutrition

Nutrition has been shown to be important for pressure ulcer prevention, in that populations with poor nutritional status have higher rates of pressure ulcer incidence. The loss of body fat reserves reduces the natural padding over bones, increasing the vulnerability to pressure and soft tissue breakdown [38]. A large retrospective cohort study of 2,420 adult nursing home residents with a stay of 14 or more days and with a risk of developing a pressure ulcer documented that an unintentional weight loss at any body mass index increased the chance of developing a pressure ulcer by 147 % [39]. Maintenance of adequate hydration is important. Well-hydrated skin is healthier skin and thus less vulnerable to breakdown [40, 41].

There are several tools to assess nutritional status. Among these is the Subjective Global Assessment of Nutritional Status. This scale is used to identify patients at risk of nutrition-related complications using information from the patients' history and physical examination [42]. Although serum albumin levels have long been used clinically, they are a poor indicator of visceral protein status related to albumin's long half-life (12–21 days) and numerous factors that decrease albumin levels even in the presence of adequate protein intake [38]. Measurement of actual oral intake through nutrient intake studies or monitoring body weight provides more reliable data from which to make clinical decisions. The NPUAP recommends to offer individuals with nutritional and pressure ulcer risks a minimum of 30–35 kcal per kg body weight per day with 1.25–1.5 g/kg/day protein and 1 ml of fluid intake per kcal per day [43]. While we currently lack specific studies that provide statistical evidence that nutritional and fluid support helps to reduce the risk of pressure ulcer development, most evidence-based guidelines include strong recommendations for nutritional assessment and support. For example, the NPUAP/EPUAP Guidelines include the following recommendations:

1. Identify and correct factors compromising protein per cal intake consistent with overall goals of care.
2. Consider nutritional supplementation/support for nutritionally compromised persons consistent with overall goals of care.
3. If appropriate offer a glass of water when turning to keep patient/resident hydrated.
4. Multivitamins with minerals per physician's order.

Immobility

All risk assessment tools include immobility as a risk factor and the two interventions currently recommended for addressing this risk factor are routine turning and positioning, and use of pressure reducing support surfaces [38]. The risk of pressure ulcer development is compounded when the patient is older and has concurrent illnesses that impair mobility or activity [37]. Standard mattresses are filled with springs and low-density foam. Pressure reduction support surfaces (PRSS) are filled with alternative materials such as gel, fiber, and air [44]. Several clinical guidelines recommend that all people at risk for pressure ulcers should use pressure reduction support surfaces. However, the evidence to support the effectiveness of PRSS is limited [45]. The National Pressure Ulcer Advisory Panel categorizes PRSS to powered support surfaces which include alternating pressure, low-air loss, and air-fluidized mattresses and alternating pressure overlays. Non-powered support surfaces include static air, gel-filled, fiber-filled, water-filled, and high-density foam mattresses and pressure redistributing overlays other than alternating pressure overlays. Powered PRSSs generally cost 100–1,000 of dollars to rent or purchase. Nonpowered PRSS generally cost less than $300. The difference in cost and style of mattress makes it important to determine if powered PRSS is more effective than non-powered [46]. Russell in 2003 performed an unblinded randomized prospective trial to determine whether a viscoelastic polymer foam mattress was superior to a standard hospital mattress for pressure ulcer prevention and to analyze the cost-effectiveness in comparison with standard hospital mattresses. A significant decrease in the incidence of blanching erythema and nonsignificant decrease in nonblanching erythema were found in patients allocated to the experimental group. To prevent nonblanching erythema the number needed to treat was 41.9 and the NNT was 11.5 to prevent any erythema. Patients with blanching or nonblanching erythema were significantly less mobile than participants with normal skin and more likely to have worsening mobility ($P < 0.001$) [47]. Comfort in 2008 performed a literature review to examine hospitals that utilized the Braden scale to identify at-risk patients and providing pressure-reducing surfaces to those found to be at risk. He found that although the programs put in place by the hospitals were not precisely the same, they could expect to reduce the odds that a patient will develop a pressure ulcer somewhere between a factor of 2 and 5 [48]. Xakellis, working at a 77-bed long-term care facility, provided inexpensive 2- and 4-in. foam overlays to those patients determined to be at risk for pressure ulcers based on a Braden Scale assessment. They used a staged approach providing overlay alone, turning schedule alone, or both turning schedule and overlay depending on the level of risk identified. This approach was successful in reducing the 6-month incidence rate from 23 % pre-protocol (16 of 69) to 5 % post-protocol (3 of 63) [49]. Rich performed a secondary analysis from prospective cohort study to evaluate the association between pressure-redistributing support surface (PRSS) use and incident pressure ulcers in older adults with hip fracture. Full-body examination for pressure ulcers, bed-bound status, and PRSS userecorded as none, powered, or non-powered. Incident pressure ulcers stage II or higher were observed in 4.2 % of visits after no PRSS use, 4.5 % of visits after powered PRSS use, and 3.6 % of visits after non-powered PRSS use. This study found that in a high-risk population there is little or no preventive effect of PRSS use in nonbed-bound patients at risk of pressure ulcers [45].

A recent Cochrane Review found good evidence of the superiority of high-specification foam over standard hospital foam, yet it was not able to determine the most effective support surface for pressure ulcer prevention or treatment. The review identified 29 pressure ulcer prevention trials and concluded that the methodologic quality was generally poor and that randomization was only adequate in only 22 % of trials. Four trials demonstrated a statistically significant reduction in the incidence and severity of pressure ulcers in high-risk patients when compared with patients on a standard foam mattress [50]. Despite the lack of compelling data, most evidence-based guidelines for pressure ulcer prevention do include a recommendation that at-risk patients be placed on a PRSS. Physiologically this makes sense, in that more conformable surfaces reduce the interface pressure over bony prominences, which translates into improved tissue perfusion.

Currently there is limited evidence to suggest that repositioning every 4 h when combined with any pressure redistributing mattress is just as effective for prevention of pressure ulcers as more frequent (every 2 h) repositioning or turning. Evidence for the optimal frequency of repositioning is lacking. Turning every 4 h in combination with the use of a viscoelastic foam redistributing mattress was shown to decrease the occurrence of pressure ulcers compared to turning every 2 or 4 h on a non-pressure redistributing mattress. Repositioning frequency should be determined by individual, activity/mobility level, and overall medical condition. In some individuals, regular turning and repositioning may not be possible because of their medical condition so consideration should be given to upgrade the support surface for these individuals. Frequent small position changes using pillows and wedges reduce pressure over bony prominences. Pad between skin surfaces such as knees that may rub together. Repositioning and use of pillows with continuous lateral rotation therapy need further research to determine its effectiveness on pressure ulcer prevention. Acute spinal cord injured patients may require more frequent turning than every 2 h due to microvascular dysfunction [51].

The NPUAP/EUPAP recommendations for pressure reduction support surfaces include:

1. Reposition bed-bound persons at least every 2 h and chair-bound persons every hour consistent with overall goals of care.
2. Use a written repositioning schedule.
3. Place at-risk persons on pressure-redistributing mattress and chair cushion surfaces.
4. Avoid using donut-type devices and sheepskin for pressure redistribution.
5. Use pressure-redistributing devices in the operating room for individuals assessed to be at high risk for pressure ulcer development.
6. Use pillows or foam wedges to keep bony prominences, such as knees and ankles, from direct contact with each other. Pad skin subjected to device-related pressure and inspect regularly.
7. Avoid positioning directly on the trochanter when using the side-lying position; use the 30° lateral inclined position.
8. Institute a rehabilitation program to maintain or improve mobility/activity status.

Friction and Shear

Friction can cause injury to the individuals skin from movement of the skin on the bed linens. Friction injuries can also develop in individuals who are in pain but are not able to process the meaning of the sensation of pain (those with confusion or dementia). Rubbing the heels on the bed is a commonly seen friction injury, which can quickly lead to superficial tissue damage on the heels. Shear stress is the "force per unit area exerted parallel to the plane of interest." Shear strain is the distortion or deformation of tissue as a result of shear stress. Friction is necessary for shear to occur and shear forces can damage the skin internally which is likely to occur when a resident must sit up in bed and then slides down [38, 52].

Exposure to Excess Moisture

Skin moisture from incontinence can be a risk factor for pressure ulcer development. The etiology of the incontinence should be identified and eliminated if possible. Moisture can arise from perspiration, wound exudates, urine, and/or feces. Sweat is not immediately toxic to skin but can result in epithelial injury through several mechanisms. Sweat between skin folds creates a warm moist environment and promotes growth of several forms of bacteria and yeast [53]. Normal skin pH is acidic at 4–6.5, which helps protect the skin against microorganism invasion. Frequent use of soap can alter skin pH to an alkaline state, leaving it more vulnerable to microorganism invasion. Skin that is water logged from continual wetness is more easily subjected to breakdown, injured by friction, permeable to irritating substances, and able to be colonized by microorganisms than normal skin as well as pressure ulcer deterioration. Exposure to urine or diarrhea damages the skin and increases the risk of pressure ulcers. Urine is absorbed by keratinocytes, and when these cells are softened, they cannot provide protection from pressure injury. Urine contains urea, and ammonia can damage the skin. In an incontinent individual with a urinary tract infection, urine will also be alkaline and injurious to the skin [38]. Diarrhea strips the outer layer of skin, and the exposed dermis cannot tolerate pressure. Diarrheal fluids are caustic and can damage the skin quickly. When urine is present in combination with feces, which contains bacteria and harsh gastrointestinal enzymes, the damage can be even quicker and more severe. In addition to this chemical irritation, the mechanical irritation from cleaning the individual can compound the damage [38]. The Wound Ostomy and Continence Nurses Society in 2010 published guidelines that recommend cleansing skin gently at each time of soiling with pH-balanced cleansers. The use of perineal skin cleansers has been found to be more effective for the prevention and treatment of incontinence-associated dermatitis (IAD) than traditional soap and water. Bar soap tends to dry the skin and create an alkaline pH on the epidermal skin surface increasing the risk of tissue injury. Vigorous cleaning can also lead to erosion of the epidermis. Smoothly woven disposable cloths are preferred over washcloths, which can increase friction at the skin's surface. Products with known irritants such as fragrance and alcohol should be avoided. Another cleaning option is the use of no-rinse cleansing foam. The WOCN also recommends using incontinence skin barriers such as creams, ointments, pastes, and film-forming skin protectants as needed to protect and maintain intact skin while avoiding products with humectants (urea, glycerin, alpha hydroxyl acids, and lactic acid). These products retain water in the skin, but with IAD the skin is over hydrated and does not need the added moisture from these products. The use of a skin protectant (i.e., dimethicone, liquid clear film barrier, petroleum, or zinc oxide) is recommended for individuals with frequent fecal incontinence or double urinary and fecal incontinence to protect against IAD.

Prevention of Heel Ulcerations

Epidemiologic data suggest that the heel is the second most common site behind the sacrum for pressure ulcers [54]. Heel pressure ulcers can cost $2,000–$30,000 to treat [55]. Prevalence data from more than 85,000 patients reveal that heel pressure ulcers account for 23.7 % of ulcers seen in acute care facilities, 22.5 % of those seen in long-term acute care facilities, and 22.9 % of those seen in long-term care facilities [56]. Okuwa identified three risk factors for lower extremity pressure ulceration in the elderly (1) low ankle-brachial index, (2) duration of time a patient is confined to bed, and (3) male gender. An ankle-brachial index was associated with a 2.27 LR (likelihood ratio) for developing a pressure ulcer [57]. The heel is one of the most difficult anatomical areas to effectively off-load pressure because of its small surface area and high tissue-interface pressure [58]. Specialized foam and sheepskin overlays were superior to standard hospital mattresses in preventing ulceration. However, none of the available bed surfaces provide complete pressure relief in the heel region [59]. Vanderwee and coinvestigators compared an alternating air overlay surface with a viscoelastic foam mattress. 447 patients admitted to acute care facilities in Belgium were randomly allocated to alternating air overlay surface and use of an air cushion when sitting or a viscoelastic foam mattress and use of the same air cushion when sitting plus patient repositioning every 4 h. More patients on the viscoelastic foam support surface plus turning program developed heel pressure ulcers than those managed on the alternating air surface overaly. The relationship remained after a logistic regression analysis that adjusted for length of stay, inpatient unit, method of assessment of pressure ulcer risk, and prevention protocol variables [60].

Many studies have been done comparing the effectiveness of pressure relief boots vs. standard hospital pillows for prevention of heel pressure sores. Tymec in 1997 evaluated 52 patients and found that patients using a boot-shaped air cushion were more likely to develop a heel pressure ulcer than patients using pillows [61]. In a comparison between heel protector made of siliconized hollow fibers with an ordinary pillow in 30 elderly patients (mean age 82 years), the pillow was more effective at reducing pressure on the heel [62]. The above studies suggested that pillows were more effective than boots for prevention of heel pressure ulcers. The types of pillows used in the above studies were standard hospital foam pillows. Heyneman compared a wedge-shaped cushion constructed from viscoelastic foam to a standard foam pillow. Patients managed with the wedge-shaped cushion had a significantly lower incidence of heel pressure ulcer than those managed with standard foam pillows (Fisher exact test $P=0.03$) [63].

Boots are another category of heel protection devices. Junkin in 2009 suggests that boot-type devices are most likely to stay on the feet and that they support the foot in a neutral position, reducing the risk of foot-drop. There are two categories of boots: those with and those without a brace. The brace acts as an orthotic to prevent foot-drop and rotation of the leg. These devices are often referred to as podus or AFO (ankle-foot-orthosis) boots. Nevertheless, a wound care expert panel strongly supports observations that placing a brace on patients increases their risk of pressure ulcer. Orthotic boots are not an attractive alternative for prevention of heel pressure ulcer. Prevention of heel pressure ulcers relies on the physical therapists in fitting the boot with a brace (AFO) [46].

Boots have also been designed expressly for the purpose of preventing pressure ulcers on heels and ankle malleoli. These devices are made of foam, some are plastic filled with air, and some are fiber filled or made of a synthetic sheepskin material. Clinical experience reveals strengths and limitations associated with each product.

For example, foam boots tend to be warm and make it more difficult to move easily in bed but are relatively more inexpensive. Air-filled plastic boots are light, helping with bed mobility. The clinician must monitor and add more air if needed to maintain appropriate air pressure. Fiber-filled boots incorporate fiber wicks to take away heat and moisture. Some brands are covered with a slick surface that is easy to clean and assit patient bed mobility [46].

Overall Recommendations

The NPUAP recommends interventions including, but not limited to, turning patient every 2 h, avoiding wrinkles in the linen under a patient, avoiding excessive linen between the patient and the bed, and identifying and managing any sources of moisture. Special padding may be considered for the intra-operative period if the surgical procedure is expected to be long, or special mattresses can be ordered to ensure patients are immediately placed on a bed that minimizes risk of skin deterioration [46]. Rich summarized interventions recommended for prevention of pressure ulcers in 2009 article. Recommendations with clinical evidence included using an instrument such as the Braden or Norton scales, pressure-reducing devices such as overlays or mattresses, avoidance of exposure of skin to moisture from urinary or fecal incontinence, reduction of shear forces by limiting the head of the bed to an angle below 30°, and regular repositioning of immobile patients. Most of these recommendations are based on primarily expert opinion except for the use of pressure reducing devices which includes systematic reviews of randomized controlled trials [64].

Rich performed a cross-sectional study of 792 hospitalized patients over age 65 to examine adherence to pressure ulcer prevention guidelines and to determine the frequency and correlates of recording pressure ulcers in the patient record. The research nurse evaluated patients on hospital day 3 to determine the use of preventive devices, presence of pressure ulcers, and risk of pressure ulcers (Norton scale). Data on additional risk factors were obtained from the admission nursing assessment. They found that only 15 % of patients had any preventative devices in use at the time of the examination. 51 % of high-risk patients (Norton score ≤14) had a preventative device. High risk of pressure ulcers was associated with use of preventative devices (OR 41.8) whereas the type and stage of pressure ulcer were not. Documentation of a pressure ulcer was present for only 68 % of patients who had a pressure ulcer according to the researcher examination. Limitation of this study was that the data were collected between 1998 and 2001 and the emphasis on pressure ulcer prevention may have changed since that time [64]. A comprehensive pressure ulcer prevention protocol can be costly both in equipment needs as well as additional manpower. A summary of recommendations for pressure ulcer prevention includes:

1. Complete a Risk Assessment Instrument for Pressure Ulcers (Braden/Norton Scale) on admission and weekly in an inpatient setting. Complete a Risk Assessment Instrument on first visit as an outpatient and with any significant change in condition.

2. Use pressure reduction mattresses and cushions as indicated.
3. Minimize the amount of chronic moisture exposure from urinary or fecal incontinence or sweat.
4. Use of pressure reduction devices including pillows or boots for reduction of pressure on the heel.
5. Optimize nutritional status including protein intake and hydration.
6. Remind and/or assist patients in repositioning at least every 4 h and in high-risk patients every 2 h.

References

1. National Pressure Ulcer Advisory Panel (NPUAP). Pressure ulcer stages revised. Washington, DC: NPUAP; 2007.
2. Baugh N, Zuelzer H. Wounds in surgical patients who are obese. Am J Nurs. 2007;107(6): 40–50.
3. Directors, National Pressure Ulcer Advisory Panel. Pressure ulcers in America: prevalence, incidence, and implications for the future. Adv Skin Wound Care. 2001;14:208–15.
4. Centers for Medicare and Medicaid Services. Medicare and Medicaid Move aggressively to encourage greater patient safety in hospitals and reduce never events. 2008. https://www.cms.gov/apps/media/press/release.asp? Accessed 5 Jan 2012.
5. Dimond B. Legal and ethical issues in advanced practice. In: Castledine G, McGee P, editors. Advanced nursing practice. Oxford: Blackwell; 2003. p. 184–99.
6. NICE. Pressure ulcer prevention. London: NICE; 2003.
7. Bethell E. Wound care for patients with darkly pigmented skin. Nurs Stand. 2005;41–49.
8. Matas A, Sowa MG. Eliminating the issue of skin color in assessment of the blanch response. Adv Skin Wound Care. 2001;14(4):180–8.
9. Pancorbo-Hidalgo PL, Garcia-Fernandez FP, Lopez-Medina IM. Risk assessment scales for pressure ulcer prevention: a systematic review. J Adv Nurs. 2006;54(1):94–110.
10. Papanikolaou P, Lyne P. Risk assessment scales for pressure ulcers: a methodological review. Int J Nurs Stud. 2007;44(2):285–96.
11. Bergstrom N, Braden BJ. The Braden scale for predicting pressure sore risk. Nurs Res. 1987;36(4):205–10.
12. Magnan MS, Maklebust J. The effect of web-based Braden Scale training on the reliability of Braden subscale ratings. J Wound Ostomy Continence Nurs. 2008;36(1):199–208.
13. Bergstrom N, Braden B. A prospective study of pressure sore risk among institutionalized elderly. J Am Geriatr Soc. 1992;40(8):747–58.
14. Lyder CH, Yu C. Validating the Braden Scale for the prediction of pressure ulcer risk in blacks and Latino/Hispanci elders: a pilot study. Ostomy Wound Manage. 1998;44(3A Suppl): 42S–9.
15. Gosnell D. An assessment tool to identify pressure sores. Nurs Res. 1973;22:55–9.
16. Norton D. An investigation of geriatric nursing problems in hosital. London: National Corporation for the Care of Old People; 1962.
17. Waterlow J. Pressure sores: a risk assessment card. Nurs Times. 1985;81:49–55.
18. Ramstadius B. Preventing instituion acquired pressure ulcers. Aust Nurs J. 2000;7(10):34.
19. Salzberg C, Byrne DW. Predicting and preventing pressure ulcers in adults with paralysis. Adv Wound Care. 1998;11(5):237–46.
20. Bolton L. Which pressure ulcer risk assessment scales are valid for use in the clinical setting? J Wound Ostomy Continence Nurs. 2007;34(4):368–81.
21. Fogerty MD, Abumrad NN. Risk factors for pressure ulcers in acute care hospitals. Wound Rep Regen. 2008;16(1):11–8.

22. Cowan L, Stechmiller JK. Enhancing Braden pressure ulcer risk assessment in acutely ill veterans. Wound Repair Regen. 2012;20(2):137–48.
23. Jalali R, Rezaie M. Predicting pressure ulcer risk: comparing the predictive validity of 4 scales. Adv Skin Wound Care. 2005;18:92–7.
24. Webster J, Coleman K. Pressure ulcers: effectiveness of risk-assessment tools. A randomized controlled trial (the ULCER trial). BMJ Qual Saf. 2011;20:297–306.
25. Karadag M, Gümüskaya N. The incidence of pressure ulcers in surgical patients: a sample hospital in Turkey. J Clin Nurs. 2006;15:413–21.
26. Walton-Greer P. Prevention of pressure ulcers in the surgical patient. AORN J. 2009;89: 538–52.
27. Bales I. A comparison between the use of intravenous bags and the heellift suspension boot to prevent pressure ulcers in orthopedic patients. Adv Skin Wound Care. 2012;25:125–31.
28. Lindgren M, Unosson M. Immobility - a major risk factor for development of pressure sores among adult hospitalized patients: a prospective study. Scand J Caring Sci. 2004;18:57–64.
29. Tschannen D, Bates O. Patient-specific and surgical characteristics in the development of pressure ulcers. Am J Crit Care. 2012;21:116–24.
30. Schoonhoven L, Defloor T. Incidence of pressure ulcers due to surgery. J Clin Nurs. 2002; 11:479–87.
31. Pham B, Stern A. Preventing pressure ulcers in long-term care: a cost-effectiveness analysis. Arch Intern Med. 2011;171:1839–47.
32. Bergquist S, Frantz R. Pressure ulcers in community-based older adults receiving home health care: prevalence, incidence and associated risk factors. Adv Wound Care. 1999;12:339–51.
33. Bergquist S. Pressure ulcer prediction in older adults receiving home health care: implications for use with the OASIS. Adv Skin Wound Care. 2003;16:132–9.
34. Shaughnessy PW, Hittle DF. Improving patient outcomes of home health care: findings from two demonstration trials of outcome-based quality improvement. J Am Geriatr Soc. 2002;50: 1354–64.
35. Center for Medicare and Medicaid Services (CMS). 2011. http://www.cms.gov/HomeHealthQualityInits/06_OASISC.asp
36. Hill-Brown S. Reduction of pressure ulcer incidence in the home healthcare setting: a pressure-relief seating cushion project to reuce the number of community-acquired pressure ulcers. Home Healthc Nurse. 2011;29:575–9.
37. Henoch I, Gustafsson M. Pressure ulcers in palliative care: development of a hospice pressure ulcer risk assessment scale. Int J Palliat Nurs. 2003;9:474–84.
38. Langemo D, Black J. Pressure ulcers ini individuals receiving palliative care: a National Pressure Ulcer Advisory Panel white paper. Adv Skin Wound Care. 2010;23:59–72.
39. Horn SD, Bender SA. The national pressure ulcer long-term care study: pressure ulcer development in long-term care residents. J Am Geriatr Soc. 2004;52:359–67.
40. Bossingham MJ, Carnell NS. Water balance, hydration status, and fat-free mass hydration in younger and older adults. Am J Clin Nutr. 2005;81:1342–50.
41. Schols JM, De Groot CP. Preventing and treating dehydration in the elderly during periods of illness and warm weather. J Nutr Health Aging. 2009;13:150–7.
42. Reilly HM. Screening for nutritional risk. Proc Nutr Soc. 1996;55:841–53.
43. National Pressure Ulcer Advisory Panel. The role of nutrition in pressure ulcer prevention and treatment: NPUAP White Panel. 2009. http://www.npuap.org/wp-content/uploads/2012/03/Nutrition-White-Paper-Website-Version.pdf
44. Anderson J, Hanson D. The evolution of support surfaces. Adv Skin Wound Care. 2006;19: 130–2.
45. Rich S, Shardell M. Pressure-redistribution support surface use and pressure ulcer incidence in elderly hip fracture patients. J Am Geriatr Soc. 2011;59:1052–9.
46. National Pressure Ulcer Advisory Panel. Pressure ulcer prevention points. National Pressure Ulcer Advisory Panel. 2007. http://www.npuap.org/PU_Prev_Points.pdf Accessed 20 Aug 2012.
47. Russell L, Reynolds TM. Randomized clinical trial comparing 2 support surfaces: results of the prevention of pressure ulcers study. Adv Skin Wound Care. 2003;16:317–27.

48. Comfort E. Reducing pressure ulcer incidence through braden scale risk assessment and support surface use. Adv Skin Wound Care. 2008;16:330–4.
49. Xakellis GC, Frantz RA. Cost effectiveness of an intensive pressure ulcer prevention protocol in long-term care. Adv Wound Care. 1998;11:22–9.
50. Cullum N, Deeks J. Beds, mattresses and cushions for pressure sore prevention and treatment. Cochrane Database Syst Rev. 2000;2:CD001735.
51. Wound Ostomy and Continence Nurses Society (WOCN). Guideline for prevention and management of pressure ulcers, WOCN clinical practice guideline, vol. 2. Mount Laurel, NJ: Wound Ostomy and Continence Nurses Society (WOCN); 2010. 96 p.
52. NPUAP. Terms and definitions related to support surfaces. Washington, DC: NPUAP; 2007.
53. Copson D. Management of tissue excoriation in older patients with urinary or fecal incontience. Nurs Stand. 2006;21:57–66.
54. Whittington K, Briones R. National prevalence and incidence study: 6-year sequential acute care data. Adv Skin Wound Care. 2004;17:490–4.
55. Young Z, Evans A. Nosocomial pressure ulcer prevention. J Nurs Adm. 2003;33:380–3.
56. Vanglider C, Macfarlane GD. Results of nine international pressure ulcer prevalence surveys: 1989–2005. Ostomy Wound Manage. 2008;54:40–54.
57. Okuwa M, Sanada H. A prospective cohort study of lower-extremity pressure ulcer risk among bedfast older adults. Adv Skin Wound Care. 2006;19:391–7.
58. Lyman V. Successful heel pressure ulcer prevention program in a long-term care setting. J Wound Ostomy Continence Nurs. 2009;36:616–21.
59. Reddy M, Gill SS. Preventing presure ulcers: a systematic review. JAMA. 2006;296:974–84.
60. Vanderwee K, Grypdonck MH. Effectiveness of alternating presure air mattress for the prevention of pressure ulcers. Age Ageing. 2005;34:261–7.
61. Tymec AC, Pieper B. A comparison of two pressure-relieving devices on the prevention of heel pressure ulcers. Adv Wound Care. 1997;10:39–44.
62. De Keyser G, Dejaeger E. Pressure-reducing effects of heel protectors. Adv Wound Care. 1994;7:30–4.
63. Heyneman A, Vanderwee K. Effectiveness of two cushions in the prevention of heel pressure ulcers. Worldviews Evid Based Nurs. 2009;6:114–20.
64. Junkin J, Gray M. Are pressure redistribution surfaces or heel protection devices effective for preventing heel pressure ulcers. J Wound Ostomy Continence Nurs. 2009;36:602–8.

Other Useful Pressure Ulcer Prevention Resources

AHRQ Toolkit–Preventing Pressure Ulcers in Hospitals. http://www.ahrq.gov/research/ltc/pressureulcertoolkit/

AHRQ Guideline Synthesis on Preventing Pressure Ulcers. http://www.guideline.gov/syntheses/synthesis.aspx?id=25078

National Pressure Ulcer Advisory Panel. http://www.npuap.org/

IHI How to Guide Reducing Pressure Ulcers. http://www.ihi.org/knowledge

Implementation Guide to Prevention of Hospital Acquired Pressure Ulcers (HAPU). http://hrethen.org/images/phocadownload/hapu_final_508.pdf

Chapter 4
Assessment and Documentation of Pressure Ulcers

Jan Kottner and Kathrin Raeder

Abstract Pressure ulcer assessment includes the correct diagnosis, classification, and wound assessment. Pressure ulcers are caused by compression of skin and/or subcutaneous fat and/or muscle tissue between hard internal body structures and hard external devices or support surfaces. Pressure ulcers are classified according to their depth and kinds of involved tissues. Differentiating pressure ulcer from other skin or tissue lesions is difficult and accurate classification is challenging. Pressure ulcer wound assessments further include the determination of location, size, tissue types and their quality, possible undermining, kind and amount of exudates, odor, edge, periwound appearance, and pain. Standardized tools and scores are available for wound assessment and/or predicting of healing.

Keywords Assessment • Classification • Etiology • Pressure ulcer • Wound

Assessment and Documentation of Pressure Ulcers

Correct and precise pressure ulcer (PU) assessment is a prerequisite for accurate communication, documentation, and treatment decisions. Because PU diagnoses and classifications also have reimbursement, legal, and quality evaluating consequences,

J. Kottner (✉)
Department of Dermatology and Allergy, Clinical Research Center for Hair and Skin Science, Charité-Universitätsmedizin Berlin, Charitéplatz 1, 10117 Berlin, Germany
e-mail: jan.kottner@charite.de

K. Raeder
Department of Nursing Science, Charité Universitätsmedizin Berlin, Augustenburger Platz 1, 13353 Berlin, Germany
e-mail: kathrin.raeder@charite.de

D.R. Thomas and G.A. Compton (eds.), *Pressure Ulcers in the Aging Population: A Guide for Clinicians*, Aging Medicine 1, DOI 10.1007/978-1-62703-700-6_4, © Springer Science+Business Media New York 2014

the importance of valid diagnostic statements cannot be overemphasized. Unfortunately PU diagnostic in the clinical practice is not easy because a number of questions need to be answered within the diagnostic process, e.g., Is it a PU? If "yes," what category is it? If "no," what else can it be? How do I measure the PU size? Is this PU worsening or healing? This chapter aims to provide some guidance how such a complex task might be managed at the bedside. However, there are still many unresolved problems and new developments within the field of PU diagnostics that are briefly mentioned as well, because compared to many other fields of medicine and healthcare things we take for granted today will be outdated tomorrow. This is not negative but rather the normal course of science and clinical practice development.

Is it a Pressure Ulcer?

According to the latest definition in the "Pressure Ulcer Prevention and Treatment Clinical Practice Guideline" provided by the National Pressure Ulcer Advisory Panel (NPUAP) and the European Pressure Ulcer Advisory Panel (EPUAP) in 2009: "A pressure ulcer is localized injury to the skin and/or underlying tissue usually over a bony prominence, as a result of pressure, or pressure in combination with shear. A number of contributing or confounding factors are also associated with pressure ulcers; the significance of these factors is yet to be elucidated" [1]. From this definition three important consequences follow:

- PUs are not necessarily skin injuries. The two skin layers epidermis and dermis might be damaged or might be intact. In the latter case subdermal tissue structures like subcutaneous fat, muscle tissue, or supporting structures like bones or joints might be affected only. In clinical practice this may cause problems, because as long as the skin is intact the real degree of tissue injury is unknown.
- PUs are defined by their etiology: pressure, or pressure in combination with shear. In reality both loads pressure and shear cannot occur alone because within loaded tissues compression, shear and tensile stresses always occur simultaneously [2]. The more important point is that the etiology must be known to name a skin injury as PU. In other words, when one is not entirely sure that prolonged mechanical tissue deformations were responsible for the injury one cannot be sure that this wound is really a PU.
- Our knowledge about PU development is clearly limited and it is likely that future research will change our current understanding of the phenomenon. This means that we are faced with uncertainties within PU prevention and treatment including diagnostic and prognostic statements about PU wounds.

What does all this mean for clinical practice? PU diagnostics always start with a sound assessment of the whole person. Among others, impairments in mobility and/or sensory perception are the strongest predictors for PU development

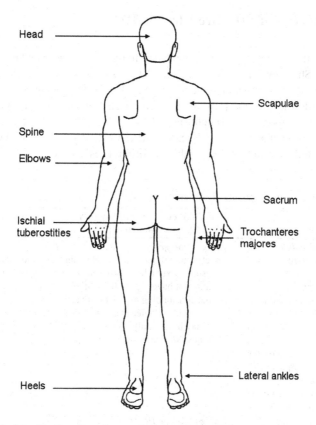

Head

Spine

Elbows

Ischial
tuberostities

Heels

Scapulae

Sacrum

Trochanteres
majores

Lateral ankles

Fig. 4.1 Typical predilection sites of pressure ulcer occurrence

[3–5]. Therefore hospital patients who underwent long diagnostic or operating procedures, unconscious persons, persons with long transfer times (e.g., admissions from emergency departments), SCI patients, geriatric patients, or nursing home residents with high degrees of care dependency are more likely to show PUs than mobile, active, and independent persons. Having a history of resolved PUs is also a very strong hint that a new PU might have had developed [4, 6]. Another important cue for PU identification is the anatomic location. Pressure ulcers due to impaired mobility often occur at so-called predilection sites. Among others the sacral region, the ischial tubrosities, the trochanteres majores, and the heels are most often affected [7–9] because due to anatomic structures, body build, movements, and contact patterns with underlying surfaces (e.g., wheal-chairs) tissues at these predilection sites are more susceptible for compression injuries than other skin areas (Fig. 4.1).

Device-related PUs occur at regions, where medical equipment presses, rubs, or pushes against the body surface, e.g., compression devices, tubes, casts, catheters, and comparable diagnostic or therapeutic devices [10, 11].

What Category of Pressure Ulcer Is It?

PUs are classified according to their depth and to the kinds of affected tissues. In the 1970s Darell Shea developed the first formal PU classification system at the University of Miami primarily for treatment decisions but also for improving the precision of clinical records and research [12]. Since then this classification was adapted several times resulting in more than 20 published classifications [13, 14]. Today the current PU classifications in the ICD-10 [15] and the NPUAP/EPUAP [1] are used worldwide (Table 4.1). Both systems are comparable but differences also occur.

Table 4.1 Currently used pressure ulcer classifications

ICD-10 Version: 2010 [15]	National Pressure Ulcer Advisory Panel/European Pressure Ulcer Classification 2009 [1]
L89.0 Stage I decubitus ulcer and pressure area Definition The ulcer appears as a defined area of persistent redness (erythema) in lightly pigmented skin, whereas in darker skin tones, the ulcer may appear with persistent red, blue, or purple hues, without skin loss Incl.: Decubitus [pressure] ulcer limited to erythema only	*Category/Stage I: Non-blanchable erythema* Intact skin with non-blanchable redness of a localized area usually over a bony prominence. Darkly pigmented skin may not have visible blanching; its color may differ from the surrounding area. The area may be painful, firm, soft, warmer, or cooler as compared to adjacent tissue. Category I may be difficult to detect in individuals with dark skin tones. May indicate "at-risk" persons
L89.1 Stage II decubitus ulcer and pressure area Incl.: Decubitus [pressure] ulcer with: • Abrasion • Blister • Partial thickness skin loss involving epidermis and/or dermis • Skin loss NOS	*Category/Stage II: Partial thickness* Partial thickness loss of dermis presenting as a shallow open ulcer with a red pink wound bed, without slough. May also present as an intact or open/ruptured serum-filled or sero-sanginous-filled blister. Presents as a shiny or dry shallow ulcer without slough or bruising[a]. This category should not be used to describe skin tears, tape burns, incontinence-associated dermatitis, maceration, or excoriation
L89.2 Stage III decubitus ulcer and pressure area Definition Decubitus [pressure] ulcer with full thickness skin loss involving damage or necrosis of subcutaneous tissue extending to underlying fascia	*Category/Stage III: Full thickness skin loss* Full thickness tissue loss. Subcutaneous fat may be visible but bone, tendon, or muscle is *not* exposed. Slough may be present but does not obscure the depth of tissue loss. *May* include undermining and tunneling. The depth of a Category/Stage III pressure ulcer varies by anatomical location. The bridge of the nose, ear, occiput, and malleolus do not have (adipose) subcutaneous tissue and Category/Stage III ulcers can be shallow. In contrast, areas of significant adiposity can develop extremely deep Category/Stage III pressure ulcers. Bone/tendon is not visible or directly palpable

(continued)

Table 4.1   (continued)

ICD-10 Version: 2010 [15]	National Pressure Ulcer Advisory Panel/European Pressure Ulcer Classification 2009 [1]
L89.3 Stage IV decubitus ulcer and pressure area Definition Decubitus [pressure] ulcer with necrosis of muscle, bone, or supporting structures (i.e., tendon or joint capsule)	*Category/Stage IV: Full thickness tissue loss* Full thickness tissue loss with exposed bone, tendon, or muscle. Slough or eschar may be present. Often includes undermining and tunneling. The depth of a Category/Stage IV pressure ulcer varies by anatomical location. The bridge of the nose, ear, occiput, and malleolus do not have (adipose) subcutaneous tissue and these ulcers can be shallow. Category/Stage IV ulcers can extend into muscle and/or supporting structures (e.g., fascia, tendon, or joint capsule) making osteomyelitis or osteitis likely to occur. Exposed bone/muscle is visible or directly palpable
L89.9 Decubitus ulcer and pressure area, unspecified Incl.: Decubitus [pressure] ulcer without mention of stage	*Unstageable/ Unclassified: Full thickness skin or tissue loss—depth unknown* Full thickness tissue loss in which actual depth of the ulcer is completely obscured by slough (yellow, tan, gray, green, or brown) and/or eschar (tan, brown, or black) in the wound bed. Until enough slough and/or eschar are removed to expose the base of the wound, the true depth cannot be determined, but it will be either a Category/Stage III or IV. Stable (dry, adherent, intact without erythema or fluctuance) eschar on the heels serves as "the body's natural (biological) cover" and should not be removed Suspected deep tissue injury—depth unknown Purple or maroon localized area of discolored intact skin or blood-filled blister due to damage of underlying soft tissue from pressure and/or *shear*. The area may be preceded by tissue that is painful, firm, mushy, boggy, warmer, or cooler as compared to adjacent tissue. Deep tissue injury may be difficult to detect in individuals with dark skin tones. Evolution may include a thin blister over a dark wound bed. The wound may further evolve and become covered by thin eschar. Evolution may be rapid exposing additional layers of tissue even with optimal treatment

[a]Bruising indicates deep tissue injury

Category I Pressure Ulcer

Compared to the other categories the conceptualization of category I PUs is most difficult. It is defined as persisting localized (non-blanchable) skin redness (Table 4.1, Fig. 4.2). In healthy conditions non-nociceptive external loads on the skin lead to vasodilation of the dermal mircovessels which is called pressure-induced vasodilation [16]. The increased blood flow is regarded as protecting the tissue since the deleterious effects of ischemia are prevented or delayed. The occurrence of

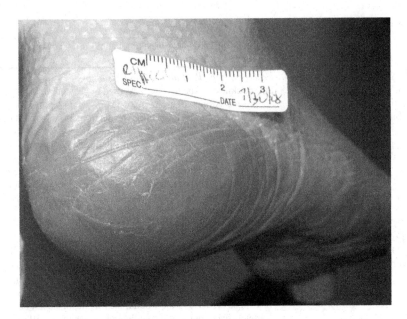

Fig. 4.2 Heel category I pressure ulcer (NPUAP copyright and used with permission)

pressure-induced vasodilation in aged hospital patients in various lying positions beneath bony prominences could be recently demonstrated in superficial as well as in deeper tissues [17]. This is a physiologic reaction, but if the localized erythema persists after longer periods of offloading (e.g., after 30 min or more) or under slight finger press, it is assumed that pathologic skin damage has already occurred [18, 19]. Recently petechial dots and telangietic streaks in category I PUs were described indicating pathologic vasodilation and hemorrhage due to ischemia [20]. However, because the skin is still intact, the point at which category I PUs become irreversible is unknown [21], and most erythema resolve after offloading, it is considered not appropriate to talk about a real ulcer. Instead category I PUs should be regarded as important warning signs indicating that subjects are of urgent need for preventive actions [22]. Compared to younger persons the pressure-induced vasodilation in older subjects might be impaired or even lacking [23]. This is one reason why older immobile persons are greater PU risk.

In clinical practice the diagnosis of category I PUs is difficult, because a non-blanchable erythema must be reliably detected. To test for blanchability the finger ("finger method") or a small transparent device ("disc method") can be used to slightly press on the suspected skin area. Which method enhances reliability and precision is unknown so far [24, 25], but empirical evidence suggests that category I PU identification in general contains large amounts of measurement error [14, 26, 27].

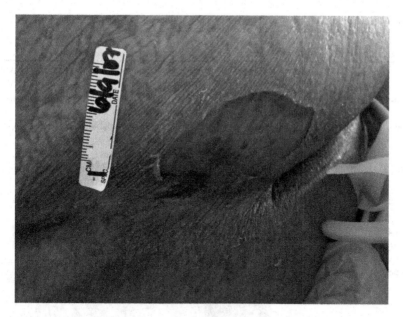

Fig. 4.3 Sacral category II pressure ulcer, open ruptured blister (NPUAP copyright and used with permission)

Category II Pressure Ulcers

This category comprises epidermal and/or dermal injuries or serum-filled blisters that may rupture (Table 4.1, Fig. 4.3). Since the epidermis and dermis are comparably thin tissue layers these wounds are always shallow. Fresh exposed dermis appears wet and reddish. Because category II PUs are real skin damages they are easier to detect than category I PUs. Unfortunately clinicians are faced with another still unsolved problem here: the differentiation between category II PUs and other skin lesions. Per definition PUs are caused by pressure and shear. That means that only skin lesions should be named PUs when these loads were the etiological factors. Empirical evidence and clinical experiences suggest that most superficial skin lesions within the context of immobility and care dependency are moisture and/or friction related [28, 29]. Above all the incontinence-associated dermatitis (IAD) [30, 31] plays a significant role in geriatric care settings. IAD or other friction-related skin injuries like skin tears should not be labeled as PU. On the other hand the current version of the ICD-10 is not that clear regarding this etiologic issue (see NPUAP/EPUAP description in Table 4.1).

When detecting superficial skin lesions there are various cues helping to decide whether this might be a category II PU or moisture-related injury like IAD. Above all clinical signs like anatomic location, shape, and color should be taken into

Table 4.2 Distinguishing category II pressure ulcers from other skin lesions adapted from [32, 33]

Defining characteristic	Pressure ulcer	Incontinence-associated dermatitis
Cause	Pressure and/or shear must be present	Moisture must be present (e.g., shining, wet skin caused by urinary incontinence or diarrhea)
Location	Likely to occur over a bony prominence	May occur over a bony prominence, but pressure and shear should be excluded as causes
Shape	Limited to one spot, circular with regular shape	Diffuse, different superficial spots, spread to other areas not affected by pressure
Edges	Distinct edges	Diffuse or irregular edges
Color	If redness is non-blanchable, this is most likely a pressure ulcer category I	Blanchable or non-blanchable erythema, redness not uniformly distributed, pink or white surrounding skin due to maceration

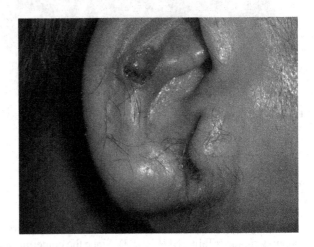

Fig. 4.4 Category III pressure ulcer at the ear (NPUAP copyright and used with permission)

account in the assessment process (Table 4.2) [32, 33]. While category II PUs may be covered by eschar they never contain slough or other necrotic material. If there is necrotic tissue or slough it is not a category II PU. As long as only the superficial dermal layer (stratum papillare) is affected the healing process leads to full restoration of original functional skin without scars (restitutio ad integrum).

Category III Pressure Ulcers

These are full thickness wounds affecting the cutis and/or the subcutaneous fat tissue. The anatomic boundary is the deep fascia meaning that muscle, bones, or joints are not involved and they are neither visible nor directly palpable (Table 4.1). Subcutaneous fat in wounds has a pale yellow or yellow-brown waxy appearance. Depending on the anatomic location category III PUs may be deep (e.g., trochanteric PUs in obese subjects) or shallow at skin areas, where the subcutaneous fat is absent (e.g., at the ear, Fig. 4.4) or very thin (e.g., in underweight subjects).

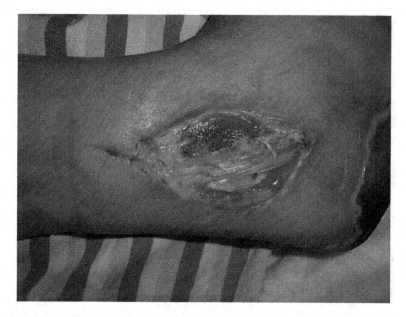

Fig. 4.5 Category IV pressure ulcer at the lateral ankle with visible tendon (NPUAP copyright and used with permission)

Healing times for category III PUs are much longer than for superficial wounds [34] and except the epidermis injured tissues are replaced by nonfunctional scar tissue. The wound may be covered by slough or other necrotic material and undermining is possible. In case of impaired wound healing the wound edges are typically raised, thickened, or rolled, indicating that it is rather unlikely that re-epithlization occurs without special therapeutic interventions.

Category IV Pressure Ulcers

These wounds are severe tissue injuries affecting dermal and/or subdermal structures like subcutaneous fat, muscle, tendons, joints, or bones. Their appearance is similar to category III PUs, but muscle tissue or supporting structures are visible or directly palpable (Fig. 4.5). Again, these ulcers can be shallow at skin areas where there is no subcutaneous tissue (e.g., at the heels).

Suspected Deep Tissue Injury

Although not new, the concept of Deep Tissue Injuries (DTIs), which are pressure/shear injuries under intact skin, gained much attention in the last 10 years

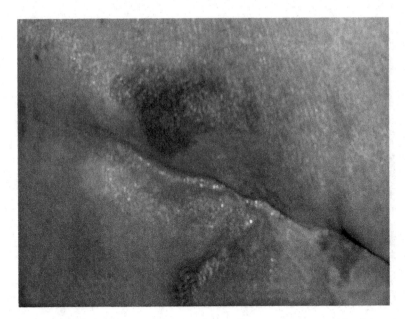

Fig. 4.6 Suspected deep tissue injury (DTI) at the sacral area (NPUAP copyright and used with permission)

[35]. As early as 1942 Groth distinguished between superficial PUs evolving in the skin and deep PUs evolving in the skeletal muscle [36]. The background is that different tissue layers have different susceptibilities to sustained deformation injuries. For instance skeletal muscle and/or subcutaneous fat are much more vulnerable when compressed than the skin layers. Consequently pressure injuries occur first in deeper tissues under a more or less healthy skin. After the injury there are two possibilities: the damaged area is small and necrotic tissue and fluids are reabsorbed and the area is replaced by scar tissue. On the other hand the size of the damaged area might be non-absorbable and undermining and progression of the necrosis takes place and eventually breaks through the skin surface [37]. This mechanism is also called the inside-out or bottom-up pathway of PU development [29].

Because comparable with category I PUs the skin is intact, the accuracy of clinical judgment is challenged. Recent study results suggest indeed that category I PUs and DTIs are likely being confused [27, 38, 39]. Imaging techniques like for instance ultrasonography show good results in diagnosing subcutaneous injuries even before other clinical signs emerge [40], but these technical devices are usually not available at the bedside. Macroscopically skin areas above suspected DTIs look purple, maroon, or even black (see description in Table 4.1, Fig. 4.6) and they typically occur at the heels, the sacral region, and hips [38, 41].

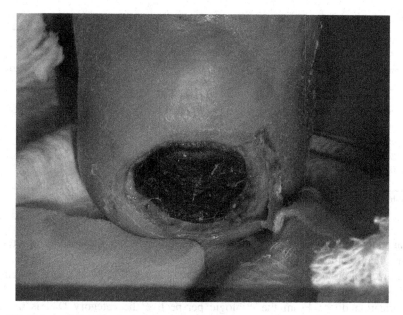

Fig. 4.7 Unstageable pressure ulcer at the heel (NPUAP copyright and used with permission)

Unstageable Pressure Ulcers

Deep PUs covered by slough or eschar are classified as "Unstageable" as long as the extent of ulcer depth is unknown (Fig. 4.7). Unstageable PUs are always category III or IV PUs.

Current Problems of Pressure Ulcer Classification

There are several conceptual and practical problems within available PU definitions and category descriptions. A minor but still discussed issue is the numbers I to IV used for PU staging. Increasing numbers might suggest a linear course of PU development from skin redness to deep category IV PUs. A large body of evidence and clinical experience indicate that this is not the case. For instance there seem to be etiological differences between superficial category II and deep category III and IV PUs [42, 43]. The microclimate factors skin surface moisture and skin temperature are likely to affect the skin eventually leading to superficial macerations, abrasions, or excoriations while compression and shear are likely to produce deep tissue injuries like category III and IV with or without full thickness skin loss. Different etiologies obviously lead to different types of tissue trauma [28, 29] that might

Table 4.3 Recent suggestions for alternative pressure ulcer classifications (examples)

Current pressure ulcer categories	Beeckman et al. [45]	Kottner et al. [28]	Sibbald et al. [29]
Category I	Warning sign for potential tissue breakdown[a]	Warning sign for potential tissue breakdown[a]	Excluded from the current system until nature is fully understood
Category II	Superficial ulcer	Superficial ulcer	Superficial skin change
Category III	Deep pressure ulcer	Deep pressure ulcer	Deep pressure ulcer
Category IV			
Unstageable			
Deep tissue injury		Warning sign potential full thickness loss[a]	

[a]Requiring urgent preventive measures like complete offloading

occur independently from each other and that are subsumed under one umbrella term called PU [44].

A practical problem is the non-comparability of current PU classification systems. For instance descriptions of category II PUs within the ICD-10 and NPUAP/EPUAP classification differ. From the etiologic perspective the category DTI is useful because this very type of PU corresponds well with our current understanding of PU development. However, this category is propagated in the USA only—not in Europe [1]. This limits international communication and comparability of PU figures. The same is true for the category unstageable. Furthermore, according to the recent category I to IV descriptions DTIs cannot be classified in Europe at all. In the previous EPUAP classification system a category IV PU was defined as "Extensive destruction of tissue necrosis, or damage to muscle, bone or supporting structures with or without full-thickness skin loss" [19]. Consequently DTIs could be classified as category IV in this previous system. Because the important words "with or without" were deleted in the new classification this is no longer possible. In the literature there are several new ideas how to change the current PU classification system (Table 4.3) [28, 29, 45]. Despite their differences available proposals have two things in common: [1] reduction of complexity and [2] clear differentiation from non-pressure-related skin damages like IAD [46]. In face of these existing suggestions and the problems within the current classification changes seem to be highly likely in the future.

Pressure Ulcer Wound Assessment

Despite its importance, PU classification provides only minor guidance for wound assessment and subsequent therapeutic decisions and evaluations. Important features characterizing PU wounds include location, size, tissue types and their quality, possible undermining, kind and amount of exudates, odor, PU edges, periwound appearance, and pain [34, 47, 48].

Pressure Ulcer Size

The quickest and easiest way to measure PU size is the determination of length, width, and depths. Length and width can be measured with disposable rulers or comparable devices and are documented in millimeters or centimeters. Wound length can be defined as the largest distance between any two points of the wound margin and width as the largest distance between another two points on a second line crossing the length line in a right angle. Alternatively, length can also be determined along a line within the largest distance in a wound parallel from head to foot. Width is the line perpendicular to the length. Because wounds do not re-epithelize at equal rates along wound edges the head to foot and perpendicular measurements are believed being more accurate [49], but study results suggest that the simple length x width method is more reliable [50]. Training is important and always the same methods should be applied under the same conditions to ensure comparability [51]. The depth of a PU may be estimated by inserting a sterile cotton swab or stick into the deepest point in the wound. The largest drawbacks of these simple measurements are that varying wound shapes limit accuracy and reproducibility. Planimetric methods, e.g., computerized via digital photography or manual via tracing sheets, provide more accurate estimations of wound areas and can be considered as reference standard for wound measurement today [52]. Today, various 2- or 3D photographic wound assessment technologies are available for wound photography and planimetry that can be implemented in clinical practice [52–54].

Types and Qualities of Exposed Tissues

Among others the type of visible tissues in the wound is determined by the anatomical PU depth. Category II PUs are shallow and the dermis appears usually wet and red or pink. Subcutaneous fat in category III PUs is pale yellow, waxy, globular and oily, but dry fat turns to yellow-brown in the open wound [55]. Yellowness in PUs may also indicate the presence of slough or fibrinous tissue that may be confused with subcutaneous fat. Exposed skeletal muscle in category IV PUs is shiny and deep red that might be confused with granulation tissue. Tendon (Fig. 4.5) and bone appear as palpable and hard structures within deep in category IV PUs. Necrotic tissue may be leathery, mostly flat, dry, and black or brown or thick, moist, spongy, and brown, gray, or yellow. The necrosis or slough may mask the true size and depths of the wounds. Slough usually adheres to the wound and cannot be washed away or wiped off which distinguishes it from pus.

Undermining

Undermining might occur in deep category III and IV PUs and means that the wound under the skin is larger than visible at the skin surface. Undermining is a characteristic of the inside-out mechanism of PU development because tissue destruction in DTIs usually starts beneath intact skin especially near the bone because loads are highest near bony prominences. Extensive deep lesions with a small skin window typically form hourglass-shaped necroses [56]. Undermining is evaluated by inserting a probe under the skin. The real area of the wound under the skin can be documented using diagrams (e.g., clock face like) [57] or imaging techniques like ultrasound [58].

Exudate

Exudate has the function to clean and to moisturize wounds. Heavy drainage may indicate an infection. Exudate amount is estimated by the frequency of dressing changes and/or the observed moisture in the wound. Exudate amounts can be classified according the Pressure Ulcer Scale for Healing (PUSH) as "none," "light," "moderate," or "heavy" [59]. Other classifications exist, for instance in the Pressure Sore Status Tool [60] or the DESIGN-R tool [61], but descriptions are similar.

Odor

Conspicuous odor might be caused by necrotic tissue, by specific treatments, or by increased bacterial loads. Wound infection typically is associated with putrid smell but distinguishing different odors (sweetish, putrid, feculent …) is difficult. Practical instruments on how to evaluate or to quantify odor objectively are lacking [62, 63]. The latest guideline of the German Society for Wound Healing [64] recommends the documentation of simple categorisations like "inconspicuous odor" or "conspicuous odor" for example.

Wound Edge

The wound edge can be described as macerated, xerotic, hyperkeratotic, vitality, or anemic. In full thickness PUs wound edges are often thickened and rolled indicating that normal re-epithelization will not take place [55].

Does This Pressure Ulcer Heal?

Evaluation of PU healing is important because it guides the clinician through therapy. Wound healing can be divided into three phases: inflammation, tissue formation including granulation and re-epithelization, and tissue remodeling including scarring. The function of inflammation is to prepare the wound bed for healing by removing necrotic tissue and debris and to recruit and activate fibroblasts for tissue buildup. Under normal conditions this is a self-limiting process, but in chronic wounds like some deep PUs there is a continuing upregulation of inflammation leading to non-healing and chronic wounds [65]. The non-healing deep PU is typically covered with gel-like yellow slough or dry brown or black eschar. Beefy reed shiny granulation tissue indicates the granulation phase. However, the presence of granulation tissue is a prerequisite for wound healing but this that does not necessarily indicate soon PU wound closure, especially when the granulation tissue looks unhealthy and pale [55, 66]. Re-epithelization of PUs usually begins from the wound edge when activated keratinocytes move across the newly formed regenerated tissue. The newly epithelized surface consists of a fragile cell layer that is flat, thin, and lighter than the surrounding skin. Epidermal thickening starts at the wound edges and later in the center.

Compared to younger persons the wound healing phases in aged individuals are delayed or even impaired. If the person is healthy and the wound is in optimal conditions no functional detriments occur [67]. Unfortunately for the majority of older PU patients with numerous baseline impairments this does not apply.

Tools for standardized assessment of PU healing are available [1, 34, 61, 68]. Among those the Pressure Ulcer Scale for Healing (PUSH) developed by the NPUAP is widely used in Northern America [59, 69]. The characteristics wound surface area, amount of exudates, and visible tissue type in the ulcer are scored resulting in an overall sum score regarded as predictive for PU healing. Numerous studies investigated the validity of PUSH scores and it is regarded as useful tool in clinical practice [68]. However, comparable to other standardized scores (e.g., PU risk scale scores) also the PUSH score seems to be only moderately related to clinical judgment [70]. Due to the complexity of wound healing summative scale scores are only crude overall predictors for healing [71].

References

1. National Pressure Ulcer Advisory Panel, European Pressure Ulcer Advisory Panel. Pressure ulcer prevention and treatment. Washington, DC: National Pressure Ulcer Advisory Panel; 2009.
2. Takahashi M, Black J, Dealey C, Gefen A. Pressure in context. Pressure, shear, friction and microclimate in context A consensus document. London: Wounds International; 2010.
3. Lindgren M, Unosson M, Fredrikson M, Ek AC. Immobility—a major risk factor for development of pressure ulcers among adult hospitalized patients: a prospective study. Scand J Caring Sci. 2004;18(1):57–64. Epub 2004/03/10.
4. Nonnemacher M, Stausberg J, Bartoszek G, Lottko B, Neuhaeuser M, Maier I. Predicting pressure ulcer risk: a multifactorial approach to assess risk factors in a large university hospital population. J Clin Nurs. 2009;18(1):99–107. Epub 2009/01/06.
5. Allman RM, Goode PS, Patrick MM, Burst N, Bartolucci AA. Pressure ulcer risk factors among hospitalized patients with activity limitation. JAMA. 1995;273(11):865–70. Epub 1995/03/15.

6. Berlowitz DR, Brandeis GH, Morris JN, Ash AS, Anderson JJ, Kader B, et al. Deriving a risk-adjustment model for pressure ulcer development using the minimum data set. J Am Geriatr Soc. 2001;49(7):866–71. Epub 2001/08/31.
7. Vandenkerkhof EG, Friedberg E, Harrison MB. Prevalence and risk of pressure ulcers in acute care following implementation of practice guidelines: annual pressure ulcer prevalence census 1994–2008. J Healthc Qual. 2011. doi: 10.1111/j.1945-1474.2010.00127.x. Epub 2011/11/09.
8. VanGilder C, MacFarlane G, Meyer S, Lachenbruch C. Body mass index, weight, and pressure ulcer prevalence: an analysis of the 2006–2007 International Pressure Ulcer Prevalence Surveys. J Nurs Care Qual. 2009;24(2):127–35. Epub 2009/03/17.
9. Vanderwee K, Defloor T, Beeckman D, Demarre L, Verhaeghe S, Van Durme T, et al. Assessing the adequacy of pressure ulcer prevention in hospitals: a nationwide prevalence survey. BMJ Qual Saf. 2011;20(3):260–7. Epub 2011/01/07.
10. Jaul E. A prospective pilot study of atypical pressure ulcer presentation in a skilled geriatric nursing unit. Ostomy Wound Manage. 2011;57(2):49–54. Epub 2011/02/26.
11. Skillman J, Thomas S. An audit of pressure sores caused by intermittent compression devices used to prevent venous thromboembolism. J Perioper Pract. 2011;21(12):418–20. Epub 2012/01/24.
12. Shea JD. Pressure sores: classification and management. Clin Orthop Relat Res. 1975;112:89–100. Epub 1975/10/01.
13. Reid J, Morison M. Classification of pressure sore severity. Nurs Times. 1994;90(20):46–50. Epub 1994/05/18.
14. Kottner J, Raeder K, Halfens R, Dassen T. A systematic review of interrater reliability of pressure ulcer classification systems. J Clin Nurs. 2009;18(3):315–36. Epub 2009/02/05.
15. WHO. ICD-10 Version. 2010. http://apps.who.int/classifications/icd10/browse/2010/en
16. Fromy B, Abraham P, Saumet JL. Non-nociceptive capsaicin-sensitive nerve terminal stimulation allows for an original vasodilatory reflex in the human skin. Brain Res. 1998;811(1–2): 166–8. Epub 1998/11/07.
17. Kallman U, Bergstrand S, Ek AC, Engstrom M, Lindberg LG, Lindgren M. Different lying positions and their effects on tissue blood flow and skin temperature in older adult patients. J Adv Nurs. 2012;69(1):133–44. Epub 2012/04/11.
18. Witkowski JA, Parish LC. Histopathology of the decubitus ulcer. J Am Acad Dermatol. 1982;6(6):1014–21. Epub 1982/06/01.
19. Dealey C, Lindholm C. Pressure ulcer classification. In: Romanelli M, editor. Science and practice of pressure ulcer management. London: Springer; 2006.
20. Inui S, Ikegawa H, Itami S. Dermoscopic evaluation of erythema associated with pressure ulcers. Int J Dermatol. 2011;50(8):945–7. Epub 2011/07/26.
21. Nixon J, Cranny G, Bond S. Skin alterations of intact skin and risk factors associated with pressure ulcer development in surgical patients: a cohort study. Int J Nurs Stud. 2007;44(5):655–63. Epub 2006/04/25.
22. Vanderwee K, Grypdonck M, Defloor T. Non-blanchable erythema as an indicator for the need for pressure ulcer prevention: a randomized-controlled trial. J Clin Nurs. 2007;16(2):325–35. Epub 2007/01/24.
23. Fromy B, Sigaudo-Roussel D, Gaubert-Dahan ML, Rousseau P, Abraham P, Benzoni D, et al. Aging-associated sensory neuropathy alters pressure-induced vasodilation in humans. J Invest Dermatol. 2010;130(3):849–55. Epub 2009/09/04.
24. Vanderwee K, Grypdonck MH, De Bacquer D, Defloor T. The reliability of two observation methods of nonblanchable erythema, Grade 1 pressure ulcer. Appl Nurs Res. 2006;19(3):156–62. Epub 2006/08/01.
25. Kottner J, Dassen T, Lahmann N. Comparison of two skin examination methods for grade 1 pressure ulcers. J Clin Nurs. 2009;18(17):2464–9. Epub 2009/08/22.
26. Sterner E, Lindholm C, Berg E, Stark A, Fossum B. Category I pressure ulcers: how reliable is clinical assessment? Orthop Nurs. 2011;30(3):194–205. quiz 6–7. Epub 2011/05/21.
27. Bruce TA, Shever LL, Tschannen D, Gombert J. Reliability of pressure ulcer staging: a review of literature and 1 institution's strategy. Crit Care Nurs Q. 2012;35(1):85–101. Epub 2011/12/14.

28. Kottner J, Balzer K, Dassen T, Heinze S. Pressure ulcers: a critical review of definitions and classifications. Ostomy Wound Manage. 2009;55(9):22–9. Epub 2009/10/03.
29. Sibbald RG, Krasner DL, Woo KY. Pressure ulcer staging revisited: superficial skin changes and deep pressure ulcer framework(c). Adv Skin Wound Care. 2011;24(12):571–80. quiz 81–2. Epub 2011/11/22.
30. Langemo D, Hanson D, Hunter S, Thompson P, Oh IE. Incontinence and incontinence-associated dermatitis. Adv Skin Wound Care. 2011;24(3):126–40. quiz 41–2. Epub 2011/02/18.
31. Gray M, Beeckman D, Bliss DZ, Fader M, Logan S, Junkin J, et al. Incontinence-associated dermatitis: a comprehensive review and update. J Wound Ostomy Continence Nurs. 2012;39(1):61–74. Epub 2011/12/24.
32. Defloor T, Schoonhoven L, Fletcher J, Furtado K, Heyman H, Lubbers M, et al. Statement of the European Pressure Ulcer Advisory Panel–pressure ulcer classification: differentiation between pressure ulcers and moisture lesions. J Wound Ostomy Continence Nurs. 2005; 32(5):302–6. discussion 6. Epub 2005/10/20.
33. Zulkowski K. Perineal dermatitis versus pressure ulcer: distinguishing characteristics. Adv Skin Wound Care. 2008;21(8):382–8. quiz 9–90. Epub 2008/08/06.
34. Australian Wound Management Association. Pan Pacific clinical practice guideline for the prevention and management of pressure injury. Osborne Park: Cambridge Media; 2012.
35. Ankrom MA, Bennett RG, Sprigle S, Langemo D, Black JM, Berlowitz DR, et al. Pressure-related deep tissue injury under intact skin and the current pressure ulcer staging systems. Adv Skin Wound Care. 2005;18(1):35–42. Epub 2005/02/17.
36. Groth K-E. Klinische Beobachtungen und experimentelle Studien über die Entstehung des Decubitus. Acta Chir Scand. 1942;87 Suppl 76:198–200.
37. Aoi N, Yoshimura K, Kadono T, Nakagami G, Iizuka S, Higashino T, et al. Ultrasound assessment of deep tissue injury in pressure ulcers: possible prediction of pressure ulcer progression. Plast Reconstr Surg. 2009;124:540–50. Epub 2009/08/01.
38. VanGilder C, MacFarlane GD, Harrison P, Lachenbruch C, Meyer S. The demographics of suspected deep tissue injury in the United States: an analysis of the International Pressure Ulcer Prevalence Survey 2006–2009. Adv Skin Wound Care. 2010;23(6):254–61. Epub 2010/05/22.
39. Young DL, Estocado N, Landers MR, Black J. A pilot study providing evidence for the validity of a new tool to improve assignment of national pressure ulcer advisory panel stage to pressure ulcers. Adv Skin Wound Care. 2011;24(4):168–75. Epub 2011/03/23.
40. Yabunaka K, Iizaka S, Nakagami G, Aoi N, Kadono T, Koyanagi H, et al. Can ultrasonographic evaluation of subcutaneous fat predict pressure ulceration? J Wound care. 2009; 18(5):192, 4, 6. passim. Epub 2009/05/15.
41. Kottner J, Dassen T, Lahmann N. Prevalence of deep tissue injuries in hospitals and nursing homes: two cross-sectional studies. Int J Nurs Stud. 2010;47(6):665–70. Epub 2009/12/08.
42. Berlowitz DR, Brienza DM. Are all pressure ulcers the result of deep tissue injury? A review of the literature. Ostomy Wound Manage. 2007;53(10):34–8. Epub 2007/11/06.
43. Lahmann NA, Kottner J. Relation between pressure, friction and pressure ulcer categories: a secondary data analysis of hospital patients using CHAID methods. Int J Nurs Stud. 2011;48(12):1487–94. Epub 2011/08/16.
44. Kottner J, Gefen A. Incidence of pressure ulcers as primary outcomes in clinical trials: a comment on McInnes et al. (2012). Int J Nurs Stud. 2012;49(3):372–4.
45. Beeckman D, Schoonhoven L, Fletcher J, Furtado K, Gunningberg L, Heyman H, et al. EPUAP classification system for pressure ulcers: European reliability study. J Adv Nurs. 2007;60(6):682–91. Epub 2007/11/28.
46. Beeckman D, Schoonhoven L, Fletcher J, Furtado K, Heyman H, Paquay L, et al. Pressure ulcers and incontinence-associated dermatitis: effectiveness of the pressure ulcer classification education tool on classification by nurses. Qual Saf Health Care. 2010;19(5):e3. Epub 2010/07/31.
47. Mastronicola D, Romanelli M. Clinical and instrumental assessment of pressure ulcers. In: Romanelli M, editor. Science and practice of pressure ulcer management. London: Springer; 2006.

48. Weir D. Pressure ulcers: assessment, classification, and management. In: Krasner DL, Rodeheaver GT, Sibbald RG, editors. Chronic wound care: a clinical source book for healthcare professionals. 4th ed. Malver, PA: HMP Communications; 2007.
49. Hermanns JF, Petit L, Hermanns-Le T, Pierard GE. Analytic quantification of phototype-related regional skin complexion. Skin Res Technol. 2001;7(3):168–71. Epub 2001/09/14.
50. Rijswijk LV, Catanzaro J. Wound assessment and documentation. In: Krasner DL, Rodeheaver GT, Sibbald RG, editors. Chronic wound care: a clinical source book for healthcare professionals. 4th ed. HMP Communications: Malver, PA; 2007.
51. Panfil EM, Linde E. Valid and reliable methods for describing pressure sores and leg ulcer–a systematic literature review. Pflege. 2007;20(4):225–47. Epub 2007/11/21.
52. Ahn C, Salcido RS. Advances in wound photography and assessment methods. Adv Skin Wound Care. 2008;21(2):85–93. quiz 4–5. Epub 2008/03/20.
53. Sprigle S, Nemeth M, Gajjala A. Iterative design and testing of a hand-held, non-contact wound measurement device. J Tissue Viability. 2012;21(1):17–26. Epub 2011/09/29.
54. Bradshaw LM, Gergar ME, Holko GA. Collaboration in wound photography competency development: a unique approach. Adv Skin Wound Care. 2011;24(2):85–92. quiz 3–4. Epub 2011/01/12.
55. Black J, Baharestani M, Black S, Cavazos J, Conner-Kerr T, Edsberg L, et al. An overview of tissue types in pressure ulcers: a consensus panel recommendation. Ostomy Wound Manage. 2010;56:28–44. Epub 2010/04/29.
56. Ohura T, Ohura N. Pathogenetic mechanisms and classification of undermining in pressure ulcers—elucidation of relationship with deep tissue injuries. Wounds. 2006;18(12):329–39.
57. Stotts N. Assessing a patient with a pressure ulcer. In: Morison MJ, editor. The prevention and treatment of pressure ulcers. London: Mosby; 2001.
58. Ueta M, Sugama J, Konya C, Matsuo J, Matsumoto M, Yabunaka K, et al. Use of ultrasound in assessment of necrotic tissue in pressure ulcers with adjacent undermining. J Wound Care. 2011;20(11):503–4, 6, 8. passim. Epub 2012/01/14.
59. National Pressure Ulcer Advisory Panel. Pressure Ulcer Scale for Healing (PUSH) PUSH Tool 3.0. National Pressure Ulcer Advisory Panel. 1998 [cited 2012]. http://www.npuap.org/PDF/push3.pdf
60. Bates-Jensen B. The pressure sore status tool: an outcome measure for pressure sores. Top Geriatr Rehabil. 1994;9(4):17–34.
61. Sanada H, Iizaka S, Matsui Y, Furue M, Tachibana T, Nakayama T, et al. Clinical wound assessment using DESIGN-R total score can predict pressure ulcer healing: pooled analysis from two multicenter cohort studies. Wound Repair Regen. 2011;19(5):559–67. Epub 2011/11/19.
62. Sussman C, Bates-Jensen B. Wound care: a collaborative practice manual: a collaborative practice manual for health professionals. Philadelphia, PA: Lippincott William & Wilkins; 2007.
63. Deutsches Netztwerk für Qualitätsentwicklung in der Pflege. [Expert Standard for People with Chronic Wounds]. Osnabrück, Germany2009.
64. Deutsche Gesellschaft für Wundheilung. Lokaltherapie chronischer Wunden bei Patienten mit den Risiken periphere arterielle Verschlusskrankheit, Diabetes mellitus, chronische venöse Insuffizienz 2012. http://www.awmf.org/uploads/tx_szleitlinien/091-001l_S3_Lokaltherapie_chronischer_Wunden_2012-06.pdf
65. Menke NB, Ward KR, Witten TM, Bonchev DG, Diegelmann RF. Impaired wound healing. Clin Dermatol. 2007;25(1):19–25. Epub 2007/02/06.
66. Wyffels JT, Edsberg LE. Granulation tissue of chronic pressure ulcers as a predictive indicator of wound closure. Adv Skin Wound Care. 2011;24(10):464–73. Epub 2011/09/20.
67. Ranzer MJ, DiPietro LA. Impaired wound repair and delayed angiogenesis. In: Farage MA, Miller KW, Maibach HI, editors. Textbook of aging skin. Berlin: Springer; 2010. p. 897–906.
68. Weier D. Pressure ulcers: assessment, classification, and management. In: Krasner DL, Rodeheaver GT, Sibbald RG, editors. Chronic wound care: a clinical source book for healthcare professionals. 4th ed. Malver, PA: HMP Communications; 2007.

69. Thomas DR, Rodeheaver GT, Bartolucci AA, Franz RA, Sussman C, Ferrell BA, et al. Pressure ulcer scale for healing: derivation and validation of the PUSH tool. The PUSH Task Force. Adv Wound Care. 1997;10(5):96–101. Epub 1997/11/18.
70. George-Saintilus E, Tommasulo B, Cal CE, Hussain R, Mathew N, Dlugacz Y, et al. Pressure ulcer PUSH score and traditional nursing assessment in nursing home residents: do they correlate? J Am Med Dir Assoc. 2009;10(2):141–4. Epub 2009/02/04.
71. Falanga V, Saap LJ, Ozonoff A. Wound bed score and its correlation with healing of chronic wounds. Dermatol Ther. 2006;19(6):383–90. Epub 2007/01/04.

Chapter 5
General Principles of Pressure Ulcer Management

David R. Thomas

Abstract Despite considerable research in management of pressure ulcers over the last decades, substantial issues remain unresolved. Pressure reduction is thought to be critical in healing of pressure ulcer. With the possible exception of air-fluidized beds, one type of pressure-reducing device has not been shown to be superior to another. Nutritional support is a cornerstone of clinical care and should be optimized in all persons, including persons with pressure ulcers, consistent with medical goals and patient wishes. Revisions in the staging system for pressure ulcers have resulted in more precision for clinical description and may help guide choice of therapy. However, new categories of staging may be more difficult for non-wound care specialists. Diagnosing clinical infection in pressure ulcers remains problematic and rests on careful clinical observation. The Pressure Ulcer Scale for Healing tool adequately assesses pressure ulcer status and has proved sensitive to change over time.

Keywords Pressure ulcer • Chronic wound • Pressure reduction • Pressure ulcer nutrition • Wound assessment • Pressure ulcer staging • PUSH tool • Wound infection

Pressure ulcers can be considered rare, affecting only about 0.5 % of the total population. In acute healthcare settings, the prevalence and incidence of pressure ulcers have changed little over the past 2 decades [1]. In a state-wide survey in acute hospital settings, the incidence of pressure ulcers varied from 7.0 to 8.3 per 100,000 population, but did not change from 1987 to 2000 [2]. In a voluntary convenience sample among acute hospital patients, the pressure ulcer incidence remained stable from 1999 to 2004 (8 % versus 7 %, respectively) [3]. In a hospital setting, the point

D.R. Thomas, M.D., F.A.C.P., A.G.S.F., G.S.A.F. (✉)
Division of Geriatric Medicine, Saint Louis University,
1402 South Grand Blvd. M238, Saint Louis, MO 63104, USA
e-mail: thomasdr@slu.edu

D.R. Thomas and G.A. Compton (eds.), *Pressure Ulcers in the Aging Population:*
A Guide for Clinicians, Aging Medicine 1, DOI 10.1007/978-1-62703-700-6_5,
© Springer Science+Business Media New York 2014

prevalence of pressure ulcers was 24 % in 2002 and 23 % in 2006, despite shorter lengths of stay in 2006. When Grade 1 pressure ulcers were excluded, the prevalence rates increased from 8 % in 2002 to 12 % in 2006. This increase in pressure ulcers occurred despite an increase in interventions including turning and repositioning and the use of a pressure-reducing device (25 % in 2002 versus 41 % in 2006) [4]. The distribution of pressure ulcers clusters in two groups, peaking first in younger, mostly neurologically impaired persons, and again in older persons. The cluster in the geriatric population accounts for about 70 % of all pressure ulcers [5].

Acute wounds proceed to healing through a well-researched sequential progression. Pressure ulcers, like other chronic wounds (diabetic ulcers, venous stasis ulcer, and arterial ulcers), fail to proceed through an orderly and timely process to produce anatomical or functional integrity.

Normally, fibroblasts and epithelial cells grow rapidly in skin tissue cultures, covering 80 % of in vitro surfaces within the first 3 days. In contrast, biopsy specimens from pressure ulcers usually do not grow until much later, covering only 70 % of surfaces by 14 days [6]. The result is slow clinical healing.

In a home care setting, about 75 % of stage 2 pressure ulcers healed in 8 weeks, but only 17 % of stage 3 or 4 pressure ulcers healed in that time [7]. In a nursing home setting, 23 % of stage 2 pressure ulcers remained unhealed at 1 year, and 48 % of stage 4 pressure ulcers are unhealed at 1 year. At 2 years, 8 % of stage 2 pressure ulcers, 29 % of stage 3 pressure ulcers, and 38 % of stage 4 pressure ulcers remained unhealed [8]. In 19,981 long-term care residents with pressure ulcers, 45 % of stage 2 ulcers healed and 31 % of stage 4 ulcers healed over 6-month follow-up period [9]. The median days to healing for stage 3 or stage 4 pressure ulcers in a nursing home setting was 140 days [10]. The considerable length of time to healing increases the morbidity and cost of treating pressure ulcers and is often frustrating to the patient and caregivers.

Pressure ulcers occur in persons with multiple comorbidities. The chief among these is immobility. In hospital settings, bedfast immobility increased the risk of developing a pressure ulcers by 23-fold, outweighing all other variables [11].

The risk of developing a pressure ulcer in a hospital setting is highest in patients with a hip fracture and among patients in the intensive care unit. Fifteen percent of patients undergoing hip surgery developed a pressure ulcer during their acute hospital stay. By 32 days after initial hospital admission, the cumulative incidence was 36 % [12].

In the intensive care setting (ICU), pressure ulcer incidence ranged from 4 to 12 % [13]. Subjects who developed a pressure ulcer had a higher severity of illness, including sepsis, hemodynamic instability, mechanical ventilation, use of vasopressors, sedation, use of parenteral nutrition, and requiring insulin therapy for diabetes. Risk factors included higher body temperature, tachycardia or bradycardia, hyperkalemia, acidosis, elevated creatinine, elevated glucose, and a higher C-reactive protein. However, subjects who developed a pressure ulcer did not differ in age, body mass index, or treatment days in the hospital before ICU treatment [14].

Patients undergoing surgery frequently acquire intraoperative pressure ulcers, with a range from as low as 12 % to as high as 66 % [15, 16]. Reduced hemoglobin, high creatinine, altered level of consciousness, frequency of repositioning, and number of vasoactive infusions are significantly associated with pressure ulcer development at different time points in the first 3 days after a surgical procedure [17, 18]. Cardiovascular surgery is associated with a particularly high incidence of pressure ulcers, ranging from 5 % [19] to 30 %, though to be due to longer intraoperative duration and hemodynamic instability [20, 21]. Finally, pressure ulcers also occur frequently at the end of life.

General Principles of Pressure Ulcer Management

General treatment of pressure ulcers can be divided into broad categories: improving the general condition of the patient, pressure reduction and repositioning, general nutritional support, assessing the wound, and measuring progress toward healing.

Managing Patient Comorbidities

Comorbid conditions, especially those resulting in immobility or paralysis, or reduced tissue perfusion, such as hypoxia due to respiratory or cardiac disease, greatly increase the risk of developing pressure ulcers. In theory, persons who are at high risk for developing pressure ulcers can be identified and increased effort can be directed to preventing ulcers in these persons.

Considerable effort has been directed toward risk assessment. The classical risk assessment scale is the Norton Score. Patients are classified using five risk factors graded from one to four. Scores range from 5 to 20, with higher scores indicating lower risk. In the initial study, 48 % of patients who scored less than 12 developed pressure ulcers, compared with only 5 % of those who scored above 18. The generally accepted at-risk score is 14 or less and patients with scores below 12 are at particularly high risk.

The Braden Scale is commonly used for risk assessment instrument in the USA. This instrument assesses six items, including sensory perception, moisture exposure, physical activity, mobility, nutrition, and friction/shear force. Each item is ranked from one (least favorable) to three or four (most favorable) for a maximum total score of 23. The choice of a cutpoint affects the prediction score. Generally accepted scores of 18–16 or less indicate a high risk.

Risk assessment logically directs attention to the highest risk patients in hospital settings. However, a systematic review found no decrease in pressure ulcer incidence that could be attributed to the use of an assessment scale, despite an increase in intensity of interventions [22].

Careful management of patient comorbidities is a goal of medical therapy, but whether modification of extrinsic risk factors can improve healing of pressure ulcers has not been demonstrated.

Reduce Pressure, Friction, and Shear

The most frequently recommended intervention for prevention and treatment of pressure ulcers is frequent repositioning by physically turning the patient. The exact frequency of turning and positioning has not been studied and recommendations vary by country. In the USA, an arbitrary 2 h is recommended. Whether this is effective is controversial. In prevention trials, patients who were turned and positioned every 2 h failed to show a decrease in the incidence of pressure ulcers [23, 24]. No randomized, controlled trials have been done evaluating turning and repositioning for the treatment of pressure ulcers.

A number of physical devices have been developed to reduce pressure, friction, and shear forces. The aim is to reduce surface interface pressure to below capillary closing pressure of 32 mm/Hg. These devices are classified into three groups, chiefly for reimbursement purposes. Group 1 devices include support surfaces designed as a replacement for a standard hospital or home mattress or as an overlay placed on top of a standard mattress. Products in this category include replacement mattresses, pressure pads, and mattress overlays (foam, air, water, or gel). Group 2 support surfaces are similar replacement mattresses or overlay products. Products in this category include powered air flotation beds, powered pressure-reducing air mattresses, and non-powered advanced pressure-reducing mattresses. Group 3 support surfaces are complete bed systems which use the circulation of filtered air through silicone beads, commonly known as air-fluidized beds.

While there is clear evidence that pressure reduction leads to a decrease in pressure ulcer incidence, only about 22 controlled trials have examined the effect of pressure reduction on the healing of pressure ulcers.

Five studies which compared air-fluidized beds with other surfaces all reported better healing in terms of reduction in pressure ulcer size or stage with the use of air-fluidized beds.

In four trials comparing different brands and types of alternating pressure beds, there was no evidence of differences in healing or reduction in ulcer size among the various beds. The evidence in three trials comparing alternating pressure beds with other types of beds was also inconclusive. No evidence of differences in outcomes with low-air-loss beds compared with foam surfaces was observed in three studies, or in a single study that with low-air-loss beds compared with low-air-loss overlays. A meta-analysis directly comparing different devices for improved healing has not shown a difference among devices [25].

The conceptual model of pressure ulcers suggests that relieving tissue interface pressure should aid in healing. However, no study has demonstrated that one type of device is superior to another, with the possible exception of air-fluidized beds. The choice of a pressure-reducing device should be based on patient comfort, ease of use, durability, and cost. Reimbursement for air-fluidized beds is limited by third-party payors.

Development of ischial ulcers due to confinement in a wheelchair is common. Two small trials have evaluated alternating pressure cushions used in wheelchairs with other types of cushions. One study randomized 44 community-dwelling wheelchair users with spinal cord injuries who had stage 2 or 3 pressure ulcers to either an alternating pressure cushion or a standard foam cushion. At 30-day follow-up, better rates of healing measured as reduction in wound area, days to 30 % wound closure, and probability of wound closure within 30 days were observed in the group using the alternating pressure cushion [26]. The second study of 25 hospital or nursing home residents compared an alternating pressure cushion to a dry floatation wheelchair cushion. There was no difference in pressure ulcer rate of healing between groups [27].

Address Nutritional Status

Caloric requirements in persons with pressure ulcers suggest that 30 kcal/kg/day is a reasonable target. This clinical estimate is derived from the premise that persons under stress may require higher energy intake. Most clinical observations using nutrition prediction formulas, adjusted for stress, confirm this estimate.

An optimum dietary protein intake in patients with pressure ulcers is unknown, but may be higher than current adult recommendations of 0.8 g/kg/day. Half of the chronically ill elderly persons are unable to maintain nitrogen balance at this level [28]. Increasing protein intake beyond 1.5 g/kg/day may not increase protein synthesis and may cause dehydration [29]. A reasonable protein requirement is therefore between 1.2 and 1.5 g/kg/day. Specific amino acids such as arginine and branched-chain amino acids have not demonstrated an effect on pressure ulcer healing [30].

Nutritional interventions for the healing of pressure ulcers rest on the theory that undernourished patients do not ingest sufficient energy, proteins, vitamins, or minerals to provide for adequate wound healing. However, the results of nutritional interventions in pressure ulcer treatment have been uniformly disappointing [30]. Reaching a target of 30 kcal/kg per day, or increasing protein intake to 1.5 g/kg/day, did not seem to produce any significant effect on wound healing in a nutritional intervention trial [31].

Nutritional supplementation may provide benefit in terms of weight gain. However, the effects of nutritional supplementation are not dramatic, and it is not clear whether nutritional supplementation is beneficial to all patients or only to those with evidence of nutritional deficiencies [32]. The chapter on nutritional intervention in pressure ulcers describes the evidence in greater detail.

Nutritional interventions for treatment of pressure ulcer fall broadly into three categories. These include mixed nutritional supplementation consisting of hypercaloric formulas and vitamins with or without protein supplementation, protein or amino acid supplementation with or without additional calories and vitamin supplementation, and specific nutrient supplementation with vitamins or minerals such as ascorbic acid (vitamin C) or zinc.

The deficiency of several vitamins has significant effects on wound healing. However, supplementation of vitamins to accelerate wound healing is controversial. High doses of vitamin C have not been shown to accelerate wound healing [33]. In a 12-week study of 88 patients who received either 10 or 500 mg of ascorbic acid twice daily, the healing rates and the healing velocity of their pressure ulcers were not different in the higher dosed group [34].

Zinc supplementation has not been shown to accelerate healing except in zinc-deficient patients [35]. High serum zinc levels interfere with healing and supplementation above 150 mg/day may interfere with copper metabolism [36].

Failure to ingest adequate energy or protein is common in the population who develop pressure ulcers. The causes include general debility, comorbid conditions, or the anorexia/cachexia syndrome. Addressing nutritional intake is important in all persons. There does not appear to be a specific regimen that improves healing of pressure ulcers.

In persons who are unable or unwilling to meet protein-energy requirements orally, enteral tube feeding is often recommended. In a study of enteral tube feedings in long-term care, 49 patients were followed for 3 months [37]. Patients received 1.6 times basal energy expenditure daily, 1.4 g of protein per kilogram per day, and 85 % or more of their total recommended daily allowance. At the end of 3 months, there was no difference in number or healing of pressure ulcers.

In an observational study of nursing home residents referred to the hospital for a percutaneous endoscopic gastroscopy (PEG), persons who did not have a pressure ulcer at the time of PEG insertion ($n = 1,124$) were 2.3 times more likely to develop a new pressure ulcer (95 % CI, 2.0–2.7). In those subjects who had a pressure ulcer at the time of PEG insertion ($n = 452$), the ulcer was 30 % less likely to heal (odds ratio 0.70, 95 % CI, 0.6–0.9) [38]. There are several possibilities for this unexpected observation, but the data suggest that incidence or healing of pressure ulcers is independent of enteral tube feeding and that the effectiveness of enteral feeding in pressure ulcers is not established. Whether this is due to poor effect of feeding or adverse selection of sicker patients is not clear.

Assessing the Ulcer

Several differing scales have been proposed for assessing the severity of pressure ulcers by clinical staging. The most common staging system, recommended by the National Pressure Ulcer Task Force and nursing home guidelines, derives from a modification of the Shea Scale [39]. Under this schematic, pressure ulcers are divided into four clinical stages. The staging system for pressure ulcers relies solely on a description of the depth of the wound. The area of the wound and other wound characteristics are not considered in the clinical staging system.

The staging system classifies pressure ulcers by the visible layers of damaged tissue from the surface toward the bone. This often leads to the false assumption that there is an orderly progression of an ulcer from stage 1 to stage 4. However, it is clear that pressure ulcers do not always progress in the top-to-bottom manner. Current research clearly demonstrates that a bottom-to-top pathogenesis is commonplace. This evolutionary process in the understanding of tissue injury has led to the expansion of the classification system into six stages in the USA (see Table 5.1).

Table 5.1 Clinical staging of pressure ulcers

	NPUAP	EPUAP
Stage/category I	Intact skin with non-blanchable redness of a localized area usually over a bony prominence. Darkly pigmented skin may not have visible blanching; its color may differ from the surrounding area	Intact skin with non-blanchable redness of a localized area usually over a bony prominence. Darkly pigmented skin may not have visible blanching; its color may differ from the surrounding area. The area may be painful, firm, soft, warmer, or cooler as compared to adjacent tissue. Category I may be difficult to detect in individuals with dark skin tones. May indicate "at-risk" persons
Stage/category II	Partial thickness loss of dermis presenting as a shallow open ulcer with a red pink wound bed, without slough. May also present as an intact or open/ruptured serum-filled blister	Partial thickness loss of dermis presenting as a shallow open ulcer with a red pink wound bed, without slough. May also present as an intact or open/ruptured serum-filled or sero-sanginous-filled blister. Presents as a shiny or dry shallow ulcer without slough or bruising. This category should not be used to describe skin tears, tape burns, incontinence-associated dermatitis, maceration, or excoriation
Stage/category III	Full-thickness tissue loss. Subcutaneous fat may be visible but bone, tendon, or muscle is not exposed. Slough may be present but does not obscure the depth of tissue loss. May include undermining and tunneling	Full-thickness tissue loss. Subcutaneous fat may be visible but bone, tendon, or muscle is not exposed. Slough may be present but does not obscure the depth of tissue loss. May include undermining and tunneling. The depth of a Category/Stage III pressure ulcer varies by anatomical location. The bridge of the nose, ear, occiput, and malleolus do not have (adipose) subcutaneous tissue and Category/Stage III ulcers can be shallow. In contrast, areas of significant adiposity can develop extremely deep Category/Stage III pressure ulcers. Bone/tendon is not visible or directly palpable
Stage/category IV	Full-thickness tissue loss with exposed bone, tendon, or muscle. Slough or eschar may be present on some parts of the wound bed. Often include undermining and tunneling	Full thickness tissue loss with exposed bone, tendon, or muscle. Slough or eschar may be present. Often includes undermining and tunneling. The depth of a Category/Stage IV pressure ulcer varies by anatomical location. The bridge of the nose, ear, occiput, and malleolus do not have (adipose) subcutaneous tissue and these ulcers can be shallow. Category/Stage IV ulcers can extend into muscle and/or supporting structures (e.g., fascia, tendon, or joint capsule) making osteomyelitis or osteitis likely to occur. Exposed bone/muscle is visible or directly palpable

(continued)

Table 5.1 (continued)

	NPUAP	EPUAP
Suspected deep tissue injury	Purple or maroon localized area of discolored intact skin or blood-filled blister due to damage of underlying soft tissue from pressure and/or shear. The area may be preceded by tissue that is painful, firm, mushy, boggy, warmer, or cooler as compared to adjacent tissue	Purple or maroon localized area of discolored intact skin or blood-filled blister due to damage of underlying soft tissue from pressure and/or shear. The area may be preceded by tissue that is painful, firm, mushy, boggy, warmer, or cooler as compared to adjacent tissue. Deep tissue injury may be difficult to detect in individuals with dark skin tones. Evolution may include a thin blister over a dark wound bed. The wound may further evolve and become covered by thin eschar. Evolution may be rapid exposing additional layers of tissue even with optimal treatment
Unstageable	Full-thickness tissue loss in which the base of the ulcer is covered by slough (yellow, tan, gray, green, or brown) and/or eschar (tan, brown, or black) in the wound bed	Full-thickness tissue loss in which actual depth of the ulcer is completely obscured by slough (yellow, tan, gray, green, or brown) and/or eschar (tan, brown, or black) in the wound bed. Until enough slough and/or eschar are removed to expose the base of the wound, the true depth cannot be determined, but it will be either a Category/Stage III or IV. Stable (dry, adherent, intact without erythema or fluctuance) eschar on the heels serves as "the body's natural (biological) cover" and should not be removed

A comparison of the National Pressure Ulcer Advisory Panel (NPUAP) and the European Pressure Ulcer Advisory Panel (EPUAP) clinical staging systems. In the U SA, convention is to use the term "stage" while in Europe the term "category" is preferred. Adapted from European Pressure Ulcer Advisory Panel and National Pressure Ulcer Advisory Panel (2009) Prevention and treatment of pressure ulcers: quick reference guide. Washington DC: National Pressure Ulcer Advisory Panel

This staging system for pressure ulcers has several limitations. The primary difficulty lies in the inability to distinguish progression between stages. Pressure ulcers do not progress absolutely through stage 1 to stage 4, but may appear to develop from "the inside out" as a result of the initial injury. Surface changes in pressure ulcers are often labeled as a stage 1 when in fact there is a deep tissue injury.

Muscle tissue is more highly susceptible to tissue damage than either fat or skin. In many cases, the changes visible at the surface of the tissue are minor compared to the damage occurring at the deeper layers of muscle. This differential tissue susceptibility suggests that a number of factors are involved in the development of pressure ulcers, including the type of pressure load and biochemical changes in the tissue due to reperfusion injury or tissue susceptibility [1].

Healing of a stage 4 pressure ulcer does not progress through stage 3 to stage 1, but rather healing develops by contraction and scar tissue formation. Thus, "reverse staging," which describes a healing wound as a proceeding to a lower stage, is inaccurate and the staging system cannot be used to describe healing. Since clinical staging reflects only the depth of the wound, ulcers in which the depth cannot be determined because of eschar are defined as "unstageable."

Clinical staging of pressure ulcers has become more complex and accuracy between stages is subject to observer skills. Deep tissue injury accounted for 9 % of all staged ulcers in 2009, a higher number than either stage 3 or stage 4 pressure ulcers [40].

Managing Infection

Colonization of pressure ulcers with bacteria is common and unavoidable. All chronic wounds become colonized, initially with skin organisms, followed in 48 h by gram-negative bacteria. The diagnosis of a wound infection requires two essential criteria, that is, the presence of bacteria in the wound AND evidence that the bacteria is producing tissue damage (usually in the form of an inflammatory response).

The presence of bacteria in a wound can be described in three forms. Wound bacteria can represent contamination (in the wound transiently, not growing), colonization (established in the wound but with no adverse effect), or infection (established in the wound and damaging the tissue and delaying healing) [41].

Greater than 10^5 organisms may persist for months or years in chronic wounds without apparent clinical effect. The presence of microorganisms alone (colonization) does not indicate an infection in pressure ulcers. The diagnosis of infection in chronic wounds must be made on the basis of clinical signs. However, the only two useful signs of clinical infection are advancing cellulitis and increasing pain [42].

A foul odor is often reported as a clinical sign of infection, but this is often misleading if the odor is coming from the wound dressing rather than from the ulcer itself. A foul odor coming from the ulcer usually signifies anaerobic organisms [43].

Noninfected pressure ulcers and venous stasis ulcers routinely grow varying combinations of *Staphylococcus aureus*, coagulase-negative *Staphylococcus* and *Enterococcus* species, gram-negative bacilli such as *Escherichia coli* and *Pseudomonas aeruginosa*, or anaerobic bacteria representing up to 30 % of isolates) [44, 45].

Peptococci, Bacteroides species, or Clostridia are found in over half of worsening or stationary ulcers, but were absent in healing pressure ulcers. Staphylococci and enterococci were frequently isolated from rapidly healing ulcers. In worsening pressure ulcers, *Pseudomonas aeruginosa* and *Providencia* species were found in 88 and 34 % of ulcers, respectively, compared with 0 % of stationary wounds and 7 % of rapidly healing ulcers [46, 47]. On the basis of these findings, *P. aeruginosa* and *Providencia* species should not be regarded as simple colonization.

Occlusive dressings may increase the number of bacteria in a wound (colonization), but very rarely cause a clinical infection. In a systematic review of 36 studies comparing infection rates under occlusive dressings to gauze or impregnated gauze, infection rates were 2.6 % for occlusive dressings and 7.1 % for non-occlusive gauze [48].

Growth of bacteria from wounds is not synonymous with infection, and treatment based on microbiological results alone is not warranted. It is therefore inappropriate to culture all wounds. Cultures should be taken only from wounds that are clinically suspected to be infected.

No gold standard for infection in chronic wounds exists, making clinical decisions in their management problematic. Clinical criteria of advancing cellulitis, increasing pain not explained by other factors, and delay in progress toward healing seem to indicate a possible wound infection and provide concrete reasons to consider obtaining a culture. The mechanism for obtaining a culture is not certain, but data suggest that sampling by the Levine technique may be the best trade-off. Routine surface swab cultures are likely to be more confusing than helpful [49].

Measuring Progress Toward Healing

A weekly clinical assessment of a pressure ulcer to assess healing is reasonable. Generally recommended measurements include length and width, type of tissue, amount of exudate, and changes in the surrounding skin. No single measure of a wound characteristic has been useful in measuring healing [50].

The Pressure Ulcer Status for Healing (PUSH) tool was developed and validated to measure healing of pressure ulcers. The tool measures three components, including size, exudate amount, and tissue type, to arrive at a numerical score for ulcer status. In clinical development and validation studies, the PUSH tool adequately assesses pressure ulcer status and proved sensitive to change over time [51, 52]. The PUSH tool is shown in Table 5.2.

Summary

Despite considerable research in management of pressure ulcers over the last decades, substantial issues remain unresolved. Careful management of patient comorbidities is a goal of medical therapy, but whether modification of extrinsic risk factors can improve healing of pressure ulcers has not been demonstrated. As with all patients, careful attention to diabetic control, heart failure, and renal insufficiency are goals of therapy.

There is a clear benefit of pressure-reducing devices in prevention of pressure ulcers compared to standard hospital mattresses. It is reasonable to conclude that pressure-reducing devices may improve healing of pressure ulcers, but with the possible exception of air-fluidized beds, one type of device has not been shown to be superior to another.

Table 5.2 PUSH tool version 3.0

Patient name: _____ Patient ID#: _____

Ulcer location: _____ Date: _____

DIRECTIONS: Observe and measure the pressure ulcer. Categorize the ulcer with respect to surface area, exudate, and type of wound tissue. Record a sub-score for each of these ulcer characteristics. Add the sub-scores to obtain the total score. A comparison of total scores measured over time provides an indication of the improvement or deterioration in pressure ulcer healing

	0	1	2	3	4	5	
Length × width	$0\ cm^2$	$<0.3\ cm^2$	0.3–$0.6\ cm^2$	0.7–$1.0\ cm^2$	1.1–$2.0\ cm^2$	2.1–$3.0\ cm^2$	Sub-score
		6	**7**	**8**	**9**	**10**	
		3.1–$4.0\ cm^2$	4.1–$8.0\ cm^2$	8.1–$12.0\ cm^2$	12.1–$24.0\ cm^2$	$>24.0\ cm^2$	
Exudate amount	None	Light	Moderate	Heavy			Sub-score
Tissue type	Closed	Epithelial tissue	Granulation tissue	Slough	Necrotic tissue		Sub-score
							Total score

Length × width: Measure the greatest length (head to toe) and the greatest width (side to side) using a centimeter ruler. Multiply these two measurements (length times width) to obtain an estimate of surface area in square centimeters (cm²). Caveat: Do not guess! Always use a centimeter ruler and always use the same method each time the ulcer is measured

Exudate amount: Estimate the amount of exudate (drainage) present after removal of the dressing and before applying any topical agent to the ulcer. Estimate the exudate (drainage) as none, light, moderate, or heavy

Tissue type: This refers to the types of tissue that are present in the wound (ulcer) bed. Score as a "4" if there is any necrotic tissue present. Score as a "3" if there is any amount of slough present and necrotic tissue is absent. Score as a "2" if the wound is clean and contains granulation tissue. A superficial wound that is reepithelializing is scored as a "1." When the wound is closed, score as a "0"

4—*Necrotic tissue (eschar)*: black, brown, or tan tissue that adheres firmly to the wound bed or ulcer edges and may be either firmer or softer than surrounding skin

3—*Slough*: yellow or white tissue that adheres to the ulcer bed in strings or thick clumps, or is mucinous

2—*Granulation tissue*: pink or beefy red tissue with a shiny, moist, granular appearance

1—*Epithelial tissue*: for superficial ulcers, new pink or shiny tissue (skin) that grows in from the edges or as islands on the ulcer surface

0—*Closed/resurfaced*: the wound is completely covered with epithelium (new skin)

PUSH Tool Version 3.0. Adapted from Stotts et al. [52]

Nutritional therapy should be addressed in concert with overall nutritional goals. Clinical estimates for caloric requirements in persons with pressure ulcers suggest that 30 kcal/kg/day and 1.2–1.5 g/kg/day of protein is a reasonable target. Specific nutritional supplements, supertherapeutic doses of vitamin C and zinc, have not been shown to be clearly effective in healing. Percutaneous endoscopic gastrostomy tube feeding has not improved outcome, and paradoxically may increase mortality risk.

Revisions in the staging system for pressure ulcers have resulted in more precision for clinical description and may help guide of choice of therapy. However, new categories of staging may be more difficult for non-wound care specialists.

Diagnosing clinical infection in pressure ulcers remains problematic and rests on careful clinical observation. The decision to treat a pressure ulcer with antibiotics is currently difficult for most clinicians.

Monitoring the progress of a pressure ulcer over time depends on clinical experience. The Pressure Ulcer Scale for Healing tool adequately assesses pressure ulcer status and has proved sensitive to change over time.

References

1. Thomas DR. Does pressure cause pressure ulcers? An inquiry into the etiology of pressure ulcers. J Am Med Dir Assoc. 2010;11(6):397–405.
2. Scott JR, Gibran NS, Engrav LH, Mack CD, Rivara FP. Incidence and characteristics of hospitalized patients with pressure ulcers: state of Washington, 1987 to 2000. Plast Reconstr Surg. 2006;117(2):630–4.
3. Whittington KT, Briones R. National prevalence and incidence study: 6-year sequential acute care data. Adv Skin Wound Care. 2004;17:490–4.
4. Gunningberg L, Stotts NA. Tracking quality over time: what do pressure ulcer data show? Int J Qual Health Care. 2008;20:246–53.
5. Whittington K, Patrick M, Roberts JL. A national study of pressure ulcer prevalence and incidence in acute care hospitals. J Wound Ostomy Continence Nurs. 2000;27:209–15.
6. Seiler WO, Stahelin HB, Zolliker R, et al. Impaired migration of epidermal cells from decubitus ulcers in cell culture: a cause of protracted wound healing? Am J Clin Pathol. 1989;92:430–4.
7. Ferrell BA, Osterweil D, Christenson P. A randomized trial of low-air-loss beds for treatment of pressure ulcers. JAMA. 1993;269:494–7.
8. Brandeis GH, Morris JN, Nash DJ, et al. The epidemiology and natural history of pressure ulcers in elderly nursing home residents. JAMA. 1990;264:2905–9.
9. Berlowitz DR, Brandeis GH, Anderson J, Brand HK. Predictors of pressure ulcer healing among long-term care residents. J Am Geriatr Soc. 1997;45:30–4.
10. Cullum N, Deeks J, Sheldon TA, Song F, Fletcher AW. Beds, mattresses and cushions for pressure sore prevention and treatment. Nurs Times. 2001;97:41.
11. Shahin ES, Meijers JM, Schols JM, Tannen A, Halfens RJ, Dassen T. The relationship between malnutrition parameters and pressure ulcers in hospitals and nursing homes. Nutrition. 2010;26(9):886–9.
12. Baumgarten M, Margolis DJ, Orwig DL, et al. Pressure ulcers in elderly patients with hip fracture across the continuum of care. J Am Geriatr Soc. 2009;57:863–70.
13. Shahin ESM, Dassen T, Halfens RJG. Pressure ulcer prevalence and incidence in intensive care patients: a literature review. Nurs Crit Care. 2008;13:71–9.
14. Compton F, Hoffmann F, Hortig T, et al. Pressure ulcer predictors in ICU patients: nursing skin assessment versus objective parameters. J Wound Care. 2008;17:417–24.

15. Jesurum J, Joseph K, Davis JM, Suki R. Balloons, beds, and breakdown. Effects of low-air-loss therapy on the development of pressure ulcers in cardiovascular surgical patients with intra-aortic balloon pump support. Crit Care Nurs Clin North Am. 1996;8:423–40.
16. Schultz A, Bien M, Dumond K, Brown K, Myers A. Etiology and incidence of pressure ulcers in surgical patients. AORN J. 1999;70:434–47.
17. Feuchtinger J, Halfens RJG, Dassen T. Pressure ulcer risk factors in cardiac surgery: a review of the research literature. Heart Lung. 2005;34:375–85.
18. Scott SM, Mayhew PA, Harris EA. Pressure ulcer development in the operating room. AORN J. 1992;56:242–50.
19. Lewicki LJ, Mion L, Splane KG, et al. Patient risk factors for pressure ulcer during cardiac surgery. AORN J. 1997;65:933–42.
20. Stordeur S, Laurent S, D'Hoore W. The importance of repeated risk assessment for pressure sores in cardiovascular surgery. J Cardiovasc Surg. 1998;39:343–9.
21. Papantonio CJ, Wallop JM, Kolodner KB. Sacral ulcers following cardiac surgery: incidence and risk factors. Adv Wound Care. 1994;7:24–36.
22. Pancorbo-Hidalgo PL, Garcia-Fernandez FP, Lopez-Medine IM, Alvariex-Nieto C. Risk assessment scales for pressure ulcer prevention: a systematic review. J Adv Nurs. 2006;54:94–110.
23. Lyder CH, Preston J, Grady JN, Scinto J, Allman R, Bergstrom N, Rodeheaver G. Quality of care for hospitalized medicare patients at risk for pressure ulcers. Arch Intern Med. 2001;161:1549–54.
24. Rich SE, Margolis D, Shardell M, Hawkes WG, Miller RR, Amr S, Baumgarten M. Frequent manual repositioning and incidence of pressure ulcers among bed-bound elderly hip fracture patients. Wound Repair Regen. 2011;19(1):10–8.
25. Cullum N, Deeks J, Sheldon TA, Song F, Fletcher AW. Beds, mattresses and cushions for pressure sore prevention and treatment. Cochrane Database Syst Rev 2004;2:[no page #].
26. Makhsous M, Lin F, Knaus E, et al. Promote pressure ulcer healing in individuals with spinal cord injury using an individualized cyclic pressure-relief protocol. Adv Skin Wound Care. 2009;22(11):514–21.
27. A randomised controlled trial comparing the healing of pressure sores upon two pressure-redistributing seat cushions. Proceedings of the 7th European European Conferences on Advances in Wound Management; 1997 Nov 18–20; Harrogate, UK.
28. Gersovitz M, Motil K, Munro HN, et al. Human protein requirements: assessment of the adequacy of the current recommended dietary allowance for dietary protein in elderly men and women. Am J Clin Nutr. 1982;35:6–14.
29. Long CL, Nelson KM, Akin Jr JM, et al. A physiologic bases for the provision of fuel mixtures in normal and stressed patients. J Trauma. 1990;30:1077–86.
30. Thomas DR. Improving the outcome of pressure ulcers with nutritional intervention: a review of the evidence. Nutrition. 2001;17:121–5.
31. Cereda E, Gini A, Pedrolli C, Vanotti A. Disease-specific, versus standard, nutritional support for the treatment of pressure ulcers in institutionalized older adults: a randomized controlled trial. J Am Geriatr Soc. 2009;57(8):1395–402.
32. Langer G, Knerr A, Kuss O, Behrens J, Schlömer GJ. Nutritional interventions for preventing and treating pressure ulcers. Cochrane Database Syst Rev. 2003;(4):CD003216. doi:10.1002/14651858.CD003216.
33. Vilter RW. Nutritional aspects of ascorbic acid: uses and abuses. West J Med. 1980;133:485.
34. ter Riet G, Kessels AG, Knipschild PG. Randomized clinical trial of ascorbic acid in the treatment of pressure ulcers. J Clin Epidemiol. 1995;48:1453–60.
35. Sandstead HH, Henriksen LK, Greger JL, et al. Zinc nutriture in the elderly in relation to taste acuity, immune response, and wound healing. Am J Clin Nutr. 1982;36(5 Suppl):1046–59.
36. Thomas DR. The role of nutrition in prevention and healing of pressure ulcers. Clin Geriatr Med. 1997;13:497–512.
37. Henderson CT, Trumbore LS, Mobarhan S, et al. Prolonged tube feeding in long-term care: nutritional status and clinical outcomes. J Am Coll Nutr. 1992;11:309.

38. Teno JM, Gozalo P, Mitchell SL, Kuo S, Fulton AT, Mor V. Feeding tubes and the prevention or healing of pressure ulcers. Arch Intern Med. 2012;172(9):697–701.
39. National Pressure Ulcer Advisory Panel. Pressure ulcers: incidence, economics, risk assessment. Consensus development conference statement. Decubitus. 1989;2:24–8.
40. VanGilder C, MacFarlane GD, Harrison P, Lachenbruch C, Meyer S. The demographics of suspected deep tissue injury in the United States: an analysis of the international pressure ulcer prevalence survey 2006–2009. Adv Skin Wound Care. 2010;23:254–6.
41. Casadevall A, Pirofski LA. Host-pathogen interactions: basic concepts of microbial commensalism, colonization, infection, and disease. Infect Immun. 2000;68:6511e6518.
42. Cutting KF, White RJ, Maloney P, Harding KD. Clinical identification of wound infection: a Delphi approach. In: EWMA, editor. Position document: identifying criteria for wound infection. London: MEP Ltd; 2005.
43. Sapico FL, Ginunas VJ, Thornhill-Joynes M, et al. Quantitative microbiology of pressure sores in different stages of healing. Diagn Microbiol Infect Dis. 1986;5:31–8.
44. Sopata M, Luczak J, Ciupinska M. Effect of bacteriological status on pressure ulcer healing in patients with advanced cancer. J Wound Care. 2002;11:107e110.
45. Hansson C, Hoborn J, Moller A, et al. The microbial flora in venous leg ulcers without clinical signs of infection: repeated culture using a validated standardized microbiological technique. Acta Derm Venereol. 1995;75:24e30.
46. Daltrey DC, Rhodes B, Chattwood JG. Investigation into the microbial flora of healing and non-healing decubitus ulcers. J Clin Pathol. 1981;34:701–5.
47. Seiler WO, Stahelin HB, Sonnabend W. Effect of aerobic and anaerobic germs on the healing of decubitus ulcers. Schweiz Med Wochenschr. 1979;109:1594–9.
48. Hutchinson JJ, McGuckin M. Occlusive dressings: a microbiological and clinical review. Am J Infect Control. 1990;18:257–68.
49. Thomas DR. When is a chronic wound infected? J Am Med Dir Assoc. 2012;13:5–7.
50. Thomas DR. Existing tools: are they meeting the challenges of pressure ulcer healing? Adv Wound Care. 1997;10:86–90.
51. Thomas DR, Rodeheaver GT, Bartolucci AA, et al. Pressure ulcer scale for healing: derivation and validation of the PUSH tool. Adv Wound Care. 1997;10:96–101.
52. Stotts N, Rodeheaver G, Thomas DR, et al. An instrument to measure healing in pressure ulcers: development and validation of the pressure ulcer scale for healing (PUSH). J Gerontol A Biol Sci Med Sci. 2001;56:M795–9.

Chapter 6
Local Wound Treatment in Pressure Ulcer Management

David R. Thomas

Abstract The specific treatment goals for a pressure ulcer involve a variety of modalities aimed at improving the local wound environment and promoting healing. A key component in pressure ulcer healing is maintaining a moist wound environment. Moisture occlusive dressings can be divided into broad categories of polymer films, polymer foams, hydrogels, hydrocolloids, alginates, and biomembranes. Advanced wound dressings are demonstrably more effective than traditional gauze dressings. Head-to-head comparison of various advanced dressings has not demonstrated any single superior product. Therefore, most local ulcer treatments should be chosen on the basis of specific wound characteristics, ease of use, and cost. Because of slow healing, a number of adjunctive modalities have been tried in the management of pressure ulcers. Few high-quality trials are available, but most trials have not produced remarkable benefits. Wound debridement is necessary for clinically infected wounds, but the usefulness of serial debridement is disputable. Surgical closure of a pressure ulcer depends on patient age and comorbid conditions, but in general has shown a high recurrence rate.

Keywords Pressure ulcer • Wound dressings • Vacuum-assisted closure • Growth factors • Debridement • Infection • Surgical therapy

The specific treatment goals for a pressure ulcer involve a variety of modalities aimed at improving the local wound environment and promoting healing. These include wound cleansing, topical wound dressings, and a variety of adjunctive therapies. In addition, treatment is aimed at providing a clean wound environment and

D.R. Thomas, M.D., F.A.C.P., A.G.S.F., G.S.A.F. (✉)
Division of Geriatric Medicine, Saint Louis University,
1402 South Grand Blvd. M238, Saint Louis, MO 63104, USA
e-mail: thomasdr@slu.edu

D.R. Thomas and G.A. Compton (eds.), *Pressure Ulcers in the Aging Population: A Guide for Clinicians*, Aging Medicine 1, DOI 10.1007/978-1-62703-700-6_6, © Springer Science+Business Media New York 2014

protecting the wound from contamination. Additional considerations include wound debridement and surgical repair.

The choice of a specific treatment modality may be difficult. Historically, pressure ulcer treatment has been based on a trial-and-error process. Numerous case reports have been published, but few randomized, controlled quality trials are available. A systematic review of published trials on topical wound dressings for pressure ulcers up to 2003 found only 21 published randomized controlled trials. This contrasts with over 2,500 wound care products marketed in the USA. One of the reasons for this discrepancy is that topical wound care treatments are considered medical devices. Medical devices must be shown to be safe, but proof of efficacy is not required before marketing.

One of the most commonly used dressing for pressure ulcers at hospital discharge is dry gauze [1]. The use of dry gauze persists despite clear data suggesting that it results in delayed healing. Compared with wet-to-dry gauze dressings, moist dressings are clearly superior. Moist wound healing allows experimentally induced wounds to resurface up to 40 % faster than air-exposed wounds [2].

The concept of a moist wound environment led to the development of occlusive dressings. The term "occlusive" describes the rate of transmission of water vapor from the wound to the external atmosphere. The degree to which dressings dry the wound can be measured by the moisture vapor transmission rate (MVTR). An MVTR of less than 35 g of water vapor per square meter per hour (g m^2/h) is required to maintain a moist wound environment. Woven gauze has an MVTR of 68 g m^2/h and impregnated gauze has an MVTR of 57 g m^2/h. In comparison, hydrocolloid dressings have an MVTR of 8 g m^2/h [3].

Occlusive dressings can be divided into broad categories of polymer films, polymer foams, hydrogels, hydrocolloids, alginates, and biomembranes. Each has several advantages and disadvantages. The available agents differ in their properties of permeability to water vapor and wound protection. Understanding these differences is the key to planning for wound management in a particular patient [4]. A schematic for comparative qualities among available agents is shown in Table 6.1.

Most of the occlusive dressings produce pain relief. Only absorbing granules fail to reduce pain. Polymer films are impermeable to liquid but permeable to gas and moisture vapor. Because of low permeability to water vapor, these dressings are not dehydrating to the wound. Non-permeable polymers such as polyvinylidine and polyethylene can trap water vapor resulting in maceration of normal skin. Polymer films do not absorb exudate and may leak, particularly when the wound is highly exudative. Most films have an adhesive backing that may remove epithelial cells when the dressing is changed.

Hydrocolloid dressings are complex layered dressings. They are more impermeable to moisture vapor and are highly adherent to the skin. Although their adhesiveness to surrounding skin is higher than that of some surgical tapes, these dressings are non-adherent to wound tissue and do not interfere with epithelialization of the wound. Excessive exudate may overcome the adhesiveness of the dressing and leak,

Table 6.1 Comparison of occlusive wound dressings

	Moist saline gauze	Polymer films	Polymer foams	Hydrogels	Hydrocolloids	Alginates, granules	Biomembranes
Pain relief	+	+	+	+	+	±	+
Maceration of surrounding skin	±	±	−	−	−	−	−
O_2 permeable	+	+	+	+	−	+	+
H_2O permeable	+	+	+	+	−	+	+
Absorbent	+	−	+	+	±	+	−
Damage to epithelial cells	±	+	−	−	−	−	−
Transparent	−	+	−	−	−	−	−
Resistant to bacteria	−	−	−	−	+	−	+
Ease of application	+	−	+	+	+	+	−

Sources: Adapted from Helfman T, Ovington L, Falanga V. Occlusive dressings and wound healing. Clin Dermatol 1994;12:121–127, and Witkowski JA, Parish LC. Cutaneous ulcer therapy. Internat J Dermatol 1986;25:420–426

requiring frequent dressing changes. The use of an absorptive dressing such as calcium alginate under the hydrocolloid dressing may be necessary.

Hydrogels are three-layer hydrophilic polymers that are insoluble in water but absorb aqueous solutions. They are poor bacterial barriers and are non-adherent to the wound. Because of their high specific heat, these dressings are cooling to the skin, aiding in pain control and reducing inflammation. Most of these dressings require a secondary dressing to maintain the hydrogel in the wound.

Alginates are complex polysaccharide dressings that are highly absorbent. This high absorbency is particularly suited to exudative wounds. Alginates are non-adherent to the wound but when allowed to dry in non-exudative wounds may allow damage to the epithelial tissue when the dressing is removed. Alginates can be used under a number of dressings to control exudate, including hydrocolloids.

Hydrocolloid dressings and biomembranes do not allow bacteria on the surface of the dressing to penetrate to the wound. This is particularly useful when a patient has fecal or urinary incontinence. Biomembranes are tissue-derived dressings designed to cover the wound and are thought to provide potential wound healing factors.

The dressings differ in the ease of application. This difference is important in pressure ulcers in unusual locations or when used by nonprofessionals in home care settings. Adherent occlusive dressings may be left in place until the adhesion is compromised and wound fluid is leaking, a period of days to 1 week.

Hydrocolloid Dressings

A meta-analysis of five clinical trials comparing a hydrocolloid dressing with a dry dressing demonstrated that treatment with a hydrocolloid dressing resulted in a statistically significant improvement in the rate of pressure ulcer healing (odds ratio 2.6) [5]. Hydrocolloid dressings demonstrated higher healing rates compared with moist gauze in four of the five trials.

In another systematic review, hydrocolloid wound dressings were superior to saline dressings in six trials. On the other hand, in five trials comparing other treatment modalities (dextranomer beads, paraffin gauze, polyurethane dressing, and amorphous hydrogel) with saline gauze, no differences in rate of healing were observed. In nine trials comparing hydrocolloid dressings with various other advanced dressings, no difference was observed between the intervention and comparison groups. A trial comparing two different polyurethane dressings showed no difference in healing rate [6].

This data suggest that hydrocolloid dressings are more effective compared to traditional dry or moist gauze, but that there is little difference in head-to-head comparisons of other advanced dressings.

Dextranomer Polysaccharide

Dextranomer polysaccharide is an anhydrous, porous bead or paste that is highly hydrophilic and rapidly absorbs exudate from a wound. In clinical trials, dextranomer paste was inferior to alginate dressings in producing wound area reduction after 8 weeks in patients with stage 3 and 4 pressure ulcers [7] and inferior to a hydrogel dressing in wound surface area reduction after 3 weeks (35 % vs. 7 %) [8]. These two trials suggest that dextranomer paste may be inferior to other topical pressure ulcer treatments.

Topical Collagen Dressings

Topical application of collagen showed no difference in complete healing compared with a hydrocolloid dressing (51 % vs. 50 %) over an 8-week follow-up. Collagen was more expensive and offered no major benefits to patients otherwise eligible for hydrocolloid treatment [9]. The healing rate of a collagen plus a protease modulating matrix (Promogran) did not differ in trials in which the comparator was an iodine-containing solution covered by gauze [10]. A collagen-polyvinylpyrrolidone dressing was not superior to placebo in another trial [11].

Radiant Heat Dressings

Radiant heat dressings incorporate a noncontact heating element into an occlusive dressing. In a trial comparing a radiant heat dressing with a hydrocolloid dressing, no difference in complete wound healing was observed, although the rate of closure was higher [12]. In another trial where the comparator was an alginate dressing, no difference in complete healing over a 6-week period was observed (6 % vs. 4 %) [13]. Two additional trials compared radiant heat dressing with other dressings, including gauze, alginate, foam, hydrocolloid, and hydrogel dressings [14, 15]. In all three trials that reported complete healing, no difference was found between radiant heat dressing and comparators.

Topical Phenytoin

Topical phenytoin has been used in pressure ulcers, usually limited to stage 1 or 2. The results are inconsistent. One 8-week trial observed more complete healing of stage 1 and 2 pressure ulcers with hydrocolloid compared to phenytoin (74 % vs. 40 %) [16]. Another trial in stage 2 pressure ulcers demonstrated a shorter time to complete wound healing with phenytoin compared with either a hydrocolloid dressing or a topical antibiotic ointment (35 vs. 52 vs. 54 days) [17]. However, the healing times in this trial were quite long for a stage 2 ulcer. A trial comparing phenytoin solution with saline gauze in stage 2 pressure ulcers reported nonsignificant differences for reduction in wound volume (48 % vs. 36 %) and PUSH scores.

Biological Agents

A number of growth factors have been demonstrated to mediate the healing process, including transforming growth factor alpha and beta, epidermal growth factor, platelet-derived growth factor, fibroblast growth factor, interleukins 1 and 2, and tumor necrosis factor alpha [18]. Accelerating healing in chronic wounds by using these acute wound factors is an attractive hypothesis.

Platelet-derived growth factor (PDGF) improves the rate of complete healing of stage 3 and 4 pressure ulcers (23 % vs. 0 %) over 16 weeks of follow-up compared to placebo gel [19]. Another trial [20] demonstrated no difference in wound healing (38 % vs. 14 %) at 5 months after treatment with PDGF compared to placebo. Other trials have not shown improvement in complete healing rates [21], although an improved time to closure of wounds has been shown with PDGF-BB [22] and basic fibroblast growth factor [23].

Complete healing of stage 3 and 4 pressure ulcers was observed at 1 year after a 35-day active treatment phase of a four-arm clinical trial comparing the effect of sequentially applied topical granulocyte-macrophage/colony-stimulating factor and basic fibroblast growth factor therapy to each cytokine applied alone and to placebo vehicles. There were no significant differences of patients experiencing complete healing from day 36 over the next 12 months among the four treatment groups [24]. A cautionary increased risk of mortality secondary to malignancy has been observed in patients treated with three or more tubes of becaplermin gel in a post-marketing retrospective cohort study [25].

A small study ($N = 13$) comparing allogenic platelet gel in stage 3 and 4 pressure ulcers showed no significant difference in reduction of ulcer volume at 14 weeks compared to topical alginate or several antimicrobials [26].

Topical nerve growth factor is superior to vehicle-only treated patients for pressure ulcers of the heel. Complete healing of a pressure ulcer occurred in eight subjects in the active treatment group but in only one subject in the vehicle control group. Improvement was greater (based on wound size) in the active treatment group than in the vehicle-only group [27].

The trials of topical growth factors are limited by using only vehicle or placebo controls. Only one trial has used usual or standard care in the comparator group. The development of wound healing factors is still in its infancy but shows great promise [28].

Dermal Replacement or Grafts

No difference in complete wound healing (11 % vs. 13 %), ulcer area reduction (50 % vs. 34 %), ulcer volume reduction (41 % vs. 17 %), or wound infections (17 % vs. 19 %) has been observed comparing fibroblast-derived dermal replacement (Dermagraft) treatment with no dermal replacement [29].

Vacuum-Assisted Closure

Vacuum-assisted closure (VAC), also referred to as Negative Pressure Wound Treatment (NPWT) and Topical Negative Pressure (TNP), has been used in both acute and chronic wounds. The rationale for negative pressure includes removal of excessive wound fluid and bacteria, wound volume reduction, and mechanical stimulation of granulation and epithelial growth.

An updated systematic review [30] identified only 15 publications of 13 randomized clinical trials that included acute wounds, skin grafts, mixed chronic wounds, pressure ulcers, and diabetic wounds. Excluding acute wounds, seven randomized controlled trials have compared vacuum-assisted closure in various types of chronic wounds. Of the five non-pressure ulcer treatment trials, only one trial reported a greater reduction in wound volume (but not complete healing) favoring topical negative pressure [31].

Only two randomized controlled trials on pressure ulcers have been reported. A total of 22 patients who had 35 stage 3 or 4 pressure ulcers were randomized to the vacuum-assisted closure device or a system of wound gel products for 6 weeks. Two patients in the vacuum-assisted closure group and two patients in the wound gel group showed complete healing. There was no difference in reduction in ulcer volume between groups [32].

Vacuum-assisted closure was compared with gauze moistened with Ringer's solution in a small trial of pressure ulcer treatment in spinal cord injured patients. The time to reach 50 % of the initial wound volume was 27 days in the vacuum-assisted group and 28 days in the moist gauze-treated group [33].

A retrospective cohort study in 86 spinal cord injury patients with a stage 3 or 4 pressure ulcer who were treated with negative pressure wound treatment were matched by wound surface area size to non-NPWT-treated subjects. Over a period of 4 weeks, no differences were observed in NPWT-treated wounds that were healing compared to standard care (70 % vs. 67 %) or in NPWT-treated wounds that were not healing compared to standard care (30 % vs. 33 %). No change in wound surface area was observed between groups [34].

There is a lack of good quality date evaluating topical negative pressure in the treatment of chronic wounds in terms of wound healing, quality of life, pain, and costs.

Adjuvant Therapies

Electrical Stimulation

Electrical stimulation therapy delivers direct electric current high-voltage pulsed currents with variable intensity (voltage) and frequency (pulses per second or Hz) to the wound using surface electrodes. The rationale for electrical stimulation is hypothesized to influence the migratory, proliferate, and synthetic functions of fibroblasts and may result in increased expression of growth factors. The voltage, electrode placement, timing, and duration of electrical stimulation are not standardized.

In a systematic review, two trials were identified evaluating electrical stimulation therapy. The first was a three-arm study of stage 2 or 3 pressure ulcers comparing electromagnetic therapy ($N=20$), a combination of sham electromagnetic therapy ($N=5$) and standard therapy, and standard therapy alone ($N=5$), over a 2-week period. Standard therapy included wound cleansing with hydrogen peroxide, talcum powder, and tetracycline ointment. In the electrical stimulation group, 85 % of the ulcers healed, while no ulcers healed in the other two arms [35].

The second study (Salzburg 1995) compared electromagnetic therapy with sham electromagnetic therapy over a 12-week period in hospitalized veterans with a stage 2 or 3 pressure ulcer. Sixty percent of stage 3 ulcers healed in the electromagnetic therapy group, compared with none in the sham group ($N=5$, relative risk 7.00, 95 % CI 0.45–108.26). Eighty four percent of stage 2 ulcers healed in the electrical stimulation group compared with 40 % in the sham therapy group (p value 0.01) [36]. The evidence for benefit for electrical stimulation therapy could not be defined or excluded on the basis of these small studies [37].

Several trials published since the last systematic review have shown mixed results. Trials have shown a reduction in wound surface area in stage 2 pressure ulcers [38], but no difference for complete healing in stage 4 [39] or stage 2–4 pressure ulcers [40].

Therapeutic Ultrasound

Two trials have compared therapeutic ultrasound with sham ultrasound [41, 42]. A third trial compared a combination of ultrasound and ultraviolet light with laser therapy and standard treatment [43]. The healing rate in the ultrasound group was 48 %, compared to 42 % in the sham group. In the second trial, the healing rate in the ultrasound group was 40 % compared to 44 % in the sham group. A pooled analysis of 128 participants in both trials found no evidence of a benefit of ultrasound on the healing rates of pressure ulcers (RR 0.97, 95 % CI 0.65–1.45) [44].

Ultrasound combined with ultraviolet therapy was compared with laser treatment alone and with standard therapy in 20 participants with spinal cord injury and pressure ulcers. After 12 weeks all ulcers had healed in the combined ultrasound/ ultraviolet treatment group. In the laser treatment group 66 % of ulcers healed, and in the standard wound care group 83 % of ulcers healed (NS).

Other Modalities

A number of other physical modalities have been advocated for treatment of pressure ulcers. These therapies include light therapy, laser therapy, hydrotherapy, vibration, shock wave, and hyperbaric oxygen. Very little published data are available to evaluate their use in the treatment of pressure ulcers. A good proportion of the trials that are available are of poor quality and do not show a positive effect on healing.

Summary

The data suggest that occlusive therapy aimed at maintaining a moist wound environment is a goal of pressure ulcer treatment. Advanced dressings, such as a hydrocolloid, are superior to dry or moist gauze dressings. Head-to-head comparison of various advanced dressings has not demonstrated any single superior product.

Several adjunctive topical treatments have been explored, but in general none are overwhelmingly superior. No doubt novel treatments will be explored in the future.

The adage that "you can put anything on a pressure ulcer, except the patient" certainly cannot be supported by the data. Indeed, some treatments demonstrate worse outcomes (or actual harms) compared to the study control treatment, despite the good theories and good intentions of the investigator. In some cases, the treatments may be equivalent to each other, but differ in ease of use, comfort, or cost to the patient.

A recent observational study of various pressure ulcer treatments illustrates this point. Over a 6-month period across several healthcare settings, treatment of pressure ulcers was evaluated. The analysis focused on complete healing as the primary outcome measure. Not surprisingly, those patients with larger ulcer size and a higher wound severity score healed less often than others. Surprisingly, the use of a pressure-relieving device, documentation of a turning schedule, or the use of nutritional supplements was associated with less likelihood of healing. Furthermore, the application of topical antiseptics, use of enzymatic debridement, and administration of antibiotics all significantly reduced the chances of healing. Pressure ulcers that healed in this study used more "modern" dressings (such as a hydrocolloid dressing), used more exudate management dressings, had fewer wound debridement (especially mechanical debridement), and had fewer changes in dressing type over the course of healing. Patients residing at a nursing home had more enzymatic debridement and more persons were given antibiotics, despite having fewer documented infections. Despite these differences in management, the rate of healing in the nursing home population was not different from that in the community-dwelling patients. The multivariate analysis of factors associated with healing demonstrated that patients having Medicaid coverage, cardiovascular disease, frequent changes of dressing type, application of a topical antiseptic, received antibiotics, or who used a pressure-relief device had a reduced likelihood of healing. Only the use of an exudate absorptive dressing was associated with an increased likelihood of healing [45]. These data are likely confounded by more severe wounds receiving more complex interventions, but no clear benefit was demonstrated for any specific modality [46].

Pressure Ulcer Debridement

Necrotic debris increases the possibility of bacterial infection and delays wound healing in animal models [47]. This delay in healing partly results from slow removal of debris by phagocytosis. Although widely recommended, it remains unclear whether wound debridement is a beneficial process that results in a greater frequency of complete wound healing. There are no studies that compared debridement with no debridement as the control in wound healing. Sixty-four percent of surgical debridement services in 2004 did not meet Medicare program requirements, resulting in approximately $64 million in improper payments [48].

The rationale for the use of debridement lies in a shorter time to a clean wound bed for improved wound healing or in anticipation of surgical therapy.

Options for debridement include sharp surgical debridement, mechanical debridement with dry gauze dressings, autolytic debridement with occlusive dressings, or application of exogenous enzymes. Surgical sharp debridement produces the most rapid removal of necrotic debris and is indicated in the presence of infection. Surgical or mechanical debridement can damage healthy tissue or fail to clean the wound completely. Mechanical debridement can be easily accomplished by letting saline gauze dry before removal, but may produce pain with removal. Remoistening of gauze dressings in an attempt to reduce pain can defeat the debridement effect.

Thin portions of eschar can be removed by occlusion under a semipermeable dressing. Enzymatic debridement can dissolve necrotic debris, but whether this produces possible harm to healthy tissue is debated. Penetration of enzymatic agents is limited in eschar and requires either softening by autolysis or cross-hatching by sharp incision prior to application. Both autolytic and enzymatic debridements require periods of several days to several weeks to achieve results.

The only enzyme product available in the USA for topical debridement is collagenase. Formerly used papain–urea and a papain–urea–chlorophyll combination is unavailable. A trial in 21 patients with pressure ulcers found a greater reduction in necrotic tissue using papain–urea (95 %) compared with collagenase (36 %) at 4 weeks, but the rate of complete healing was not different between groups [49].

A total of five trials have not shown that the use of enzymatic agents increased the rate of complete healing in chronic wounds compared with control treatment [50]. One trial showed an increase in wound size with both collagenase and the control treatment, but the increase was significantly less in the enzyme-treated group. Only one trial out of four that compared a hydrogel with a control treatment found a statistically significant difference between treatments. The single favorable trial suggested a small benefit from treatment with a hydrogel compared with a hydrocolloid dressing. In a single trial comparing different hydrogels, no statistically significant difference was seen between the two hydrogels.

Trials of other debridement agents have shown mixed results. Three trials of dextranomer polysaccharide found a statistically significant difference compared with control, but in two of those trials the control treatment was more effective. A hydrogel significantly reduced the necrotic wound area compared with dextranomer polysaccharide paste in one trial, but not in another. Dextranomer polysaccharide was not better than an enzymatic agent in two trials.

Other studies have not shown advantage of collagenase compared to fibrinolysin/deoxyribonuclease [51], comparing topical collagenase with papain/urea [49], or comparing a streptokinase/streptodornase preparation with zinc oxide [52] (see Table 6.2).

The larva of several species of fly have been used to debride wounds [63]. The larva have been shown to be as effective as traditional debriding agents in producing a clean wound. The maggots are reported to eat only necrotic tissue and apparently ignore granulating tissue.

Table 6.2 Comparison of debriding vs. other dressings for pressure ulcers

Study	Comparator	Results
Palmieri [53]	Dextranomer polysaccharide beads vs. collagen sponge	Mean time to healing (days): Dextranomer: 47 Collagen: 20 ($p < 0.001$)
Sayag [7]	Dextranomer polysaccharide beads vs. calcium alginate	Mean wound area reduction perweek (cm^2): Dextranomer: 0.27 Alginate: 2.39 ($p = 0.0001$)
Colin [54]	Dextranomer polysaccharide paste vs. hydrogel dressing	Median % reduction in nonviable tissue at 21 days: Dextranomer I: 62 Hydrogel: 74 ($p = 0.20$)
Thomas and Fear [55]	Dextranomer polysaccharide beads vs. hydrogel dressing	Clean wounds at 14 days: Dextranomer: 5 % Hydrogel: 40 % ($p = 0.008$)
Parish and Collins [56]	Dextranomer polysaccharide beads vs. collagenase debriding ointment	Healed wounds at 4 weeks: Dextranomer: 43 % Collagenase: 9 %
Lee and Ambrus [57]	Collagenase debriding ointment vs. deactivated placebo	Mean % change in wound volume: Collagenase: +13.14 Placebo: +78.79
Alvarez [49]	Collagenase debriding ointment vs. papain–urea debriding ointment	Healing time (mean time to 50 % granulation): 28 days vs. 6.8 days
Muller [58]	Collagenase debriding ointment vs. hydrocolloid	Complete wound healing: Collagenase: –92 % Hydrocolloid: –64 % ($p < 0.005$)
Pullen [51]	Collagenase debriding ointment vs. fibrinolysin and deoxyribonuclease	Decrease in necrotic wound area: Collagenase: –46.7 % Fibrinolysin and deoxyribonuclease: –36.1 % ($p = 0.11$)
Ågren and Strömberg [52]	Streptokinase/streptodornase enzyme preparation vs. zinc oxide	Median % change in wound area: Streptokinase: +18.7 % Zinc: –2.4 %
Moberg [59]	Cadexomer iodine polysaccharide powder vs. other standard dressings	Mean decrease in wound area at 3 weeks (cm^2): Cadexomer: 2.9 Control: 2.5 ($p < 0.05$)
Brown-Etris [60]	Hydrogel dressing vs. hydrocolloid dressing	Healed wounds at 10 weeks: Hydrogel: 51 % Hydrocolloid: 59 % (NS)
Darkovich [61]	Hydrogel dressing vs. hydrocolloid dressing	Mean wound area at 60 days (cm^2): Hydrogel: 3.5 Hydrocolloid: 5.5 (NS)
Mulder [62]	Hydrogel dressing vs. hydrocolloid dressing vs. saline solution and moistened gauze	Mean % reduction in wound area per week: Hydrogel: 8 Hydrocolloid: 3.3 Saline 5.1 (NS)

Surgical Considerations

The chronicity and poor healing rates of pressure ulcers make surgical repair an attractive option. Moreover, the efficacy of surgical repair of pressure ulcers is high in the short term. However, the efficacy for long-term management has been questioned, even in younger patients [64]. In a series of 40 patients selected for surgical closure of pressure ulcers, patients were divided into three subgroups. In nontraumatic, nonparaplegic elderly patients with a mean age of 73 years, 84 % of the surgically treated pressure ulcers were healed at discharge. However, 12 % of the surgically treated patients had another pressure ulcer at discharge. Within 8 months, 40 % of the surgically treated pressure ulcers recurred, and 69 % of the patients had a pressure ulcer at a different site. In patients with traumatic paraplegia, 74 % of operated pressure ulcers were healed at discharge, and 76 % of patients were free of pressure ulcers. Within 11 months, 79 % of operated ulcers recurred, and 79 % of patients had additional pressure ulcers. Only 21 % of traumatic paraplegics and 31 % of nontraumatic, nonparaplegic elderly patients remained healed after muscle-flap coverage for pressure ulcers [65].

In another series, after 10 years of follow-up in 16 surgically treated patients, only 1 patient remained alive and free of pressure ulcers [66]. Results from selected surgical series are shown in Table 6.3.

The proportion of pressure ulcers suitable for operation depends on the patient population, but normally only a low percentage are candidates for surgery. However, among selected groups of patients, such as those with spinal cord injury and deep stage 3 or 4 pressure ulcers, surgery may be indicated for the majority. If the factors contributing to the development of the pressure ulcer cannot be corrected, the chance of recurrence after surgery is very high.

No clear criteria for selecting patients with pressure ulcers for surgery exist, but decision guidelines have been developed [67]. A decision analysis demonstrated that myocutaneous flap procedures for stage 3 pressure ulcers were favorable unless the success rate for surgery was less than 30 % or the healing rate with medical therapy was less than 40 %. The added cost for the procedure was estimated at $17,000 per treatment episode compared with medical therapy [75].

In debilitated patients, debridement without subsequent reconstruction may be the optimal treatment. Surgical closure of the cleansed pressure sore is best achieved using local rotation, fasciocutaneous, or musculocutaneous flaps. Skin grafting is an option for superficial ulceration, but the long-term stability is around 30 %. Most surgeons agree that a musculocutaneous flap is superior to skin grafting, particularly in the presence of infected wounds.

Summary

The specific treatment goals for a pressure ulcer involve a variety of modalities aimed at improving the local wound environment and promoting healing. A key component in pressure ulcer healing is maintaining a moist wound environment.

Table 6.3 Selected examples of surgical repair of pressure ulcers

Study Ulcer site number	Surgical intervention	Follow-up	Results

Evans [64]
N=30
	Primary gluteal thigh
	split thickness
		Range 1–108
		months
			Recurrence
			Paraplegic patients 82 % at 18
			  months
			Recurrence at different site 64 %
			  at 20 months
			Non-paraplegic patients
			  recurrence 50 % at 36 months

Foster [67]
Ischial only
N=114
	Myocutaneous flap
	Fasciocutaneous flap
		10 months
		Range1
		  month to
		  9 years
			Healed wound by 1-month post
			  surgery:
			inferior gluteus maximus flap 94 %
			inferior gluteal thigh flap
			  93 % V–Y hamstring 58 %
			tensor fascia latae 50 %

Foster [68]
Pelvic and
  trochanteric
N=201
	Myocutaneous flap
	Fasciocutaneous flap
		12 months
		Range 1
		  month to
		  9 years
			Healed wound by 1-month = 89 %
			Ischial: 83 %
			Sacral: 91 %
			Trochanter: 93 %

Kierney [69]
Pelvic and
  trochanteric
N=158
	Primary closure Split-
	  thickness graft
	Cutaneous flap Limberg flap
	  Fasciocutaneous flap
	  Myocutaneous flap
		3.7 years
		Range 1
		  month to
		  15 years
			Recurrence rates:
			Overall patient: 25 %
			Overall pressure ulcer: 19 %
			Sacral: 12 %
			Ischial: 21 %
			Trochanter: 22 %

Yamamoto [70]
Pelvic
N=53
	Fasciocutaneous vs.
	  myocutaneous flap
		44 months	Recurrence rates: Ischial: 48.9 %
			  percent PU-free survival at 36
			  months:
			Sacral 70 % vs. ischial 50 %

Goodman [71] N=48	Various flaps	1–6 years	65 % recurrence of operated ulcers 79 % recurrent or new ulcers

Tavakoli [72]
N=27
	Cutaneous
	Musculocutaneous V–Y
	  Hamstring flap
		62 months
		Range 18–90
		  months
			Recurrence rates 48 %
			Nontraumatic spinal injury: 67 %
			Traumatic spinal injury: 41 %

Schryvers [73]
Pelvic and
  trochanteric
N=431
	Primary closure vs.
	  fasciocutaneous vs.
	  Myocutaneous flap
	  closure
		20 years	Recurrence rates:
			Ischial 34 %
			Sacral 29 %
			Trochanteric 18 %

Homma [74] Ischial only	Fasciocutaneous	77 months	Recurrence rate 30 %

Moisture occlusive dressings can be divided into broad categories of polymer films, polymer foams, hydrogels, hydrocolloids, alginates, and biomembranes. The choice of a specific type of dressing depends on the ulcer characteristics, most often the amount of exudate. Advanced wound dressings are demonstrably more effective than traditional gauze dressings. Head-to-head comparison of various advanced dressings has not demonstrated any single superior product. Therefore, most local ulcer treatments should be chosen on the basis of specific wound characteristics, ease of use, and cost.

Because of slow healing leading to frustration by the patient and caregivers, a number of differing modalities have been tried in the management of pressure ulcers. Few high-quality trials are available, but most trials have not produced remarkable benefits.

Wound debridement is necessary for clinically infected wounds, but the usefulness of serial debridement is disputable. Surgical closure of a pressure ulcer depends on patient age and comorbid conditions, but in general has shown a high recurrence rate.

References

1. Ferrell BA, Josephson K, Norvid P, Alcorn H. Pressure ulcers among patients admitted to home care. J Am Geriatr Soc. 2000;48:1165–6.
2. Eaglstein WH, Mertz PM. New method for assessing epidermal wound healing. The effects of triamcinolone acetonide and polyethylene film occlusion. J Invest Dermatol. 1978;71:382–4.
3. Bolton L, Johnson C, van Rijswijk L. Occlusive dressings: therapeutic agents and effects on drug delivery. Clin Dermatol. 1992;9:573–83.
4. Thomas DR. Issues and dilemmas in managing pressure ulcers. J Gerontol Med Sci. 2001;56:M238–340.
5. Bradley M, Cullum N, Nelson EA, et al. Systematic reviews of wound care management: dressings and topical agents used in the healing of chronic wounds. Health Technol Assess. 1999;3(17 Part 2):1–135.
6. Bouza C, Saz Z, Munoz A, Amate J. Efficacy of advanced dressings in the treatment of pressure ulcers: a systematic review. J Wound Care. 2005;14:193–9.
7. Sayag J, Meaume S, Bohbot S. Healing properties of calcium alginate dressings. J Wound Care. 1996;5(8):357–62.
8. Colin D, Kurring PA, Yvon C. Managing sloughy pressure sores. J Wound Care. 1996;5(10):444–6.
9. Graumlich JF, Blough LS, McLaughlin RG, et al. Healing pressure ulcers with collagen or hydrocolloid: a randomized, controlled trial. J Am Geriatr Soc. 2003;51:147–54.
10. Nisi G, Brandi C, Grimaldi L, et al. Use of a protease-modulating matrix in the treatment of pressure sores. Chir Ital. 2005;57(4):465–8.
11. Zeron HM, Krotzsch Gomez FE, Munoz REH. Pressure ulcers: a pilot study for treatment with collagen polyvinylpyrrolidone. Int J Dermatol. 2007;46(3):314–7.
12. Thomas DR, Diebold MR, Eggemeyer LM. A controlled, randomized, comparative study of a radiant heat bandage on the healing of stage 3–4 pressure ulcers: a pilot study. J Am Med Dir Assoc. 2005;6(1):46–9.
13. Price P, Bale S, Crook H, et al. The effect of a radiant heat dressing on pressure ulcers. J Wound Care. 2000;9(4):201–5.
14. Kloth LC, Berman JE, Nett M, et al. A randomized controlled clinical trial to evaluate the effects of noncontact normothermic wound therapy on chronic full-thickness pressure ulcers. Adv Skin Wound Care. 2002;15(6):270–6.
15. Whitney JD, Salvadalena G, Higa L, et al. Treatment of pressure ulcers with noncontact normothermic wound therapy: healing and warming effects. J Wound Ostomy Continence Nurs. 2001;28(5):244–52.
16. Hollisaz MT, Khedmat H, Yari F. A randomized clinical trial comparing hydrocolloid, phenytoin and simple dressings for the treatment of pressure ulcers. BMC Dermatol. 2004;4(1):18.
17. Rhodes RS, Heyneman CA, Culbertson VL, et al. Topical phenytoin treatment of stage II decubitus ulcers in the elderly. Ann Pharmacother. 2001;35(6):675–81.

18. Thomas DR. Age-related changes in wound healing. Drugs Aging. 2001;18:607–20.
19. Rees RS, Robson MC, Smiell JM, et al. Becaplermin gel in the treatment of pressure ulcers: a phase II randomized, double-blind, placebo-controlled study. Wound Repair Regen. 1999;7(3):141–7.
20. Mustoe TA, Cutler NR, Allman RM, et al. A phase II study to evaluate recombinant platelet-derived growth factor-BB in the treatment of stage 3 and 4 pressure ulcers. Arch Surg. 1994;129(2):213–9.
21. Robson MC, Phillips LG, Thomason A, et al. Recombinant human derived growth factor-BB for the treatment of chronic pressure ulcers. Ann Plast Surg. 1992;29:193–201.
22. Robson MC, Phillips LG, Thomason A, et al. Platelet-derived growth factor BB for the treatment of chronic pressure ulcers. Lancet. 1992;339:23–5.
23. Robson MC, Phillips LG, Lawrence WT, et al. The safety and effect of topically applied recombinant basic fibroblast growth factor on the healing of chronic pressure sores. Ann Surg. 1992;216:401–8.
24. Payne WG, Ochs DE, Meltzer DD, Hill DP, Mannari RJ, Robson LE, Robson MC. Long-term outcome study of growth factor-treated pressure ulcers. Am J Surg. 2001;181(1):81–6.
25. REGRANEX – becaplermin gel package insert. Ortho-McNeil-Janssen Pharmaceuticals, Inc. Revised: 09/2009.
26. Scevola S, Nicoletti G, Brenta F, et al. Allogenic platelet gel in the treatment of pressure sores: a pilot study. Int Wound J. 2010;7(3):184–90.
27. Landi F, Aloe L, Russo A, et al. Topical treatment with nerve growth factor for pressure ulcers: a randomized controlled trial. Ann Intern Med. 2003;139:635–41.
28. Thomas DR. The promise of topical nerve growth factors in the healing of pressure ulcers. Ann Intern Med. 2003;139:694–5.
29. Payne WG, Wright TE, Ochs D, et al. An exploratory study of dermal replacement therapy in the treatment of stage III pressure ulcers. J Appl Res. 2004;4(1):12–23.
30. Ubbink DT, Westerbos SJ, Evans D, et al. Topical negative pressure for treating chronic wounds. The Cochrane Wounds Group. Cochrane Database Syst Rev. 2008;(3):CD001898.
31. Eginton MT, Brown KR, Seabrook GR, Towne JB, Cambria RA. A prospective randomized evaluation of negative-pressure wound dressings for diabetic foot wounds. Ann Vasc Surg. 2003;17(6):645–9.
32. Ford CN, Reinhard ER, Yeh D, et al. Interim analysis of a prospective, randomized trial of vacuum-assisted closure versus the healthpoint system in the management of pressure ulcers. Ann Plast Surg. 2002;49:55–61.
33. Wanner MB, Schwarzl F, Strub B, et al. Vacuum-assisted wound closure for cheaper and more comfortable healing of pressure sores: a prospective study. Scand J Plast Reconstr Surg Hand Surg. 2003;37:28–33.
34. Ho CH, Powell HL, Collins JF, et al. Poor nutrition is a relative contraindication to negative pressure wound therapy for pressure ulcers: preliminary observations in patients with spinal cord injury. Adv Skin Wound Care. 2010;23(11):508–16.
35. Comorosan S, Vasilco R, Arghiropol M, Paslaru L, Jieanu V, Stelea S. The effect of Diapulse therapy on the healing of decubitus ulcer. Rom J Physiol. 1993;30(1–2):41–5.
36. Salzberg CA, Cooper-Vastola SA, Perez F, Viehbeck MG, Byrne DW. The effects of non-thermal pulsed electromagnetic energy on wound healing of pressure ulcers in spinal cord-injured patients: a randomized, double-blind study. Ostomy Wound Manage. 1995;41:42–4. 46, 48.
37. Olyaee Manesh A, Flemming K, Cullum NA, Ravaghi H. Electromagnetic therapy for treating pressure ulcers. Cochrane Database Syst Rev. 2006;(2):CD002930. doi:10.1002/14651858. CD002930.pub3.
38. Ahmad ET. High voltage pulsed galvanic stimulation: effect of treatment durations on healing of chronic pressure ulcers. Indian J Physiother Occup Ther. 2008;2(3):1–5.
39. Adegoke BO, Badmos KA. Acceleration of pressure ulcer healing in spinal cord injured patients using interrupted direct current. Afr J Med Med Sci. 2001;30(3):195–7.
40. Houghton PE, Campbell KE, Fraser CH, et al. Electrical stimulation therapy increases rate of healing of pressure ulcers in community-dwelling people with spinal cord injury. Arch Phys Med Rehabil. 2010;91(5):669–78.

41. McDiarmid T, Burns PN, Lewith GT, Machin D. Ultrasound in the treatment of pressure sores. Physiotherapy. 1985;71(2):66–70.
42. ter Riet G, Kessels AGH, Knipschild P. A randomized clinical trial of ultrasound in the treatment of pressure ulcers. Phys Ther. 1996;76(12):1301–11.
43. Nussbaum EL, Biemann I, Mustard B. Comparison of ultrasound/ultraviolet-C and laser for treatment of pressure ulcers in patients with spinal cord injury. Phys Ther. 1994;74(9):812–25.
44. Akbari Sari A, Flemming K, Cullum NA, Wollina U. Therapeutic ultrasound for pressure ulcers. Cochrane Database Syst Rev. 2006;(3):CD001275. doi:10.1002/14651858.CD001275. pub2.
45. Jones KR, Fennie K. Factors influencing pressure ulcer healing in adults over 50: an exploratory study. J Am Med Dir Assoc. 2007;8:378–87.
46. Thomas DR. Managing pressure ulcers: learning to give up cherished dogma. J Am Med Dir Assoc. 2007;8:347–8.
47. Constantine BE, Bolton LL. A wound model for ischemic ulcers in the guinea pig. Arch Dermatol Res. 1986;278:429–31.
48. Levinson DR. Medicare payments for surgical debridement services in 2004. May 2007: OEI-02-05-00390.
49. Alvarez OM, Fenandez-Obregon A, Rogers RS, et al. Chemical debridement of pressure ulcers: a prospective, randomized, comparative trial of collagenase and papain/urea formulations. Wounds. 2000;12:15–25.
50. Bradley M, Cullum N, Sheldon T. The debridement of chronic wounds: a systematic review. Health Technol Assess. 1999;3:1–78.
51. Pullen R, Popp R, Volkers P, et al. Prospective randomized double-blind study of the wound-debriding effects of collagenase and fibrinolysin/deoxyribonuclease in pressure ulcers. Age Ageing. 2002;31(2):126–30.
52. Ågren MS, Strömberg HE. Topical treatment of pressure ulcers. A randomized comparative trial of Varidase and zinc oxide. Scand J Plast Reconstr Surg. 1985;19(1):97–100.
53. Palmieri B. Heterologous collagen in wound healing: a clinical study. Int J Tissue React. 1992;14(Suppl):21–5.
54. Colin D, Kurring PA, Quinlan D, Yvon C. Managing sloughy pressure sores. J Wound Care. 1996;5(10):444–6.
55. Thomas S, Fear M. Comparing two dressings for wound debridement. J Wound Care. 1993;2(5):272–4.
56. Parish LC, Collins E. Decubitus ulcers: a comparative study. Cutis. 1979;23(1):106–10.
57. Lee LK, Ambrus JL. Collagenous therapy for decubitus ulcers. Geriatrics. 1975;30(5):91–8.
58. Muller E, van Leen MW, Bergemann R. Economic evaluation of collagenase-containing ointment and hydrocolloid dressing in the treatment of pressure ulcers. Pharmacoeconomics. 2001;19(12):1209–16.
59. Moberg S, Hoffman L, Grennert ML, Holst A. A randomized trial of cadexomer iodine in decubitus ulcers. J Am Geriatr Soc. 1983;31(8):462–5.
60. Brown-Etris M, Fowler E, Papen J, Stanfield J, Harris A, Tintle T, et al. Comparison and evaluation of the performance characteristics, usability and effectiveness on wound healing of Transorbent versus DuoDerm CGF. Proceedings of the 5th European Conference on Advances in Wound Management. London: Macmillan Ltd; 1996;5:151–5.
61. Darkovich SL, Brown-Etris M, Spencer M. Biofilm hydrogel dressing: a clinical evaluation in the treatment of pressure sores. Ostomy Wound Manage. 1990;29:47–60.
62. Mulder GD, Altman M, Seeley JE, Tintle T. Prospective randomized study of the efficacy of hydrogel, hydrocolloid, and saline solutionmoistened dressings on the management of pressure ulcers. Wound Repair Regen. 1993;1(4):213–8.
63. Gilead L, Mumcuoglu KY, Ingber A. The use of maggot debridement therapy in the treatment of chronic wounds in hospitalised and ambulatory patients. J Wound Care. 2012;21(2):78. 80, 82–85.
64. Evans GRD, Dufresne CR, Manson PN. Surgical correction of pressure ulcers in an urban center: is it efficacious? Adv Wound Care. 1994;7:40–6.

65. Disa JJ, Carlton JM, Goldberg NH. Efficacy of operative cure in pressure sore patients. Plast Reconstr Surg. 1992;89:272–8.
66. Goldberg NH. Outcomes in surgical intervention. Adv Wound Care. 1995;8:69–70.
67. Foster RD, Anthony JP, Mathes SJ, Hoffman WY. Ischial pressure sore coverage: a rationale for flap selection. Br J Plast Surg. 1997;50:374–9.
68. Foster RD, Anthony JP, Mathes SJ, et al. Flap selection as a determinant of success in pressure sore coverage. Arch Surg. 1997;132(8):868–73.
69. Kierney PC, Engrav LH, Isik FF, et al. Results of 268 pressure sores in 158 patients managed jointly by plastic surgery and rehabilitation medicine. Plast Reconstr Surg. 1998;102(3):765–72.
70. Yamamoto Y, Tsutsumida A, Murazumi M, et al. Long-term outcome of pressure sores treated with flap coverage. Plast Reconstr Surg. 1997;100(5):1212–7.
71. Goodman CM, Cohen V, Armenta A, et al. Evaluation of results and treatment variables for pressure ulcers in 48 veteran spinal cord injured patients. Ann Plast Surg. 1999;42:665–72.
72. Tavakoli K, Rutkowski S, Cope C, et al. Recurrence rates of ischial sores in para- and tetraplegics treated with hamstring flaps: an 8-year study. Br J Plast Surg. 1999;52(6):476–9.
73. Schryvers OI, Stranc MF, Nance PW. Surgical treatment of pressure ulcers: 20-year experience. Arch Phys Med Rehabil. 2000;81(12):1556–62.
74. Homma K, Murakami G, Fujioka H, Fujita T, Imai A, Ezoe K. Treatment of ischial pressure ulcers with a posteromedial thigh fasciocutaneous flap. Plast Reconstr Surg. 2001;108:1990–6.
75. Siegler EL, Lavizzo-Mourey R. Management of stage III pressure ulcers in moderately demented nursing home residents. J Gen Intern Med. 1991;6:507–13.

Chapter 7
Surgical Management of Pressure Ulcers

Dean P. Kane

Abstract The surgeon is an essential team member in the management of stage III and IV pressure ulcers. In some settings the wound team is led by a general surgeon or a plastic surgeon. The surgeon's involvement can range from conservative bedside debridement to myocutaneous advancement flaps by a reconstructive plastic surgeon. Surgical consultation can add value to the care process by advising the team as to the proper timing and extent of wound debridement and to assess the potential for wound coverage. The intent of this chapter is to introduce the generalist wound care provider to the role of the surgeon and to a range of surgical treatment options. These include patient selection for debridement, secondary healing, or reconstruction.

Keywords Pressure ulcers • Surgery • Debridement • Reconstruction • Flap

Introduction

A pressure ulcer is an injury localized to the skin and/or underlying tissue over a bony prominence that occurs as a result of pressure in conjunction with or without shear or friction [1, 2]. Pressure ulcers can also result from poorly fitting casts or appliances. They can occur in soft tissue areas due to the pressure effects of a foreign object such as a medical device. Because muscle and subcutaneous tissue are more susceptible to pressure-induced injury than dermis and epidermis, pressure ulcers are often worse than their initial presentation. Pressure ulcers are assessed and staged at the bedside as a clinical description of the depth of observable tissue destruction [3]. Unstageable and suspected deep tissue injury are relatively new

D.P. Kane, M.D., F.A.C.S. (✉)
1 Reservoir Circle, Suite 201, Baltimore, MD 21208, USA
e-mail: deankane@drdeankane.com

D.R. Thomas and G.A. Compton (eds.), *Pressure Ulcers in the Aging Population:*
A Guide for Clinicians, Aging Medicine 1, DOI 10.1007/978-1-62703-700-6_7,
© Springer Science+Business Media New York 2014

additions to the original Shea schemata [4]. These stages are the most relevant to the wound surgeon and the team assessing potential wound magnitude.

Pressure ulcers become chronic wounds experienced by the frail and the elderly. This patient population is encumbered with increasing disease burden and lower physical reserves. High-risk patients are immobile and are often malnourished. These factors along with underlying cardiovascular, renal, and other diseases are a barrier to healing and increase the risk for surgical complication [5].

It is estimated that pressure ulcer prevalence in acute care is 15 % [6] and approximately 2.5 million patients are treated for pressure ulcers in US hospitals each year [7]. Given these statistics the role of the surgeon is evident.

Pressure Ulcers: The Surgeons Perspective

Documented wound care goes back 4,000 years. Pressure ulcers have been found in Egyptian mummies [8]. Wound craft has progressed from potions, salves, and ointments to modern science-based dressing technology and advanced surgical techniques [9]. In the last 25 years, newer dressings including hydrocolloids and alginates have complemented saline-moistened gauze. Ancient topical agents such as honey have been reintroduced [10]. Advanced biosynthetic dressings, which actively change the wound environment, have also added to the wound healing armamentarium [11].

Advanced surgical techniques including revascularization, vascularized wound coverage, and other reconstructive surgical procedures can reduce time to closure, save costs, and improve quality of life. These advances place greater challenges on the surgical wound provider to advise the pressure ulcer patient among a myriad of medical and surgical options available.

The primary cause of pressure ulcers is static pressure applied to the skin and the underlying tissues. When the pressure is greater than the capillary filling pressure, blood flow is impeded. Maintaining interface pressures below arterial capillary closing pressure of approximately 32 mmHg is considered to be the gold standard for pressure relief [12]. This does not take into count the venous capillary closing pressure of 8–12 mmHg to impede the return of flow. Sustained pressure over time, enough to disrupt blood flow, results in hypoxia, localized ischemia, and tissue acidosis, leading to cellular necrosis. Muscle has been shown to withstand pressure loads of around 50 mmHg for long periods [13]. The pressure–ischemia theory maintains that pressure sores result from constant pressure sufficient to impair local blood flow to soft tissue for an extended period. The exact amount of time is under study and varies with an individual's tissue tolerance. Experience dictates that an immobile individual should lie no more than 2 h on a bony prominence before ischemia becomes irreversible and soft tissue necrosis occurs. In the hypo-perfused, malnourished patient, necrosis can occur in as little as 20 min of pressure.

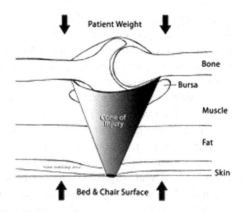

Fig. 7.1 Cone of injury concept

Pressure over a bony prominence tends to result in a cone-shaped distribution with the affected tissues located deep, adjacent to the bone–muscle interface. Thus, the extent of a deep tissue injury type pressure ulcer is often much greater than expected from the visible ulcer on the skin surface and the skin changes are just the "tip of the iceberg" [14] (see Fig. 7.1). In fact, a deep necrotic wound may be the first evidence of pressure-induced injury, rather than a gradual progression of an ulcer from the epidermis down to the bone.

The Surgical Approach to Pressure Ulcers

A pressure ulcer must be differentiated from acute wounds such as abrasions, burns, skin tears, and lacerations. Pressure ulcers are classified as chronic wounds to be differentiated from arterial ulcers, venous stasis ulcers, diabetic foot ulcers, radiation-related, burns, vasculitic, and others. An etiological diagnosis is needed to properly manage or palliate a wound. The consulting surgeon can aid in making the correct diagnosis by proper evaluation, biopsy, debridement, or obtaining tissue for culture.

When the skin is injured, its normal barrier function is breached. In the healthy immune competent host, acute wounds heal spontaneously without complications through the four normal phases of the wound healing: hemostasis, inflammation, proliferation, and remodeling [15].

Acute injuries generally have their edges revised or approximated and at times can be closed primarily. If there is no real tissue defect, direct closure is performed in their anatomic layers. Antibiotic prophylaxis and tetanus toxoid are considerations to minimize infections. Acute wounds generally heal rapidly. The injurious separation of adjacent tissues follows a natural and dynamic cascade of healing events until restoration of the defect has occurred.

In 1992 Lazarus et al. defined chronic wounds as those that "fail to progress through a normal, orderly, and timely sequence of repair or wounds that pass through the repair process without restoring anatomic and functional results" [16]. Chronic wounds may persist for months or never heal in a frail host. Wounds may fail to progress because they remain in the inflammatory phase of healing due to many intrinsic host factors and extrinsic environmental factors.

Reconstructive surgery is not indicated for patients in a catabolic state. Treating the patient's medical comorbidities and moving them from a catabolic state to that of anabolism are important to facilitate healing. These interventions include optimizing nutrition, controlling blood sugar, and treating any systemic infection. Both medical and surgical team members must optimize the comorbidities that impair healing to achieve a closed a durable defect. See Box 7.1 for a detailed list of comorbidities that need to addressed or reversed to optimize healing and prevent pressure ulcer progression. Items in bold can be modified or treated physiologically to some extent.

Infection is the most common major complication of pressure ulcers. Every pressure ulcer is colonized with bacteria. When bacterial balance is altered and microorganisms invade the surrounding tissues, cellulitis results. Pressure ulcers rarely cause bacteremia or sepsis because they are outwardly draining. Urinary tract infections or pneumonia are the primary reasons chronic pressure ulcer patients present with sepsis [17].

Pressure ulcers can be associated with a number of adverse outcomes. Infectious complications include bursitis, osteomyelitis, pyarthrosis, and abscess formation. Non infectious complications include risk for recurrent pressure ulcer, amyloidosis, fistula formation, sinus tracts, autonomic dysreflexia, heterotopic ossification, and malignant transformation of the ulcer.

Immobility is the most important host factor that contributes to pressure ulcer formation. Immobility may be permanent or transient [18]. Poor perfusion is next on the list of contributing host factors. Good nutrition, hydration, and electrolyte balance contribute to healing and need to be addressed.

Preoperatively individual host factors predisposing to pressure ulcer development should be corrected. Smokers should be encouraged to stop since continued smoking impairs wound healing and may result in higher rates flap failure, dehiscence, necrosis, and ulcer recurrence in some studies [19].

Plastic surgery consultation is considered when reconstruction will hasten the healing process, provide greater pain reduction, and/or reduce costs. The risk–benefit ratio must be clearly discussed with the patient and family. The wound must be free of necrosis and infection. Clinical observations to support readiness for surgical closure include wound contracture, healthy granulation, minimal exudate, and no cellulitis or drainage from a distal site. If these wound end-points are met, if host catabolism has been reversed, and if the patient is in a state of anabolism with appropriate protein and calorie reserves, the host is optimal for reconstruction. Correcting as many of the highlighted Box 7.1 comorbidities as practicable will minimize the risk of complications following an elective pressure ulcer excision, ostectomy, or reconstruction.

> **Box 7.1 Comorbidities Associated with Delayed Pressure Ulcer Healing**
>
> - Proximal neuropathy
> - Distal neuropathy: proprioception abnormalities, reflex spasticity, contractures, ALS, polio, spina bifida
> - Immobility associated with trauma, weakness, pain, paraplegia, quadriplegia
> - **Malnutrition** and wasting
> - **Hypoperfusion**: Congestive heart failure and hypovolemia
> - **Diabetes**
> - Diabetic associated microvascular changes including: hypoperfusion, proprioception, and sensory abnormalities
> - Venous insufficiency
> - **Arterial insufficiency**
> - Pulmonary insufficiency: low oxygen saturation
> - **Anemia**
> - **Edema**
> - **Renal insufficiency**
> - **Anti-inflammatory drugs:** NSAID's, anti-TNF RA, steroids, and other immune system modifying drugs
> - **Anticoagulants**: including NSAIDs, aspirin, and herbals

Debridement of Pressure Ulcers

Removal of non-vital, exudating, and infected tissue by wound debridement is an important element of pressure ulcer treatment [20]. Necrotic tissue promotes bacterial growth and impairs wound healing. Surgical debridement provides the host a conservation of energy by removal of necrotic and infected tissues and debris from the wound [21].

If rapid wound deterioration occurs and the wound is the source of sepsis, then emergent surgical consultation is indicated and surgical debridement with abscess drainage and removal of infected tissues are required. Systemic antibiotics are mandatory during debridement of acute wound sepsis anticipating septic shock from the acute bacteremia. At times a great deal of devitalized tissue needs to be excised. In the case of advanced age or debility the patient may not be a candidate for extensive debridement. Follow-up local care is indicated and may include staged debridement of necrotic tissue until the wound has progressed through the inflammatory stages of wound healing and has achieved a clean, granulated base with minimal bacterial colonization.

Providers should suspect bone, bursa, and/or joint infection as a source of indolent infection in poorly healing wounds [22]. Biopsy of exposed bone is recommended. If a wound involves or is adjacent to a joint or capsule, joint aspiration for

Fig. 7.2 Excision of the
pressure ulcer including
bursectomy and ostectomy of
the involved bone

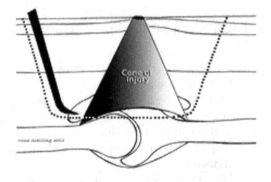

culture is advised. Debridement or excision prior to reconstruction maybe required in order to identify and reduce this as a potential source of infection. Wounds involving joints are particularly challenging. An experienced wound surgeon will be required for muscle, bursectomy, and bone and joint resection (see Fig. 7.2).

Curettage of granulation tissue in stalled wounds initiates platelet release and initiates the inflammation phase of healing. Returning a wound to the acute phase can in some cases result in an orderly sequence of inflammation, proliferation, and remodeling.

Multiple debridement techniques are available. The listed modalities are often used in combination.

1. Sharp soft tissue (skin, fat, fascia, muscle) debridement involves the use of a scalpel or scissors. This is the most rapid form of debridement. It is used to remove thick eschar and extensive necrotic tissue. The exception is patients with heel ulcers covered by a thick, dry, and noninfected eschar. Sharp debridement is not recommended at this site, because of the proximity of bone and lack of collateral perfusion for healing. Generally performed by a general or plastic surgeon, this more aggressive means of removing non-vitalized tissues is more prone to remove viable tissue and cause greater bleeding. It is performed in the operating room but may be performed at the bedside.

2. Mechanical debridement is a nonselective method of removing necrotic tissue and debris from a wound. This is most commonly done with wet-to-dry dressings. Mechanical debridement is best for wounds that contain thick exudate, slough, or loose necrotic tissue. Wet-to-dry dressings will remove nonviable tissues; caution is required to avoid maceration of healthy tissue. Pulsed lavage may be a more selective mechanical debridement. It also dilutes the concentration of bacterial or fungal burden of the wound tipping the immune balance in favor of host healing.

3. Enzymatic debridement is done with the topical application of proteolytic enzymes such as collagenase to remove necrotic tissue. The topically applied enzymes work synergistically with endogenous enzymes and wet-to-moist saline with 100 % cotton open weave gauze dressing to debride the wound. These agents may produce additional exudate.

Fig. 7.3 Sacral pressure ulcer that is incompletely healed by secondary intent

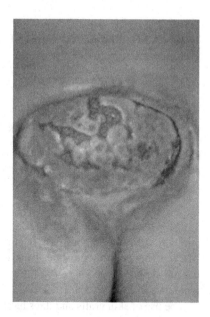

4. Autolytic debridement uses semi-occlusive transparent films, hydrocolloids, or sheet hydrogels to cover a wound so that enzymes normally present in wound tissue digest necrotic tissue. This often works best on wounds with minimal exudate. It should not be used in the presence of infection [23]. Medicinal honey may be considered for autolytic debridement of a clean wound during the process of healing.
5. Biosurgery or the use of maggots is another effective method of debridement. The larvae produce enzymes to break down dead tissue without harming healthy tissue. This can be considered when sharp debridement is contraindicated due to exposed bone, joint, or tendon.

Figure 7.3 illustrates a sacral pressure ulcer that healed by secondary intent. Maximum contracture of the wound edges and granulation has occurred. Epithelial migration and island have covered some of the granulation tissue, but the wound remains vulnerable to continued pressure, shear, friction, and soilage.

Surgical Management Beyond Debridement

Surgery is a viable option in carefully selected pressure ulcer patients, particularly when conservative interventions have failed. Since no clear criteria for patient selection and randomized controlled trials comparing operative treatments are scant, the choice of the type of closure is left to the consulting reconstructive surgeon [24]. The common practice is that the choice of technique depends on the surgeon's assessment of the patient and the site of the ulcer.

> **Box 7.2 Candidates for Surgical Intervention Are to Based on Assessment of the Following**
>
> - Etiology of the pressure ulcer
> - Anatomical site
> - Infection risk
> - Underlying medical conditions
> - Nutritional status
> - Neurological status
> - Psychosocial status

Pressure ulcer reconstruction is one of the most complex challenges to the plastic surgeon with one of the highest complication rate of all procedures performed. The risk–benefit ratio must be clearly discussed with the patient and family. Without the full support of an interdisciplinary team, pressure ulcer reconstruction has a high incidence of failure [25].

The use of skin grafts and flaps has broadened the options and improved outcomes and quality of life for well-selected pressure ulcer patients. A variety of operative options are available, often requiring staged procedures including skin grafts, skin flaps, myofasciocutaneous flaps, and free flaps [2, 26]. Patient selection is key to reconstructive surgical success. Box 7.2 lists factors that need to be considered in patient selection. Procedure selection depends upon the patient's physical condition, ulcer site, quality of life considerations, and available surgical expertise. Additional considerations include deciding the type of flap indicated for the area involved, the ability of that chosen flap to be re-harvested if the ulcer reoccurs, and donor site morbidity.

Plastic surgery consultation is considered when reconstruction will hasten the healing process, provide greater pain reduction, and/or reduce costs. There are two types of surgery beyond simple wound debridement (1) procedures that prepare the patient for healing and (2) procedures to obtain wound closure. An example of preparing a wound for healing would be the surgical exploration and unroofing of sinuses or cavities in a wound bed.

Direct Wound Closure

Direct wound closure is usually not possible for most pressure ulcers. Primary closure or approximation of wound edges may use undermining to create random adjacent flaps. These flap closures are almost always under tension and are doomed to fail. Ulcers should be free of devitalized tissue. Pressure ulcer reconstruction often necessitates radically removing underlying necrotic bone, padding of the bone stump, filling the dead space with muscle, using a large durable, covering flap, achieving adequate flap mobilization to avoid tension, and avoiding adjacent flap territories to preserve options to reconstruct other locations.

Split-Thickness Skin Grafts

Skin grafts are used for stage II and well-granulated superficial stage III wounds of non-pressure origin where wound cover without durability is needed. When large superficial injuries occur, a split-thickness skin graft is indicated to resurface the wound. Healing is rapid and stable, providing the defect with the epithelial and partial dermal components. As with many reconstructive options, a donor wound site defect remains that must heal. Split-thickness skin grafts leave behind epithelial cells in the dermal adnexal appendages, such as sweat glands and hair follicles, to repopulate the donor surface. If the donor site is void of such adnexal appendages as is seen in elderly patients with no hair-bearing thigh skin, then a secondary chronic wound at the donor site is more likely to occur. In such a case, consideration should be made for full-thickness skin grafting or expanded meshed split-thickness skin grafting to both the defect and the donor site.

It takes 3 weeks or longer of collagen formation to develop 30 % tensile strength and 6 months or longer for 90 % tensile strength in an immunocompetent patient. Wound patients are typically not immunocompetent and may require longer healing times. Clinically, those skin grafts that have initially taken but subsequently failed may have occurred due to the misconception that a taken skin graft is fully healed. When the patient is remobilized, remember the graft is not fully durable until scar or collagen anchoring of the skin graft has occurred at approximately 12 weeks.

Full-Thickness Skin Grafts

A full-thickness skin graft includes the epidermis and full-thickness dermis. On occasion, composite grafts also include underlying fat or fascia. These grafts replace a total skin deficit as might occur with a skin cancer excision on the nose. Full-thickness skin grafts will contract less and blend better due to similar texture and color if donated from surrounding redundant tissues. Due to their extra thickness and perfusion needs, full-thickness skin grafts need longer immobilization in order to survive. On occasion, epidermolysis may occur due to delayed perfusion of the epidermal layer. Because of the adnexal appendages left in the full-thickness skin grafts, reepithelialization will occur. The full-thickness donor site is closed primarily by apposition of the cut edges.

Epithelial cells migrate no more than a centimeter. If the wound is greater than 2.5 cm in diameter or is on a pressure-bearing site, the wound may heal secondarily, but without durable cover. One example of a case where a pressure ulcer may benefit from skin grafting is shown in Fig. 7.3. With completed contracture and 100 % granulation the epithelial islands cannot sustain pressure, friction, shearing, or moisture. The wound will eventually split, erode, bleed, or become infected endlessly. If the wound and the patient can tolerate it, durable surgical closure is recommended.

Flaps

A flap is defined as a transfer of skin and underlying tissue from one part of the body to another along with a blood supply. Unlike grafts, most flaps are not dependent on the recipient bed to vascularize the tissue that is transferred. A flap is the best approach to wound repair when primary repair is not appropriate and the wound bed is not amenable to grafting, as is the case with most pressure ulcers. Vascular compromise is the most common cause of flap failure however. When partial flap loss occurs, the necrotic tissue requires debridement and the residual defect is reconstructed with adjacent tissues or allowed to heal with wound care by secondary intent, contraction, and epithelialization.

Flap selection begins with an analysis of the defect location, vascularity of the wound bed, comorbidities, cosmetic significance, and functional significance. Generally, simple local and regional flaps are used if possible. More complicated flaps, such as pedicled or free flaps, are used if simpler options are not available or if a random flap will not give a better overall functional and cosmetic result.

Most pressure ulcers occur on the sacrum or heels while the patient is lying or in a partially upright position. Pressure ulcers of the trochanter occur while the patient is in a side-lying position. Pressure ulcers of the ischium occur while the patient is in a sitting position. Depending on the degree of immobility, limb contractures, and spasticity, other sites of pressure ulcers include the occiput, scapulae, elbows, knees, ankles, iliac crest, and buttocks and thus partially determine the most optimal donor site and flap option.

The choice of flap for reconstruction depends on the location of the ulcer. The most durable closures involve composite tissue and provide padding over underlying structures [27]. Many well-vascularized and durable flaps are available based on the known circulation of the region. Gluteal myocutaneous and gluteal fasciocutaneous flaps are used in the sacral region. The rectus femoris muscle flap is, at times added under the tensor fascia lata fasciocutaneous flaps, at times to pad and provide well-vascularized muscle to the bone stump in reconstructing hip ulcers. Latissimus dorsi myocutaneous and lumbar fasciocutaneous flaps can be used to cover scapula wounds.

There are several systems used to classify flaps. A commonly used method is to list flap types into categories (1) type of blood supply, (2) type of tissue to be transferred, and (3) location of donor site. The terms used to classify flaps based on the blood supply include two types: random flaps and axial flaps. Random flaps have no named, specific blood vessel to supply the flap. In this type of flap many smaller unnamed vessels supply the transferred tissue. The second type is referred to as an axial flap. It uses a specific, named blood vessel to vascularize the flap [28].

Flaps may comprise almost any component of human tissue. The tissue can be transferred as long as it has adequate blood supply. Flaps may be composed of only one type of tissue or several different types called composite flaps [29]. Flaps composed of one type of tissue include skin, fascia, muscle, bone, and viscera (i.e., omentum). Composite flaps include fasciocutaneous, myocutaneous, and tendocutaneous to name a few.

When tissue is transferred from an area adjacent to the defect is referred to as a local flap. A local flap can be further described based on its size or design. Local pivotal flaps include rotation, transposition, and interpolation. Local advancement flaps include single pedicle, bipedicle, and V-Y flaps [30]. It is beyond the scope of this chapter to explain in detail the nuances of the types and selection of flaps in reconstructive surgery in pressure ulcers. The above information is presented so the generalist can have a better grasp of the surgeon's lexicon and to allow better understanding of the case studies below.

When tissue is transferred from a site not adjacent to the defect it is referred to as a distant flap. Distant flaps may be either pedicled, which means it is transferred still attached to their original blood supply or free. Free flaps are detached from their native blood supply and then reattached to vessels at the recipient site, often using microsurgical techniques.

Reconstructive surgical techinques have evolved rapidly since WWII when pedicle flaps were in common use by military surgeons. It was not until the 1970s that a distinction was made between axial and random flaps. This fact makes reading the early literature difficult.

Random Flaps

The first level in flap wound construction complexity is that of adjacent tissue reconstruction. Flaps based on the random circulation of the subdermal capillary plexus under the skin allow for undermining and advancement or flap creation and rotation of the skin and subcutaneous tissues.

Random flaps are useful in any portion of the body from the scalp to the toes where redundancy of tissue in one direction will allow for closure of the donor site and advancement or rotation of tissues to fill the defect.

Axial Flaps

Well-vascularized composite flaps of skin, fat, fascia, muscle, and occasionally bone are used to reconstruct the larger defects created over bony prominences. The essence of modern day surgical reconstruction is to carry prefabricated tissues into the prepared wound site for repair. This may include the plumbing (vessels), electrical conduits (nerves for sensation and proprioception), insulation (subcutis, muscle, fascia), and durable cover (skin). Surgical options range from simple to complex providing the missing components according to the clinical stage of injury. This may include the foundation of the wound (bone, cartilage, muscle, or subcutaneous tissue), the walls (structure and scaffolding) of the wound, or its roof (skin).

Free Tissue Transfer

Free tissue transfer is defined as the vascular detachment of an isolated and specific region of the body followed by transfer of that tissue to another region of the body with reattachment of the divided artery and vein to an artery and vein at the graft site. The ability to transplant living tissue from one region of the body to another is a significant surgical advancement. The advantages include stable wound coverage, improved aesthetic, and minimal donor site complications. Since the introduction of free tissue transfer in the 1960s, the success rate has improved substantially and is currently 95–99 % among experienced surgeons [31, 32].

State-of-the-art techniques, including micro-revascularization, have allowed for composite tissues to be transferred from one body area, such as the face or back, to the defect site. Supple, well-vascularized fascia or muscle tissue may be transferred as a free flap to defects in the leg, which would have otherwise progressed to limb loss. This new millennium adds the challenges of allotransplanted free tissue transfers reducing rejection with the use of anti-rejection drugs and chimeric techniques, as seen in our wounded soldiers. These free tissue transfers are more technically challenging, take much longer operative times, and are not typically an option for pressure ulcer reconstructions. It is mentioned here for completeness.

When a wound is fully excised, a new acute wound has been created with removal of all infected senescent cells and tissues. Flap wound healing is hastened as the tissue components are placed in apposition at the repair site and only collagen needs to hold the wound together. Since it takes at least 6 weeks in the immunocompetent patient to achieve 60 % tensile strength, splinting and protection of the wound against stress are recommended. Since many patients have poor nutritional reserves, this author recommends no less than 12 weeks of wound support.

Heel Wounds

Posterior heel wounds are often the most difficult pressure ulcers to heal due to the end arterial blood supply based on the peroneal vessels laterally and the posterior tibial vessels medially of the foot, especially in the patient with peripheral artery disease. Once a full-thickness wound has interrupted the dermal blood supply, no collateral circulation is available and healing by secondary intent frequently fails. Debriding these types of wounds may lead to wet gangrene due to distal peripheral vascular disease. It is best to treat these ulcers conservatively.

In these cases, it is recommended the clinician "float" the heel off the bed surface. There are many devices and techniques to pressure offload the heel. The wound should also be desiccated with an antiseptic, such as povidone-iodine. Many patients with posterior heel dry gangrene will subsequently lose their limbs to wet gangrene even with frequent monitoring. Not debriding a stable, chronic, dry wound may be the best option for many of these patients. The use of a splint itself may also cause a pressure or traumatic injury.

Some heel pressure ulcer patients may benefit from coverage with a suralis fasciocutaneous flap [24, 33]. Less commonly in non-ambulatory patients, direct closure after debridement of the calcaneus can be accomplished.

Sacral Pressure Ulcers: Case Study #1

Sacral ulcers are common in patients who have been on prolonged bed rest in the supine position. Treatment involves complete ulcer excision, including the entire bursa, and conservative ostectomy. Small sacral ulcers can be reconstructed with an inferiorly based skin rotation flap with or without the superior gluteus maximus myocutaneous flap (see photos below). The use of the random skin rotation flap does not preclude later use of the gluteus muscle. When using a random skin rotation flap, designing a large and wide flap with an axis of rotation that permits tension-free closure is essential.

Case Study #1 involves an optimized sacral decubitus ulcer in a qudraplegic patient. The patient presents with a contracted, granulated, and minimally epithelialized wound prepared for ulcer excision, ostectomy, and myocutaneous flap reconstruction (see Fig. 7.4). The unstable sacral ulcer required excision of the chronic wound, ostectomy of the superficial sacral bone, and reconstruction using a left gluteal myocutaneous rotation and right gluteal myocutaneous advancement flaps. Myocutaneous flaps are the surgeon's first choice in deep pressure ulcers because the flap has sufficient bulk to fill the wound void, has good blood supply, and has a full-thickness skin cover [34]).

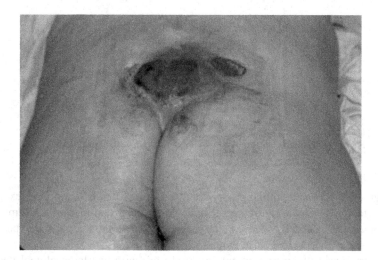

Fig. 7.4 Sacral pressure ulcer prepared for ulcer excision, ostectomy, and myocutaneous flap reconstruction

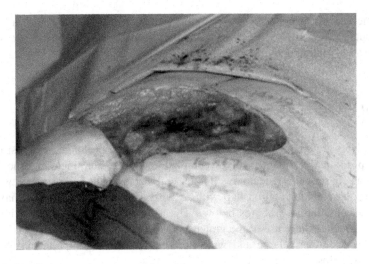

Fig. 7.5 Sacral pressure ulcer post excision with ostectomy

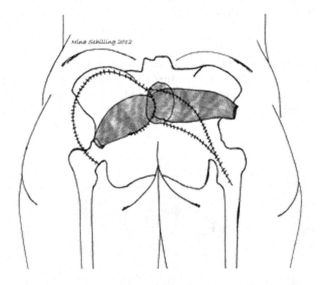

Fig. 7.6 Sacral wound defect closure with two large gluteal flaps is illustrated

Figure 7.5 shows the initial phase of the proceedure that is sacral ulcer excision with ostectomy of underlying sacral bone and gluteal flap markings. Removing the contracted ulcer edges leaves a larger defect due to the unopposed expansion of the "acute," sterile, and clean wound edges.

Illustration of the sacral wound defect closure with two large gluteal flaps is shown in Fig. 7.6. The right buttock flap diagrams a gluteal myocutaneous

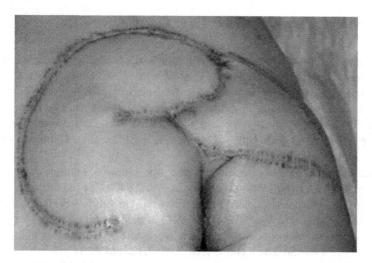

Fig. 7.7 Same patient 6 weeks postoperatively

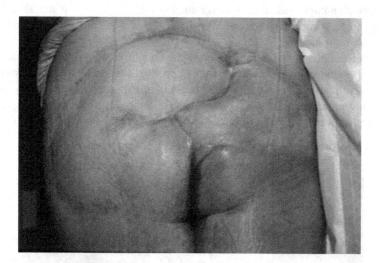

Fig. 7.8 One year post flap surgery

advancement flap. The left buttock demonstrates a gluteal myofasciocutaneous flap (Figs. 7.7 and 7.8).

Outcome in sacral decubitus ulcer patient 1-year post reconstruction demonstration complete healing without recurrence. This kind of outcome requires four elements: proper patient selection, an experienced surgeon, excellent post-op care, and a patient who can adhere to an ongoing regimen of pressure offloading.

Trochanteric Pressure Ulcer: Case Study #2

Trochanteric pressure sores are less common and are typically associated from prolonged side-lying position with less skin loss. Excisional debridement of trochanteric ulcers in preparation for flap repair involves resection of the entire bursa and greater trochanter of the femur. The tensor fascia lata myofasciocutaneous flap is the first option for reconstruction of trochanteric pressure ulcers [35]. The flap has good blood supply and the muscle is expendable. The donor site can often be closed primarily.

A patient with a right trochanteric pressure ulcer following multiple debridements and bone removal for infection is shown in Fig. 7.9. Notice the articular surface of the hip joint which is considered infected by exposure. Distally (to the right) on the leg are two healed skin graft donor sites which demonstrate failure of a partial-thickness dermal cover as reconstruction of a pressure prone area. Skin lines mark the undermined wound extent (Figs. 7.10, 7.11, 7.12, and 7.13).

The right hip wound defect reconstruction is shown in Fig. 7.14. Staples will further support the incision against tension during the healing process. The entire well-perfused, "pre-fabricated" tissue is rotated into the defect, covering the bony prominence and apposed in layers over suction drains. Closure of the TFL donor site with underlying suction drains. The donor site is also easily apposed in layers for a tensionless closure.

The above right trochanteric pressure ulcer patient failed a prior split-thickness skin graft as evidenced by the healed hypopigmented squares on the lower posterior thigh. These photos illustrate the wide excision of the ulcer and ostectomy of the underlying greater trochanter. The tensor fascia lata fasciocutaneous flap itself is lifted on a vascular pedicle with the composite skin, fat, and fascia visible.

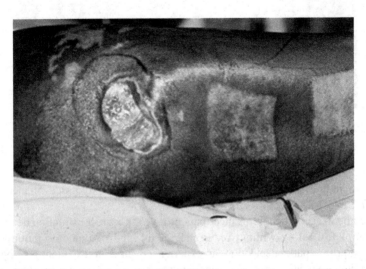

Fig. 7.9 A preoperative view of patient with a right trochanteric pressure ulcer following multiple debridements who had bone excised due to osteomyelitis

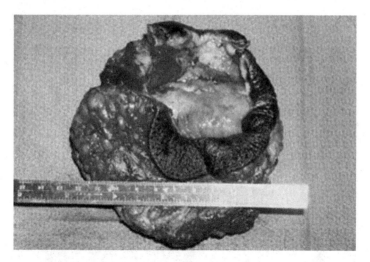

Fig. 7.10 The surgical specimen from the surgical excision of the trochanter pressure ulcer

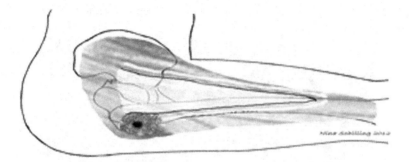

Fig. 7.11 Is an illustration of the right trochanteric wound and underlying femur. The tensor fascia lata (TFL) fasciocutaneous flap is outlined

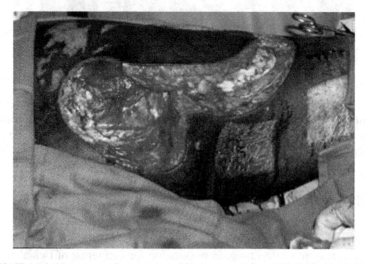

Fig. 7.12 The right hip pressure ulcer excision with ostectomy defect and incised adjacent TFL flap

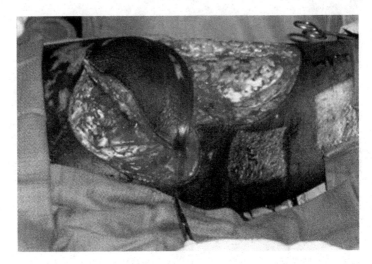

Fig. 7.13 The TFL flap is shown being rotated into the right hip wound defect

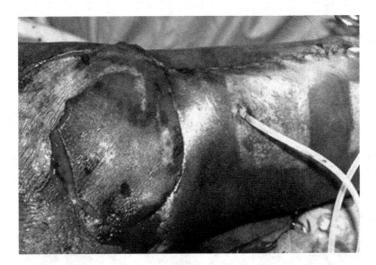

Fig. 7.14 The right hip wound defect reconstruction completed

The entire well-perfused "prefabricated" tissue is rotated into the defect, covering the bony prominence and apposed in layers over suction drains. The donor site is also easily apposed in layers for a tensionless closure.

Ischial Pressure Ulcer: Case Study #3

The ischial location is the most common location in paraplegics and others with unrelieved pressure while sitting. In preparation for flap repair of ischial wounds, aggressive resection of the ischial tuberosity may risk a contralateral ischial

Fig. 7.15 Shows a patient with a chronic left ischial tuberosity pressure ulcer that has failed to progress

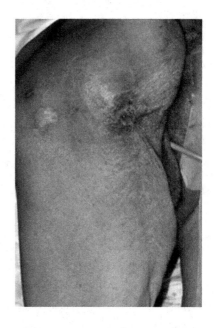

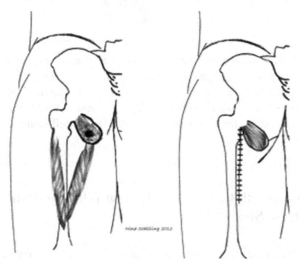

Fig. 7.16 *On Left*: ischial excisional wound with ostectomy and biceps femoris myofasciocutaneous flap on the *left*. *On right*: the flap rotation and donor site closure

pressure ulcer from increased contralateral pressure, injure the perineum creating a urethral or vaginal fistula [36], and may preclude the use of the gluteal flaps for sacral ulcer reconstruction. A rotated biceps femoris myofasciocutaneous (one of the hamstrings muscles) flap is a common first choice to fill and close an ischial pressure sore [37] (Figs. 7.15 and 7.16).

Fig. 7.17 Left ischial wound
defect and elevated biceps
femoris flap and donor site
showing the axial blood
vessels perfusing the flap

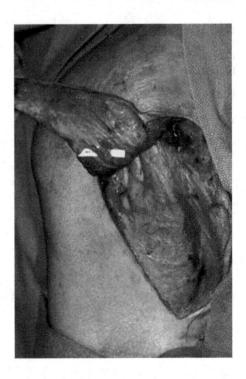

The ischial ulcer in the above case appears quite small on the outside due to contracture of the wound edges, but the undermining is wide and dangerously close to adjacent vital structures. Careful excision and ostectomy are mandatory. The biceps femoris myofasciocutaneous flap is elevated illustrating the vascular pedicle and inset without tension (Figs. 7.17 and 7.18). A well-healed reconstruction is shown in Fig. 7.19.

Femoral Disarticulation for Hip Osteomyelitis or Joint Infection: Case Study #4

Pyarthrosis of the hip joint can occur with communication of ischial or trochanteric ulcers. Often, the femoral head contains osteomyelitis, which mandates its removal. Without a femoral head prosthesis or fusion, the entire leg becomes flaccid and unstable and must be removed. A hip disarticulation is indicated with muscle coverage of the articular surface and soft tissue with a thigh filet flap over the hip defect.

In Fig. 7.20, left illustration shows a left hip pressure sore and hip pyarthrosis with (anterior) rectus femoris muscle for flap lining of the articular surface. Right illustration shows rectus muscle inset into the hip following disarticulation, curettage of the femoral articular surface, inset of the rectus femoris muscle flap, removal of the femur and distal leg, and thigh fillet flap reconstruction.

Fig. 7.18 The left biceps
femoris flap inset and donor
site closure

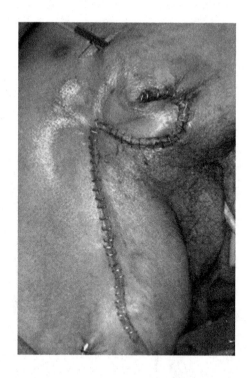

Fig. 7.19 Staples removed
from left ischial pressure
ulcer reconstruction at 12
weeks

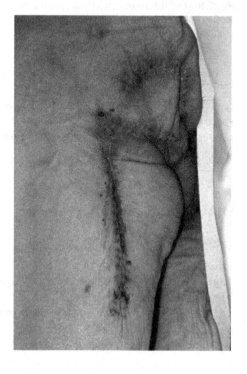

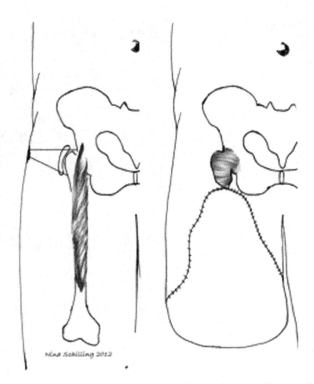

Fig. 7.20 *Left iIllustration*: a left hip pressure sore and hip pyarthrosis with rectus femoris muscle for flap lining of the articular surface. *Right Illustration*: rectus muscle inset into the hip following disarticulation

Figure 7.21 shows the postoperative state of the hip disarticulation for femoral head osteomyelitis and pyarthrosis of the hip joint. The femur and distal leg are removed. A rectus femoris or vastus lateralis muscle flap lines the excised joint space and a thigh fillet flap covers the wound. This type of surgery is aggressive but can result in a better quality of life for selected patients who otherwise have to live with a chronic infected wound.

Other Considerations

Multiple pressure sores occurred in this same patient. Excision of each ulcer, ostectomy, and reconstruction of multiple ulcers may require the use of a total thigh flap. It should be reserved as a salvage procedure when other attempts have been unsuccessful.

Some surgeons will recommend colonic or urinary diversion prior to reconstruction in patients with heavily colonized wounds from stool or urine. This is a controversial topic and recommendations are case specific [38].

Fig. 7.21 Shows the
post-operative state of the hip
disarticulation for femoral
head osteomyelitis

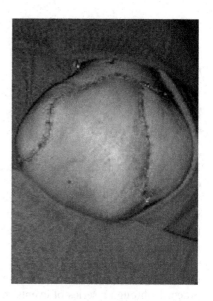

Fixed contractures and muscular spasm in spinal cord injury patients need to be addressed preoperatively. Serial casting and even surgical release of flexion contractures are at times indicated prior to surgery. Any type of traction on the suture line can result in surgical wound dehiscence. Contractures make postoperative repositioning difficult as well.

Complications

Complications following pressure sore reconstruction can be high because of patient noncompliance, seromas, hematomas, wound infections, and dehiscence. Sutures dissolve by 3–6 weeks leaving minimal wound strength across the reconstructed incision. Follow-up evaluation and monitoring for a minimum of 3 months following wound closure are essential to maintain incision integrity. Staple reinforcement across the incision line should not be removed for 3 months. Thereafter, the patient is deemed surgically stable.

Flap Failure

The complication rate of pressure ulcer reconstruction is high; poor candidates for surgery should not undergo pressure ulcer reconstruction. Patients without a good support system at home are not good candidates for pressure sore reconstruction.

> **Box 7.3 Signs of Impending Flap Failure**
>
> - Swelling (hyperpermeability)
> - Erythema (hyperemia)
> - Cyanosis (venous congestion)
> - Epidermolysis (partial-thickness necrosis)

Patients who are noncompliant with pressure offloading and local care are also poor candidates for reconstruction.

The postoperative regimen for the transition from bed rest to sitting and return to wheelchair seating must be strict and careful. Patients may need to be reevaluated by the rehabilitation team so to have all the needed adaptive equipment and training when the surgeon gives clearance.

Even with valiant attempts for wound closure, offloading, and rehabilitation, underlying problems may cause flap or skin graft failure. Flap or graft failure proceeds through a series of events that, if caught early enough, may be reversed. The cardinal signs of impending flap failure are included in Box 7.3.

Flap failure can occur due to secondary infection or compromise in blood supply. Diminished blood supply to the flap can occur due to unavoidable intrinsic vascular compromise or to unrelieved pressure to the vulnerable flap.

Rescue of failing flaps is possible but dependent on diligent observation of the wound by the attending physician and referral for immediate reevaluation by the reconstructive surgeon.

Adjunctive Therapies to Surgical Management

Moist wound healing is the best method to promote healing to occur in chronic wounds [39]. A moist, clean wound promotes epithelialization from the edges across an adequate granular base to sustain and protect the budding peripheral cells during the mid-proliferative phase of healing. A chronic wound may need serial sharp debridement to remove necrotic tissue not eliminated by autolysis or enzymatic debridement.

Negative pressure wound closure therapy can be considered for deep wounds that are clean and in bacteriologic balance. Negative pressure therapy has been found to enhance wound healing by increasing blood flow, decreasing edema, and increasing the formation of granulation tissue [40–42]. It will also decrease healing time and bacterial contamination [43]. Relative contraindications to the use of negative pressure wound therapy include infection or vascular structures adjacent to the wound base.

Hyperbaric Oxygen (HBO) Therapy may be useful for rapidly progressive cellulitis or fasciitis. The principal treatment for severe soft tissue infections such as clostridial myonecrosis, necrotizing fasciitis, and Fournier's gangrene is broad-spectrum antibiotic therapy and aggressive debridement. A number of retrospective and observational studies have evaluated the role of HBO as an adjunctive therapy for severe, life-, or limb-threatening necrotizing infection [44, 45]. There are no human randomized, controlled trials demonstrating survival benefit. But there is good survival data in clostridial infections in a dog model that demonstrated a 35 % survival increase with adjunctive HBO [46]. Adjunctive HBO may decrease mortality and limit the extent of debridement in Fournier's gangrene and necrotizing fasciitis [47].

HBO is indicated as adjunctive therapy for a group of traumatic and ischemic syndromes, including crush injuries, compartment syndromes, and vascular compromise [48]. Following surgical reconstruction, HBO may oxygenate a failing flap reconstruction and "buy" time until reperfusion is accomplished. HBO therapy may improve the survival of skin grafts and reconstructive flaps that have compromised blood flow [49]. It is unknown if prophylactic HBO therapy is efficacious in the face of flap vascular compromise.

Electrical stimulation, in which a direct current is applied to the wound, has also resulted in enhanced healing in several small studies [50, 51]. Its use is very limited and requires specialized equipment and trained personnel. Low-frequency ultrasound has also found limited use as therapy for pressure ulcers [52].

Defects found with single cell type injuries such as burns; multicellular defects such as the urethra; and hollow viscus defects such as the bladder and solid organs such as the penis, liver, and partial hearts are undergoing current trials with the use of pluripotent stem cell cloning of manufactured and cell-free organ scaffolds. Composite wound reconstruction with the use of regenerative techniques may not be too far distant.

Outcomes

In a well-conducted longitudinal study of pressure patients followed for up to 12 years 48 % of the ulcers recurred [53]. In the 36 patients who were followed 56 % were younger spinal cord injury patients. Forty-eight out of 66 ulcers ultimately healed in these 36 patients. The results were the same for musculocutaneous flaps and were comparable to those reached by closure with cutaneous flaps in this study.

Palliative Considerations in Pressure Ulcer Management

Reconstructive surgery, with the ultimate goal of hastened healing, pain reduction, durable repair, and less healthcare costs, is offered in those relatively few patients whose catabolic states have been reversed and whose wounds are of such size that they otherwise would not heal by secondary intent. A chronic wound without pain or infection in an end-stage patient is a candidate for compassionate, palliative care. Debridement and potentially painful dressing changes are not indicated. Allowing these wounds to desiccate is appropriate. Judicial use of analgesics should be considered for pain control. Antiseptics and dressings to remove exudate and suppress bioburden can be of value.

Summary

Pressure ulcers cause considerable harm to patients, hindering functional recovery, and can lead to serious infection. Pressure ulcers have also been associated with an extended length of hospital stay, sepsis, and mortality. It is estimated that nearly 60,000 US hospital patients die each year from complications due to pressure ulcers. The estimated cost of managing a single full-thickness pressure ulcer is as high as $70,000, and the total cost for treatment of pressure ulcers in the USA is estimated at $11 billion per year [54, 55].

Surgical care for pressure ulcer patients including debridement and when appropriate reconstructive surgery can save cost and shorten the time to closure. Nonetheless reconstructive surgery even in well-selected patients and by expert surgeons has a high rate of recurrence [56]. Wound surgeons are important to the care process in pressure ulcer care [53].

References

1. Black J, Baharestani MM, Cuddigan J, et al. National Pressure Ulcer Advisory Panel's updated pressure ulcer staging system. Adv Skin Wound Care. 2007;20(5):270–4.
2. Clinical practice guidelines: number 15 treatment of pressure ulcers. Rockville, MD: US Department of Health and Human Services, Agency for Health Care Policy and Research; 1994. AHCPR publication 95-06542.
3. European Pressure Ulcer Advisory panel and National Pressure Ulcer Advisory Panel. Prevention and treatment of pressure ulcers: quick reference guide. Washington, DC: National Pressure Ulcer Advisory Panel; 2009.
4. Shea JD. Pressure sores classification and management. Clin Orthop Relat Res. 1975;112: 89–100.
5. Thomas DR, Goode PS, Tarquine PH, Allman R. Hospital acquired pressure ulcers and risk of death. J Am Geriatr Soc. 1996;44:1435–40.
6. Wound, Ostomy, and Continence Nurses Society. Prevalence and incidence: a toolkit for clinicians. Glenview, IL: WOCN; 2004.
7. Reddy M, Gill SS, Rochon PA. Preventing pressure ulcers: a systematic review. JAMA. 2006;296:974–84.
8. Thompson RJ. Pathological changes in mummies. Proc R Soc Med. 1961;54:409.
9. Broughton G, Janis J, Attinger C. Reconstructive wound-healing supplement: original articles: reconstructive a brief history of wound care. Plast Reconstr Surg. 2006;117(7S):6S–11.
10. Lay-flurrie K. Honey in wound care: effects, clinical application and patient benefit. Br J Nurs. 2008;17(11):S30–6.
11. Moues CM, Heule F, Legerstee R, Hovious SER. Five millennia of wound care products: what is new? a literature review. Ostomy Wound Manage. 2009;55(3):16–32.

12. Kane DP. Chronic wound healing and chronic wound management. In: Krasner DL, Rodeheaver GT, Sibbald RG, editors. Chronic wound care: a clinical source book for healthcare professionals. 4th ed. Malvern, PA: HMP Communications; 2007. p. 11–24.
13. Gefen A. Reswick and Rogers pressure time curve for pressure ulcer risk. Part 2. Nurs Stand. 2009;23:40–4.
14. Bauer J, Phillips J. Pressure sores. MOC-PSSM CME article. Plast Reconstr Surg. 2008;121:1.
15. Singer AJ, Clark RA. Cutaneous wound healing. N Engl J Med. 1999;341:738–46.
16. Lazarus GS, Cooper DM, Knighton DR, et al. Definitions and guidelines for assessment for wounds and evaluation of healing. Arch Dermatol. 1994;130(4):489–93.
17. Reddy M, Gill SS, Wu W, Kalkar SR, et al. Does this patient have an infection of a chronic wound? JAMA. 2012;307:605–11.
18. Barbenel JC, Ferguson-Pell MW, Kennedy R. Mobility of elderly patients in bed. Measurement and association with patient condition. J Am Geriatr Soc. 1986;34:633.
19. Niazi ZB, Salzberg CA, Byrne DW, Viehbeck M. Recurrence of initial pressure ulcer in persons with spinal cord injuries. Adv Wound Care. 1997;10:38.
20. Bradley M, Cullum N, Sheldon T. The debridement of chronic wounds: a systematic review. Health Technol Assess. 1999;3:1–78.
21. The management of pressure ulcers in primary and secondary care A Clinical Practice Guideline. Royal College of Nursing, London. 2005. http://www.ncbi.nlm.nih.gov/pubmedhealth/PMH0009866/pdf/TOC.pdf. Last accessed 2/1/13.
22. Deloach ED, DiBenedetto RJ, Womble JD. The treatment of osteomyelitis underlying pressure ulcers. Decubitus. 1992;5:32–41.
23. Schultz GS, Sibbald RG, Falanga V, et al. Wound bed preparation: a systematic approach to wound management. Wound Repair Regen. 2003;11 Suppl 1:S1.
24. Sorensen JL, Jorgensen B, Gottrup F. Surgical treatment of pressure ulcers. Am J Surg. 2004;188(1A Suppl):43S–51.
25. Phillips LG, Robson MC. Pathobiology and treatment of pressure ulcerations. In: Jurkiewicz MJ, editor. Plastic surgery principle and practice. St. Louis, MO: Mosby; 1990. p. 1223.
26. Niazi ZB, Salzberg CA. Surgical management of pressure ulcers. Ostomy Wound Manage. 1997;43:44.
27. Disa JJ, Carlton JM, Goldberg NH. Efficacy of operative cure for pressure sore patients. Plast Reconstr Surg. 1992;89:272–8.
28. Mathes SJ, Nahai F. Classification of the vascular anatomy of muscles: experimental and clinical correlation. Plast Reconstr Surg. 1981;67(2):177–87.
29. Kayser MR. Selected readings in plastic surgery. Surgical Flaps. 1999;9(2):1.
30. Tobin GR, Brown GL, Derr JW, et al. V-Y advancement flaps. Reusable flaps for pressure ulcer repair. Clin Plast Surg. 1990;17(4):727–32.
31. Serletti JM, Higgins JP, Moran S, Orlando GS. Factors affecting outcome in free-tissue transfer in the elderly. Plast Reconstr Surg. 2000;106(1):66–70.
32. Kroll SS, Schusterman MA, Reece GP, et al. Choice of flap and incidence of free flap success. Plast Reconstr Surg. 1996;98(3):459–63.
33. Strauch B, Vasconex LO, Hall-Findlay EJ, Grabb WC. Grabb's encyllopedia of flapps. Boston, MA: Little Brown; 1990.
34. Rubayi S, Cousins S, Valentine WA. Myocutaneous flaps: surgical treatment of severe pressure ulcers. AORN J. 1990;52:40–55.
35. Siddiqui A, Eiedrich T, Lewis Jr VL. Tensor fascia lata V-Y reposition myocutaneous flap: clinical experience. Ann Plast Surg. 1993;31:313–7.
36. Hackler RH, Zampari TA. Urethral complications following isciectiomy in spinal cord injury patients: a urethral pressure study. J Urol. 1987;137:233–5.
37. Kroll SS, Hamilton S. Multiple and repetitive uses of the extended hamstring myocutaneous flap. Plast Reconstr Surg. 1989;84:296–302.
38. Whitney J, Phillips L, Rummana A, Barbul A, et al. Guideline for the treatment of pressure ulcers. Wound Repair Regen. 2006;14:663–79.
39. Sibbald RG, Williamson D, Orstead H, et al. Preparing the wound bed – debridement, bacterial balance and moisture balance. Ostomy Wound Manage. 2000;46(1):14–35.

40. Argenta LC, Morykwas MJ. Vacuum-assisted closure: a new method for wound control and treatment: clinical experience. Ann Plast Surg. 1997;38:563.
41. Joseph E, Hamori CA, Bergman S, et al. A prospective randomized trial of vacuum-assisted closure versus standard therapy of chronic nonhealing wounds. Wounds. 2000;12:60.
42. Mendez-Eastman S. Guidelines for using negative pressure wound therapy. Adv Skin Wound Care. 2001;14:314.
43. Bradon J, Wilhelmi J, Vistnes LM, et al. Surgical treatment of pressure ulcers. http://emedicine.medscape.com/article/1293724-overview. Last accessed 12 Dec 2012.
44. Wilkinson D, Doolette D. Hyperbaric oxygen treatment and survival from necrotizing soft tissue infection. Arch Surg. 2004;139:1339.
45. Pizzorno R, Bonini F, Donelli A, et al. Hyperbaric oxygen therapy in the treatment of Fournier's gangrene: therapeutic impact of hyperbaric oxygen. J Urol. 1997;158:837.
46. Demello FJ, Haglin JJ, Hitchcock CR. Comparative study of experimental Clostridium perfringens infection in dogs treated with antibiotics, surgery and hyperbaric oxygen. Surgery. 1973;73:936.
47. Green RJ, Dafoe DC, Raffin TA. Necrotizing fasciitis. Chest. 1996;110:219.
48. Thorn SR. Hyperbaric oxygen: its mechanism and efficacy. Plast Reconstr Surg. 2011; 127(Suppl1):131S.
49. Wang C, Schwaitzberg S, Berliner E, et al. Hyperbaric oxygen for treating wounds: a systematic review of the literature. Arch Surg. 2003;138:272.
50. Griffin JW, Tooms RE, Mendius RA, et al. Efficacy of high voltage pulsed current for healing of pressure ulcers in patients with spinal cord injury. Phys Ther. 1991;71:433.
51. Feedar JA, Kloth LC, Gentzkow GD. Chronic dermal ulcer healing enhanced with monophasic pulsed electrical stimulation. Phys Ther. 1991;71:639.
52. Flemming K, Cullum N. Therapeutic ultrasound for pressure sores. Cochrane Database Syst Rev. 2000;4:CD001275.
53. Relander M, Palmer B. Recurrence of surgically treated pressure sores. Scand J Plast Reconstr Surg Hand Surg. 1988;22:89–92.
54. Redelings MD, Lee NE, Sorvillo F. Pressure ulcers: more lethal than we thought? Adv Skin Wound Care. 2005;18(7):367–72.
55. Allman R. The impact of pressure ulcers on healthcare costs and mortality. Adv Wound Care. 1998;11(3 Suppl):2.
56. Kane DP. Surgical repair in advanced wound caring. In: Krasner DL, Rodeheaver GT, Sibbald RG, editors. Chronic wound care: a clinical source book for healthcare professionals. 4th ed. Malvern, PA: HMP Communications; 2007. p. 363–72.

Other Useful References

57. How-to guide: prevent pressure ulcers. Cambridge, MA: Institute for Healthcare Improvement; 2011. http://www.ihi.org. Last accessed 16 Dec 2012.
58. Pieper B, National Pressure Ulcer Advisory Panel (NPUAP), editors. Pressure ulcers: prevalence, incidence, and implications for the future. Washington, DC: NPUAP; 2012.
59. Stechmiller JK, Cowan L, Whitney JD, et al. Guidelines for the prevention of pressure ulcers. Wound Repair Regen. 2008;16:151.
60. Thomas DR. The new F-tag 314: prevention and management of pressure ulcers. J Am Med Dir Assoc. 2006;7:523.

Chapter 8
The Role of Nutrition in the Management and Prevention of Pressure Ulcers

David R. Thomas

Abstract Nutritional support is a cornerstone of clinical care and should be provided to all persons, including persons with pressure ulcers, consistent with medical goals and patient wishes. Whether nutrition can improve the outcome of pressure ulcers remains disputable. Energy requirements for persons with pressure ulcers are estimated empirically between 25 and 30 kcal/kg/day, but have been confirmed in studies using nutritional formulas such as the Harris–Benedict equation. The optimum amount of protein intake is not known, but likely lies between 1.2 and 1.5 g/kg/day. Higher protein intakes may be harmful and have not been associated with higher rates of healing. Supplemental amino acids and supertherapeutic supplements of vitamins and minerals have not been shown to have much effect on the healing of pressure ulcers. Clinical nutritional intervention trials suffer from small sample sizes and poor methodological design, but in general have not shown exceptional benefit in improving complete healing of pressure ulcers. Nutritional therapy will improve starvation due to lack of food, but cachexia associated with inflammatory conditions has been remarkably resistant to hypercaloric feeding.

Keywords Pressure ulcer • Chronic wound • Pressure ulcer nutrition • Malnutrition • Protein • Vitamin C • Zinc • Nutritional requirements • Nutritional assessment • Cachexia • Cytokines

Introduction and Background

In the minds of most clinicians, wound healing is intricately linked to nutrition. Severe protein-calorie undernutrition in humans alters tissue regeneration, the inflammatory reaction, and immune function [1]. Hospitalized patients defined as

D.R. Thomas, M.D., F.A.C.P., A.G.S.F., G.S.A.F. (✉)
Division of Geriatric Medicine, Saint Louis University,
1402 South Grand Blvd. M238, Saint Louis, MO 63104, USA
e-mail: thomasdr@slu.edu

D.R. Thomas and G.A. Compton (eds.), *Pressure Ulcers in the Aging Population: A Guide for Clinicians*, Aging Medicine 1, DOI 10.1007/978-1-62703-700-6_8,
© Springer Science+Business Media New York 2014

malnourished have a higher risk for death, sepsis, infections, and increased length of stay [2]. Undernourished patients are more likely to have postoperative complications than well-nourished patients [3]. After vascular surgery, hypoalbuminemia and low transferrin levels have predicted wound healing complications [4].

Experimental studies in animal models suggest a biologically plausible relationship between undernutrition and development of pressure ulcers. When pressure was applied for 4 h to the skin of well-nourished animals and malnourished animals, pressure ulcers occurred equally in both groups. However, the degree of ischemic skin destruction was more severe in the malnourished animals. At 3 days post-injury, epithelialization of the pressure lesions had occurred in normal animals, while massive necrosis of the epidermis was still present in the malnourished animals [5]. This data suggests that while pressure damage may occur independently of nutritional status, malnourished animals may have impaired healing after a pressure injury.

Further indication of a relationship between nutrition and tissue damage is suggested by the finding that mitotic activity in normal epidermis is severely depressed in mice whose food intake was reduced to 70 % of normal [6]. Dietary restriction to 60 % of normal intake in other animal models is associated with impaired collagen cross-linking 1 week after wounding [7]. Classical studies have shown that wound dehiscence occurs more commonly in dogs with chronic protein undernutrition [8].

Nevertheless, animal studies create some problems relevant to human wound healing. For example, collagen deposition differs in animals, requiring 42 days for completion compared to 88 days in humans [9]. The effects of short-term starvation is much more severe in animals than in humans [10]. Interestingly, hypoalbuminemia alone is not associated with impaired wound healing in analbuminemic rats [11].

Epidemiological Associations of Nutrition and Pressure Ulcers

Most of the data for the interaction of nutrition and pressure ulcers derive from epidemiological studies. In a prospective study of high-risk patients, undernutrition (defined by an index of biochemical and anthropometric variables) was present in 29 % of patients at hospital admission. At 4 weeks, 17 % of the undernourished patients had developed a pressure ulcer, compared to 9 % of the non-undernourished patients. Thus, patients who were undernourished at hospital admission were twice as likely to develop pressure ulcers as non-undernourished patients (RR 2.1, 95 % confidence intervals [CI] 1.1, 4.2) [12].

In a long-term care setting, 59 % of residents were diagnosed as undernourished on admission. Among these residents, 7 % were classified as severely undernourished. Pressure ulcers occurred in 65 % of these severely undernourished residents. No pressure ulcers developed in the mild-to-moderately undernourished or well-nourished groups [13].

In a 2007 study of 4,067 patients from 22 hospitals in Germany, a positive relationship was shown between the presence of a pressure ulcer and unintentional weight loss of 5–10 %, a body mass index less than 18.5 kg/m², poor nutritional intake (from the Braden Scale), and being bedfast. Being bedfast for hospitalized subjects was the most critical risk factor with an odds ratio of 23 (95 % CI 10, 52). In 2,393 patients from 29 German nursing homes, a positive association for the presence of a pressure ulcer was observed for an unintentional weight loss of 5 to greater than 10 %, a body mass index less than 20 kg/m², poor nutritional intake (from the Braden Scale), and probable inadequate nutritional intake (from the Braden Scale) [14].

Two epidemiological studies have correlated the development of pressure ulcers with dietary protein intake. In a long-term care setting, the estimated percent intake of dietary protein, but not total caloric intake, predicted development of pressure ulcers. Patients with pressure ulcers ingested 93 % of the recommended daily intake of protein compared to an intake of 119 % of the recommended protein in the non-pressure ulcer group. Only dietary intake of protein was important in this study. The total dietary intake of calories or the calculated intake of vitamins A and C, iron or zinc did not predict ulcer development [15].

In another study, impaired nutritional intake, defined as a persistently poor appetite, meals held due to gastrointestinal disease, or a prescribed diet less than 1,100 kcal or 50 g protein/day, predicted pressure ulcer development in a long-term care setting [32]. However, no other nutritional variable was univariately significant.

These epidemiological data confirms the association of select nutrition-related variables to the incidence and prevalence of pressure ulcers. In spite of these data, the association of undernutrition and pressure ulcers remains problematic. The major difficulty in defining the relationship of pressure ulcers and nutrition lies in the lack of a gold standard for the diagnosis of undernutrition.

A number of risk instruments have been developed to assess nutritional status. Examples of instruments designed to diagnose malnutrition include the Subjective Global Assessment, the Mini-Nutritional Assessment, the Malnutrition Universal Screening tool, the Nutritional Risk Screening-2002, and the Geriatric Nutritional Risk Index. These tools differ in the variables assessed, the skill needed to complete the tool, and the sensitivity and specificity of the results [16].

Despite differences among tools, all of the nutritional assessment tools perform well in identifying persons who will have future complications. Undernourished and at risk individuals identified by most of these tools have longer lengths of hospital stay, higher likelihood of intensive care stays, more acute illness, more weight loss, lower functional status, and higher mortality. Therefore, common sense suggests that repletion of nutritional status should be able to reverse these adverse outcomes. However, randomized, controlled trials have failed by and large to demonstrate an effect on these outcomes [17]. A major conceptual problem in the use of nutrition assessment instruments is whether what is being measured reflects true undernutrition or whether the measurement merely identifies sicker patients.

Despite a strong relationship of poor nutritional status to pressure ulcers, the association does not confirm that one follows the other (causality), but that both undernutrition and pressure ulcers frequently coexist in the same persons.

General Nutritional Support for Persons with Pressure Ulcers

Energy Requirements

An important question relates to whether the measured resting energy expenditure (mREE) is higher in persons with pressure ulcers. A meta-analysis of 5 trials, the mREE was 20.7 ± 0.8 in persons with a pressure ulcer ($n = 92$) vs. 23.7 ± 2.2 kcal/kg/day in the controls without a pressure ulcer ($n = 101$), suggesting a small but significant difference ($p = 0.0001$) [18]. However, 43 % of the subjects with a pressure ulcer had a spinal cord injury, perhaps accounting for the difference.

In another study of 29 older hospitalized persons with a pressure ulcer, the measured resting metabolic rate did not differ from controls and did not vary by ulcer size or severity [19]. The data suggest that a pressure ulcer may be associated with an increase in energy requirement, but the magnitude is small. Both of these trials confirmed an estimated daily caloric requirement of 25–30 kcal/kg using the Harris–Benedict equation in Table 8.1.

Various formulas, including the Harris–Benedict equation, can be used to predict caloric requirements, but controversy exists over accuracy in obese or severely undernourished individuals [20]. Other formulas have been adjusted for severely stressed hospitalized subjects [21]. The use of prediction formulas achieve almost the same results for caloric requirements as bedside clinical estimates.

Generally accepted clinical estimates of caloric requirements range from 25 kcal/kg/day for sedentary adults up to 40 kcal/kg/day for stressed adults. Stress generally includes persons with burns, pressure ulcers, cancer, infections, and other similar conditions. In general, caloric requirements can be met at 30–35 kcal/kg/day for elderly patients under moderate stress.

Protein Intake

Greater healing of pressure ulcers has been reported with a higher protein intake irrespective of positive nitrogen balance. In a small study of 12 enterally fed patients with pressure ulcers, the group who received 1.8 g/kg of protein had a 73 % improvement in pressure ulcer surface area compared to a 42 % improvement in surface area in the group receiving 1.2 g/kg of protein, despite the fact that the group that received the higher protein level began the study with larger surface area pressure ulcers (22.6 cm^2 vs. 9.1 cm^2). None of the patients in the high protein group and four

Table 8.1 Nutritional therapy for pressure ulcers		
Estimated caloric intake	30–35 Kcal/kg/day
Estimated protein intake	1.2–1.5 g/kg/day
Specific amino acids	Slight, if any, benefit
Supertherapeutic vitamin C	No demonstrated benefit
Supertherapeutic zinc	No demonstrated benefit

patients in the very high protein group had complete healing of their ulcer (relative risk of healing of 0.11, 95 % CI 0.01–1.70) [22].

The recommended daily intake of protein in adults is 0.8 g/kg/day, which is adequate for 97 % of the normal population consuming an adequate energy intake. Yet half of chronically ill elderly persons cannot maintain nitrogen balance at this level [23].

Studies in critically ill adults have shown that a protein intake of 1.2 g/kg/day of normally hydrated weight or 1.0 g/kg/day of resuscitated weight was more effective than a lower protein intake in achieving complete protein sparing in persons with severe systemic inflammatory response. However, further protein sparing cannot be demonstrated at protein intakes greater than 1.5 g/kg/day [24, 25]. The optimum daily protein intake for patients with pressure ulcers has not been defined, but may lie between 1.2 and 1.5 g/kg/day, based on the data from these and other studies. Increasing protein intake beyond 1.5 g/kg/day may not increase protein synthesis and may cause dehydration [26].

Specific Amino Acids

The association of wound healing with protein intake has led to investigation of specific amino acids in healing of pressure ulcers. Leucine seems to be important in severely ill patients. Glutamine is essential for the immune system function, but supplemental glutamine has not been shown to have noticeable effects on wound healing [27]. Arginine enhances wound collagen deposition in healthy volunteers [28, 29] but has not been effective in producing higher rates of complete healing in pressure ulcers. No trial in wound healing has demonstrated an effect of using concentrated supplements of branched-chain amino acid formulations [30].

In a trial of 26 nursing home residents with one or more pressure ulcers, subjects were randomized to receive 17 g of arginine or an oral supplement containing 0 g of arginine for 4 weeks. Although there were increases in arginine levels, no difference in immune function or pressure ulcer healing was observed [31].

Sixteen inpatients with stage 2–4 pressure ulcers were randomized to a standard hospital diet compared to a standard diet plus two high-protein/energy supplements or a standard diet plus two high-protein/energy supplements containing 9 g of arginine, 500 mg of vitamin C, and 30 mg of zinc for 3 weeks. Pressure Ulcer Scale for Healing tool scores improved in both the control and arginine/vitamin C/zinc groups but not in the protein/energy supplemented group. The major improvement in PUSH score was in the arginine/vitamin C/zinc group. The groups were not similar at baseline, and no changes in biochemical markers, oral dietary intake, or body weight were observed in any group [32].

In a study of 23 participants with 31 non-healing wounds, supplemental arginine 4.5 g was compared to supplemental arginine 9 g, and healing evaluated over 3 weeks. Most of the pressure ulcers were stage 2 (74 %) or stage 3 (19 %), with 7 % stage 4. No difference in healing rates between the two treatment groups were observed, suggesting no dose–response effect for arginine [33].

Vitamins and Minerals

The deficiency of several vitamins has significant effects on wound healing. However, supplementation of vitamins to accelerate wound healing is controversial. Vitamin C is essential for wound healing and, impaired wound healing has been observed in clinical scurvy. However, clinically impaired wound healing requires 6 months of a ascorbate-free diet [34]. In animals who are vitamin C deficient, wound healing is abnormal at 7 days but completely normal at 14 days [35].

Although nutritionally essential, there is no evidence of acceleration of wound healing by vitamin C supplementation in patients who are not vitamin C deficient [36]. The recommended daily allowance of vitamin C is 60 mg. This RDA is easily achieved from dietary sources that include citrus fruits, green vegetables, peppers, tomatoes, and potatoes. Supertherapeutic doses of vitamin C has not been shown to accelerate wound healing [37].

In a multicenter, blinded trial, 88 patients with pressure ulcers were randomized to either 10 mg or 500 mg twice daily of vitamin C. The wound closure rate, relative healing rate, and wound improvement score were not different between groups [38]. An earlier trial in acute surgical patients with pressure ulcers found an 84 % mean reduction in surface area at 1 month in patients treated with large doses of vitamin C compared to a reduction in surface area of 43 % in the control group ($p < 0.005$). Complete healing of pressure ulcers occurred in six patients in the vitamin C group versus three patients in the placebo group. The relative risk for complete healing with supplemental vitamin C was not different. (2.0, 95 % CI 0.68–5.85) [39].

Vitamin A deficiency results in delayed wound healing and increased susceptibility to infection [40]. Vitamin A has been shown to be effective in counteracting delayed healing in patients on corticosteroids [41]. Vitamin E deficiency does not appear to play an active role in wound healing [42].

Zinc was first implicated in delayed wound healing in 1967 [43]. No study has shown improved wound healing in patients supplemented with zinc who were not zinc deficient [44, 45]. In a small study of patients with pressure ulcers ($n = 10$), no effect on ulcer healing was seen at 12 weeks in zinc supplemented versus non-zinc supplemented patients [46]. Zinc levels have not been associated with development of pressure ulcers in patients with femoral neck fractures [47]. High serum zinc levels may inhibit healing, impair phagocytosis, and interfere with copper metabolism [48–50]. The recommended daily allowance for zinc is 12–15 mg, but most elderly persons' intake is 7–11 mg of zinc/day [51], chiefly from meats and cereal.

Nutritional Intervention Studies

Clinical trials have examined dietary interventions in the healing pressure ulcers. In 48 patients with stage 2 through 4 pressure ulcers who were being fed enterally, undernutrition was defined as a serum albumin below 35 g/L or body weight more than 10 % below the midpoint of the age-specific weight range. Total truncal pressure ulcer surface area showed more decrease (-4.2 cm^2 vs. -2.1 cm^2) in surface area in patients fed with the enteral formula containing 24 % protein compared to a formula containing 14 % protein. However, changes in body weight or in biochemical parameters of nutritional status did not differ between groups. The study was limited by a small sample size (only 28 patients completed the study), nonrandom assignment to treatment groups, confounding effects of air-fluidized beds, and the use of two different feeding routes [52].

In a study of enteral tube feedings in a long-term care setting, 49 patients were followed for 3 months [53]. Patients received 1.6 times basal energy expenditure daily, 1.4 g of protein/kg/day, and 85 % or more of their total recommended daily allowance. At the end of 3 months, there was no difference in number or healing of pressure ulcers.

A concentrated, fortified, collagen protein hydrolysate supplement was evaluated in 44 subjects with 75 pressure ulcers and compared to 27 subjects with 33 pressure ulcers who received a noncaloric control. At 8 weeks there was a small but statistically significant difference in the Pressure Ulcer Scale for Healing score (3.55 intervention vs. 3.22 control) [54]. The randomization process did not produce equal group size, and the number and severity of the pressure ulcers at baseline was not balanced between groups, potentially biasing the study.

In a long-term care setting, 93 tube-fed residents with a wound were compared to 57 tube-fed residents without a wound. Persons with a wound were started on an enteral tube feeding formula containing 1.25 g/protein/day, and persons without a wound were started on an enteral tube feeding formula containing 1.0 g/protein/day. At admission, only 12 % of persons with a wound and 21 % of persons without a wound had normal prealbumin levels. Over a mean follow-up of about 1 month, the amount of protein in the feeding formula was maintained or increased based on serum prealbumin levels. The serum prealbumin level normalized or increased by 8 points in 42 % of persons with a wound and in 46 % of persons without a wound. However, there was no correlation between persons who improved their serum prealbumin and those who did not based on protein intake. There was also no correlation observed between the PUSH score and improvement in serum prealbumin [55]. These data suggest that increasing protein intake, in some cases to greater than 2 g/protein/day, is not associated with greater healing of pressure ulcers. It also indicates that serum prealbumin is a poor marker of nutritional status.

Forty-three non-malnourished subjects with stage 3 or 4 pressure ulcer were evaluated in a multisite, randomized, controlled, double-blind trial. Subjects were screened to exclude malnutrition, defined as a body mass index less than 18.5 kg/m^2 for those younger than 70 years or 21 kg/m^2 for those older than 70 years. Other exclusion criteria were severe medical conditions, life expectancy shorter than 6 months, receiving palliative care, use of corticosteroids, and/or dietary restrictions such as a protein-restricted diet. Subjects were offered 200 mL of a high energy supplement enriched with arginine, antioxidants, and other micronutrients (not specified) three times daily for a maximum of 8 weeks or a non-caloric placebo, similar in taste and appearance, over the same timeframe. In the supplemented group, the mean change in wound size was 0.26 cm^2/day compared to 0.14 cm^2/day in the control group over the first 3 weeks. By 8 weeks, the mean healing rate in the supplemented group was similar to the control group (0.16 cm²/day vs. 0.15 cm²/day, respectively). In this population screened to exclude undernutrition, complete healing was observed in 6 ulcers in the supplemented group, compared to 5 ulcers in the control group by 8 weeks. No change was observed in body mass index [56].

Twenty-eight subjects older than 65 years with a stage 3–4 pressure ulcer which was present for less than 1 month were randomized to receive a standard hospital diet with no supplement ($N=15$) or a standard hospital diet plus a supplement containing 500 kcal with 34 g protein, 6 g arginine, 500 mg vitamin C, and 18 mg zinc ($N=13$). Nine subjects who were tube fed in the treatment group (69 %) received a formula containing 1,000 kcal, 55 g protein (20 %), 8 g arginine, 380 mg vitamin C, and 20 mg zinc. Nine subjects who were tube fed in the control group (60 %) received an enteral formula containing 16 % protein. All subjects were adjusted to a target of 30 Kcal/kg/day. After 12 weeks, complete pressure ulcer healing was documented for only one person in the treatment group. The PUSH score between groups was different only at week 12. The was no difference in ulcer area measured in square millimeters at any time point. The percentage of decrease in pressure ulcer area in the treatment group was greater compared to the control group at week 8 and 12. No nutritional parameter was different between groups except for the treatment group having a higher zinc level. Surprisingly, reaching a target of 30 kcal/kg/day did not affect wound healing, and no benefit from increased protein intake or independent effect of arginine or zinc was observed. These findings call into question empirically derived recommendations. In addition, no effect on wound healing measured by change in PUSH score or change in ulcer area was observed despite an increase in energy intake and protein intake over a 12 week period (controls 4.6 kcal/kg/day vs. treatment 3.1 kcal/kg/day). This data suggest that a specific nutritional formula may produce small benefits in improving pressure ulcer size. However, no specific supplemental nutritional component could account for the variation [57].

Nutrition and Prevention of Pressure Ulcers

Increasing knowledge of the complexity of wound healing has led to hypothesis that providing hypercaloric feeding in the form of nutritional supplements to patients at risk for undernutrition might lead to reversal of undernutrition and the prevention of pressure ulcers. Despite the observed epidemiological association, results of trials of nutritional intervention in prevention of pressure ulcers has been disappointing.

Controversy exists about the ability of nutritional support to reduce complications or improve wound healing [58]. Although correction of poor nutrition is part of total patient care and should be addressed in each patient, only one nutritional intervention has shown effectiveness in prevention of pressure ulcers in published studies [59].

In that trial, 672 persons older than 65 years, in the acute phase of a critical illness, received 2 oral supplements per day in addition to the standard hospital diet compared to a group receiving a standard hospital diet alone. After 15 days of follow-up, the incidence of pressure ulcers (stages 1–4) was 40 % in the nutritional intervention group compared to 48 % in the control group (relative risk 0.83, 95 % CI 0.70–0.99). The groups were randomized by ward, rather than individually, and were not comparable at baseline, with the nutritional intervention group having a lower initial pressure ulcer risk [60].

In another trial, oral nutrition supplements were given to 33 % of one group compared to 87 % of another group. There was no difference in pressure ulcer incidence (26 % vs. 20 %), pressure ulcer prevalence at discharge (15 % vs. 10 %), mortality (16 % vs. 14 %), length of stay (17.3 days vs. 17.4 days), or nosocomial infections (26 % vs. 19 %) between groups [61]. This observational study of hospitalized, critically ill patients given nutritional supplements suggests no effect on pressure ulcer incidence.

The effect of overnight supplemental enteral feeding in patients with a fracture of the hip and a high pressure ulcer risk score has been evaluated. Of the 62 patients randomized for enteral feeding, only 25 tolerated their tube for more than 1 week, and only 16 tolerated their tube for 2 weeks. No difference was found for the development of a pressure ulcer, total serum protein, serum albumin, or the severity of pressure sores after 1 and 2 weeks. Comparison of the actually tube-fed group ($n=25$ at 1 week, $n=16$ at 2 weeks) and the control group showed two to three times higher protein and energy intake ($p<0.0001$) and a significantly higher total serum protein and serum albumin after 1 and 2 weeks in the actually tube-fed group (all $p<0.001$). However, the development of pressure ulcers and severity were not significantly influenced in the per protocol tube-fed group [62]. It is possible that the lack of effect on supplemental enteral feeding was due to poor tolerance of the feedings.

In another observational trial of nursing home residents referred to the hospital for a percutaneous endoscopic gastroscopy (PEG), persons who did not have a pressure ulcer at the time of PEG insertion ($n=1,124$) were 2.3 times more likely to develop a new pressure ulcer (95 % CI, 2.0–2.7). In those subjects who had a pressure ulcer at the time of PEG insertion ($n=452$), the ulcer was 30 % less likely to heal (odds ratio 0.70, 95 % CI, 0.55–0.89) compared to controls [63]. There are several possibilities for this unexpected observation, but the data suggest that incidence or healing of pressure ulcers is independent of enteral tube feeding.

In 59 older hospitalized patients after a hip fracture, subjects were randomized to receive either a standard hospital diet alone or standard hospital diet with one additional oral nutrition supplement daily. The number of pressure ulcers during hospitalization, during rehabilitation, and after 6 months was not different between groups [64].

In 103 hospitalized patients with a hip fracture, the intervention group received one supplement daily in addition to the standard hospital diet, and the control group received the standard hospital diet plus a noncaloric water-based placebo. The incidence of stage 1–2 pressure ulcers at 2 weeks was not different between groups (55 % versus 59 % control). At 28 days, the incidence of stage 2 or higher pressure ulcer was not different in the nutritional intervention group (18 % vs. 28 %) [65].

In a study of survival among residents in long-term care with severe cognitive impairment, 135 residents were followed for 24 months [66]. The reasons for the placement of a feeding tube included the presence of a pressure ulcer. Having a feeding tube was not associated with increased survival; in fact the risk was slightly increased (OR 1.09). There was no apparent effect of the prevalence of pressure ulcers in this group of enterally fed persons.

These trials are limited by small sample size, short durations, and methodological flaws. Although limited in the power to detect important clinical differences between groups, the studies to date have not suggested an effect of nutritional interventions on the prevention of pressure ulcers.

Factors Contributing to the Nutritional Paradox

Historically, hypoalbuminemia has been a hallmark of the pediatric syndrome of kwasiokor. Until recently, serum albumin and other acute phase reactants (e.g., pre-albumin) have been used to define undernutrition. Increasingly, serum albumin and prealbumin are now recognized as acute phase reactants [67]. Physiological stress (such as surgical operations), cortisol excess, and hypermetabolic states reduce serum albumin even in the presence of adequate protein intake. Serum albumin has poor correlation with objective measures of nutritional status, suggesting that serum albumin is measuring a nonnutritional construct [68].

Inflammatory cytokines are well known for producing decreases in albumin, pre-albumin, cholesterol, transferrin, and hemoglobin. The use of these acute-phase reactants as nutritional markers could lead to overdiagnosis of undernutrition [69]. Poor nutritional status defined by these variables may indicate poor health rather than poor nutrient intake [70].

In chronic disease, cachexia is recognized as a major cause of weight loss [71]. Cachexia is a complex metabolic syndrome associated with underlying illness and characterized by loss of muscle with or without loss of fat mass. Anorexia, inflammation, insulin resistance, and increased muscle protein breakdown are frequently associated with cachexia. Moreover, cachexia is distinct from starvation, age-related loss of muscle mass, or primary medical illnesses and is associated with increased mortality [72]. Cachexia is associated with cancer [73], end-stage renal disease [74], congestive heart failure [75], AIDS [76], and rheumatoid arthritis [77], among others.

These evolving concepts have led to proposals for redefinition of nutritional constructs. Current understanding of undernutrition defines three categories: pure chronic starvation without inflammation, acute disease or major injury with inflammation, and chronic diseases or conditions that impose sustained inflammation of a mild to moderate degree [78]. One of the chief distinguishing factors is that starvation without inflammation is amenable to hypercaloric feeding in all but the terminally undernourished patients, while acute and chronic inflammatory conditions are remarkably resistant to hypercaloric feeding [79, 80].

Cytokine-mediated anorexia and weight loss are common in the population that develop pressure ulcers. A preliminary study of cytokines in patients with pressure ulcers indicates that serum interleukin-6 was not different between subjects with a pressure ulcer ($N=23$) and those without pressure ulcers ($N=17$) within 5 days of acute hospitalization. Serum interleukin-1β is elevated in patients with pressure ulcers [81].

Elevated cytokines, particularly interleukin-1α, interleukin-1β, and interleukin-6, have been observed in persons with pressure ulcers. Whether these levels change with healing, or are predictive of healing are not known. These cytokines are known to also increase in severe undernutrition. Existing studies are not clear whether the elevation is due to the presence of a pressure ulcer or due to underlying severe undernutrition. Alternatively, the elevation of cytokine levels may be a common pathway for both conditions.

Circulating serum levels of interleukin-6, interleukin-2, and interleukin-2R are higher in spinal cord injured patients compared to normal controls and highest in subjects with pressure ulcers ($N=19$). The highest concentration of cytokines were in subjects with the slowest healing pressure ulcers [82]. Among spinal injury patients with pressure ulcers ($N=19$), interleukin-6 blood levels were increased, but interleukin-1 and tumor necrosis factor were not elevated [83]. Levels of interleukin-1α are elevated in chronic wounds but low in acute wound fluid [84].

Cytokines regulate appetite directly through the central feeding drive. Interleukin-1 concentrations are elevated in elderly patients with severe undernutrition of unknown etiology [85]. Levels of interleukin-1β and interleukin-6 are increased in elderly persons without evidence of infection or cancer [86]. Interleukin-1, interleukin-6, tumor necrosis factor, interferon-γ, leukemia inhibitory factor (D-factor), and prostaglandin E_2 have all been implicated in cancer-induced severe undernutrition [87, 88]. Leptin, a central regulator of food intake and body fat mass, increases under the stress of hip operations [89], but is low in undernourished men [90].

The lack of effect of hypercaloric feeding in pressure ulcers may reflect that the underlying pathophysiology is cytokine-induced cachexia rather than simple starvation.

Conclusions

Nutritional support is a cornerstone of clinical care and should be provided to all persons, including persons with pressure ulcers, consistent with medical goals and patient wishes. Whether nutrition can improve the outcome of pressure ulcers remains disputable.

Energy requirements for persons with pressure ulcers are estimated empirically between 25 and 30 kcal/kg/day and has been confirmed in studies using nutritional formulas such as the Harris–Benedict equation. The optimum amount of protein intake is not known but likely lies between 1.2 and 1.5 g/kg/day. Higher protein intakes may be harmful and have not been associated with higher rates of healing. Supplemental amino acids and supertherapeutic supplements of vitamins and minerals have not been shown to have much effect on the healing of pressure ulcers.

Clinical nutritional intervention trials suffer from small sample sizes and poor methodological design, but in general have not shown exceptional benefit in improving complete healing of pressure ulcers. Improvements in nutritional markers, such as serum protein concentrations, nitrogen balance, and weight gain, have not usually been accompanied by clinical wound healing [91, 92].

Nutritional therapy will improve starvation due to lack of food, but cachexia associated with inflammatory conditions has been remarkably resistant to hypercaloric feeding [93]. Additional interventions besides providing adequate nutrients may be required in persons with cachexia [94].

References

1. Young ME. Malnutrition and wound healing. Heart Lung. 1988;17:60–7.
2. Dempsey DT, Mullen JL, Buzby GP. The link between nutritional status and clinical outcome: can nutritional intervention modify it? Am J Clin Nutr. 1988;47(2 Suppl):352–6.
3. Detsky AS, Baker JP, O'Rourke K, et al. Predicting nutrition-associated complications for patients undergoing gastrointestinal surgery. JPEN J Parenter Enteral Nutr. 1987;11:440–6.
4. Casey J, Flinn WR, Yao JST, et al. Correlation of immune and nutritional status with wound complications in patients undergoing vascular operations. Surgery. 1983;93:822–7.
5. Takeda T, Koyama T, Izawa Y, et al. Effects of malnutrition on development of experimental pressure sores. J Dermatol. 1992;19:602–9.
6. Bullough WS, Eisa EA. The effects of a graded series of restricted diets on epidermal mitotic activity in the mouse. Br J Cancer. 1950;4:321–8.
7. Reiser KM. Nonenzymatic glycations and enzymatic crosslinking in a model of wound healing. J Ger Dermotol. 1993;1:90–9.
8. Thompson W, Ravdin IS, Frank IL. The effect of hypoproteinemic on wound disruption. Arch Surg. 1938;26:500.
9. Levenson SM. Some challenging wound healing problems for clinicians and basic scientists. In: Dunphy JE, Van Winkle Jr W, editors. Repair and regeneration: the scientific basis for surgical practice. New York, NY: McGraw-Hill; 1969. p. 309–37.
10. Barbul A, Purtill WA. Nutrition in wound healing. Clin Dermatol. 1994;12:133–40.
11. Felcher A, Schwartz J, Schechter C, et al. Wound healing in normal and analbuminemic rates. J Surg Res. 1987;43:546.
12. Thomas DR, Goode PS, Tarquine PH, Allman R. Hospital acquired pressure ulcers and risk of death. J Am Geriatr Soc. 1996;44:1435–40.
13. Pinchcofsky-Devin GD, Kaminski Jr MV. Correlation of pressure sores and nutritional status. J Am Geriatr Soc. 1986;34:435–40.
14. Shahin ES, Meijers JM, Schols JM, Tannen A, Halfens RJ, Dassen T. The relationship between malnutrition parameters and pressure ulcers in hospitals and nursing homes. Nutrition. 2010;26(9):886–9.
15. Bergstrom N, Braden B. A prospective study of pressure sore risk among institutionalized elderly. J Am Geriatr Soc. 1992;40:747–58.
16. Thomas DR. Nutritional assessment in long term care. Nutr Clin Pract. 2008;23:383–7.
17. Koretz RL, Avenell A, Lipman TO, Braunschweig CL, Milne AC. Does enteral nutrition affect clinical outcome? A systematic review of the randomized trials. Am J Gastroenterol. 2007;102(2):412–29.

18. Cereda E, Klersy C, Rondanelli M, Caccialanza R. Energy balance in patients with pressure ulcers: a systematic review and meta-analysis of observational studies. J Am Diet Assoc. 2011;111(12):1868–76.
19. Dambach B, Salle A, Marteau C, Mouzet JB, Ghali A, Favreau AM, Berrut G, Ritz P. Energy requirements are not greater in elderly patients suffering from pressure ulcers. J Am Geriatr Soc. 2005;53(3):478–82.
20. Choban PS, Burge JC, Flanobaum L. Nutrition support of obese hospitalized patients. Nutr Clin Pract. 1997;12:149–54.
21. Ireton-Jones CS. Evaluation of energy expenditures in obese patients. Nutr Clin Pract. 1989;4:127–9.
22. Chernoff RS, Milton KY, Lipschitz DA. The effect of a very high-protein liquid formula on decubitus ulcer healing in long-term tube-fed institutionalized patients. J Am Diet Assoc. 1990;90:A–130.
23. Gersovitz M, Motil K, Munro HN, Scrimshaw NS. Human protein requirements: assessment of the adequacy of the current recommended dietary allowance for dietary protein in elderly men and women. Am J Clin Nutr. 1982;35:6–14.
24. Wolfe RR, et al. Response of protein and urea kinetics in burn patients to different levels of protein intake. Ann Surg. 1983;197:163–71.
25. Ishibashi N, Plank LD, Sando K, et al. Optimal protein requirements during the first 2 weeks after the onset of critical illness. Crit Care Med. 1998;26:1529–35.
26. Long CL, Nelson KM, Akin Jr JM, Geiger JW, Merrick HW, Blakemore WZ. A physiologic bases for the provision of fuel mixtures in normal and stressed patients. J Trauma. 1990;30:1077–86.
27. McCauley R, Platell C, Hall J, McCulloch R. Effects of glutamine on colonic strength anastomosis in the rat. JPEN J Parenter Enteral Nutr. 1991;116:821.
28. Barbul A, Lazarous S, Efron DT, et al. Arginine enhances wound healing in humans. Surgery. 1990;108:331–7.
29. Kirk SJ, Regan MC, Holt D, et al. Arginine stimulates wound healing and immune function in aged humans. Surgery. 1993;114:155.
30. McCauley C, Platell C, Hall J, McCullock R. Influence of branched chain amino acid solutions on wound healing. Aust N Z J Surg. 1990;60:471.
31. Langkamp-Henken B, Herrlinger-Garcia KA, Stechmiller JK, Nickerson-Troy JA, Lewis B, Moffatt L. Arginine supplementation is well tolerated but does not enhance mitogen-induced lymphocyte proliferation in elderly nursing home residents with pressure ulcers. JPEN J Parenter Enteral Nutr. 2000;24(5):280–7.
32. Desneves KJ, Todorovic BE, Cassar A, Crowe TC. Treatment with supplementary arginine, vitamin C and zinc in patients with pressure ulcers: a randomised controlled trial. Clin Nutr. 2005;24:979–87.
33. Leigh B, Desneves K, Rafferty J, Pearce L, King S, Woodward MC, Brown D, Martin R, Crowe TC. The effect of different doses of an arginine-containing supplement on the healing of pressure ulcers. J Wound Care. 2012;21(3):150–6.
34. Crandon JH, Lind CC, Dill DB. Experimental human scurvy. N Engl J Med. 1940;223:353.
35. Levenson SM, Upjohn HL, Preston JA, et al. Effect of thermal burns on wound healing. Ann Surg. 1957;146:357–68.
36. Rackett SC, Rothe MJ, Grant-Kels JM. Diet and dermatology. The role of dietary manipulation in the prevention and treatment of cutaneous disorders. J Am Acad Dermatol. 1993;29:447–61.
37. Vilter RW. Nutritional aspects of ascorbic acid: uses and abuses. West J Med. 1980;133:485.
38. ter Riet G, Kessels AG, Knipschild PG. Randomized clinical trial of ascorbic acid in the treatment of pressure ulcers. J Clin Epidemiol. 1995;48:1453–60.
39. Taylor TV, Rimmer S, Day B, Butcher J, Dymock IW. Ascorbic acid supplementation in the treatment of pressure sores. Lancet. 1974;2:544–6.
40. Hunt TK. Vitamin A, and wound healing. J Am Acad Dermatol. 1986;15:817–21.
41. Ehrlich HP, Hunt TK. Effects of cortisone and vitamin A on wound healing. Ann Surg. 1968;167:324.

42. Waldorf H, Fewkes J. Wound healing. Adv Dermatol. 1995;10:77–96.
43. Pories WJ, Henzel WH, Rob CG, et al. Acceleration of healing with zinc sulfate. Ann Surg. 1967;165:423.
44. Hallbrook T, Lanner E. Serum zinc and healing of leg ulcers. Lancet. 1972;2:780.
45. Sandstead SH, Henrikson LK, Greger JL, et al. Zinc nutriture in the elderly in relation to taste acuity, immune response, and wound healing. Am J Clin Nutr. 1982;36(Supp):1046.
46. Norris JR, Reynolds RE. The effect of oral zinc sulfate therapy on decubitus ulcers. J Am Geriatr Soc. 1971;19:793.
47. Goode HF, Burns E, Walker BE. Vitamin C depletion and pressure ulcers in elderly patients with femoral neck fracture. BMJ. 1992;305:925–7.
48. Goode P, Allman R. The prevention and management of pressure ulcers. Med Clin N Am. 1989;73:1511–24.
49. Rasad AS. Discovery of human zinc deficiency and studies in an experimental human model. Am J Clin Nutr. 1991;53:403–12.
50. Reed BR, Clark RAF. Cutaneous tissue repair: practical implications of current knowledge: II. J Am Acad Dermatol. 1985;13:919–41.
51. Gregger JL. Potential for trace mineral deficiencies and toxicities in the elderly. In: Bales CW, editor. Mineral homeostasis in the elderly. New York, NY: Dekker; 1989. p. 171–200.
52. Breslow RA, Hallfrisch J, Guy DG, et al. The importance of dietary protein in healing pressure ulcers. J Am Geriatr Soc. 1993;41:357–62.
53. Henderson CT, Trumbore LS, Mobarhan S, et al. Prolonged tube feeding in long-term care: nutritional status and clinical outcomes. J Am Coll Clin Nutr. 1992;11:309.
54. Lee SK, Posthauer ME, Dorner B, Redovian V, Maloney MJ. Pressure ulcer healing with a concentrated, fortified, collagen protein hydrolysate supplement: a randomized controlled trial. Adv Skin Wound Care. 2006;19(2):92–6.
55. Pompeo M. Misconceptions about protein requirements for wound healing: results of a prospective study. Ostomy Wound Manage. 2007;53(8):30–2, 34, 36–38.
56. van Anholt RD, Sobotka L, Meijer EP, Heyman H, Groen HW, Topinkova E, van Leen M, Schols JM. Specific nutritional support accelerates pressure ulcer healing and reduces wound care intensity in non-malnourished patients. Nutrition. 2010;26(9):867–72.
57. Cereda E, Gini A, Pedrolli C, Vanotti A. Disease-specific, versus standard, nutritional support for the treatment of pressure ulcers in institutionalized older adults: a randomized controlled trial. J Am Geriatr Soc. 2009;57(8):1395–402.
58. Albina JE. Nutrition and wound healing. JPEN J Parenter Enteral Nutr. 1994;18:367–76.
59. Thomas DR. The role of nutrition in prevention and healing of pressure ulcers. Clin Geriatr Med. 1997;13:497–511.
60. Bourdel-Marchasson I, Barateau M, Rondeau V, Dequae-Merchadou L, Salles-Montaudon N, Emeriau JP, Manciet G, Dartigues JF. A multi-center trial of the effects of oral nutritional supplementation in critically ill older inpatients. GAGE Group. Groupe Aquitain Geriatrique d'Evaluation. Nutrition. 2000;16(1):1–5.
61. Bourdel-Marchasson I, Barateau M, Sourgen C, et al. Prospective audits of quality of PEM recognition and nutritional support in critically ill elderly patients. Clin Nutr. 1999;18:233–40.
62. Hartgrink HH, Wille J, Konig P, et al. Pressure sores and tube feeding in patients with a fracture of the hip: a randomized clinical trial. Clin Nutr. 1998;17:287–92.
63. Teno JM, Gozalo P, Mitchell SL, Kuo S, Fulton AT, Mor V. Feeding tubes and the prevention or healing of pressure ulcers. Arch Intern Med. 2012;172(9):697–701.
64. Delmi M, Rapin CH, Bengoa JM, Delmas PD, Vasey H, Bonjour JP. Dietary supplementation in elderly patients with fractured neck of the femur. Lancet. 1990;335(8696):1013–6.
65. Houwing R, Rozendaal M, Wouters-Wesseling W, Beulens JWJ, Buskens E, Haalboom J. A randomised, double-blind assessment of the effect of nutritional supplementation on the prevention of pressure ulcers in hip-fracture patients. Clin Nutr. 2003;22(4):401–5.
66. Mitchell SL, Kiely DK, Lipsitz LA. The risk factors and impact on survival of feeding tube placement in nursing home residents with severe cognitive impairment. Arch Intern Med. 1997;157:327–32.

67. Friedman FJ, Campbell AJ. Caradoc-Davies. Hypoalbuminemia in the elderly is due to disease not malnutrition. Clin Exp Gerontol. 1985;7:191–203.
68. Covinsky KE, Covinsky MH, Palmer RM, Sehgal AR. Serum albumin concentration and clinical assessments of nutritional status in hospitalized older people: different sides of different coins? J Am Geriatr Soc. 2002;50:631–7.
69. Rosenthal AJ, Sanders KM, McMurtry CT, Jacobs MA, Thompson DD, Gheorghiu D, Little KL, Adler RA. Is malnutrition overdiagnosed in older hospitalized patients? Association between the soluble interleukin-2 receptor and serum markers of malnutrition. J Gerontol A Biol Sci Med Sci. 1998;53:M81–6.
70. Thomas DR. Loss of skeletal muscle mass in aging: examining the relationship of starvation, sarcopenia and cachexia. Clin Nutr. 2007;26(4):389–99.
71. Thomas DR. Unintended weight loss in older adults. Aging Health. 2008;4(2):191–200.
72. Evans WJ, Morley JE, Argile's J, et al. Cachexia: a new definition. Clin Nutr. 2008;10:1–7.
73. Shike M, Russell DM, Detsky AS, Harrison JE, McNeill KG, Shepherd FA, et al. Changes in body composition in patients with small-cell cancer. The effect of total parenteral nutrition as an adjunct to chemotherapy. Ann Intern Med. 1984;101:303–9.
74. Mitch WE. Mechanisms causing loss of lean body mass in kedney disease. Am J Clin Nutr. 1998;67:359–66.
75. Toth MJ, Gottlieb SS, Goran MI, Fisher ML, Poehlman ET. Daily energy expenditure in free-living heart failure patients. Am J Physiol. 1997;272:469–75.
76. Kotler DP, Wang J, Pierson RN. Body composition studies in patients with the acquired immunodeficiency syndrome. Am J Clin Nutr. 1985;42:1255–65.
77. Roubenoff R, Roubenoff RA, Cannon JG, Kehayias JJ, Zhuang H, Dawson-Hughes B, et al. Rheumatoid cachexia: cytokine-driven hypermetalboism accompanying reduced body cell mass in chronic inflammation. J Clin Invest. 1994;93:2379–86.
78. Jensen G, et al. Adult starvation and disease-related malnutrition: a proposal for etiology-based diagnosis in the clinical practice setting from the international consensus guideline committee. JPEN J Parenter Enteral Nutr. 2010;34:156–9.
79. Souba WW. Drug therapy: nutritional support. N Engl J Med. 1997;336:41–8.
80. Atkinson S, Sieffert E, Bihari D. A prospective, randomized, double-blind, controlled clinical trial of enteral immunonutrition in the critically ill. Crit Care Med. 1998;26:1164–72.
81. Matsuyama N, Takano K, Mashiko T, Jimbo S, Shimetani N, Ohtani H. The possibility of acute inflammatory reaction affects the development of pressure ulcers in bedridden elderly patients. Rinsho Byori. 1999;47:1039–145.
82. Segal JL, Gonzales E, Yousefi S, Jamshidipour L, Brunnemann SR. Circulating levels of IL-2R, ICAM-1, and IL-6 in spinal cord injuries. Arch Phys Med Rehabil. 1997;78:44–7.
83. Bonnefoy M, Coulon L, Bienvenu J, Boisson RC, Rys L. Implication of cytokines in the aggravation of malnutrition and hypercatabolism in elderly patients with severe pressure sores. Age Ageing. 1995;24:37–42.
84. Barone EJ, Yager DR, Pozez AL, Olutoye OO, Crossland MC, Diegelmann RF, Cohen IK. Interleukin-1α and collagenase activity are elevated in chronic wounds. Plas Reconstr Surg. 1998;102:1023–7.
85. Liso Z, Tu JH, Small CB, Schnipper SM, Rosenstreich DL. Increased urine IL-1 levels in aging. Gerontology. 1993;39:19–27.
86. Cederholm T, Whetline B, Hollstrom K, et al. Enhanced generation of Interleukin 1β and 6 may contribute to the cachexia of chronic disease. Am J Clin Nutr. 1997;65:876–82.
87. Noguchi Y, Yoshikawa T, Marsumoto A, Svaninger G, Gelin J. Are cytokines possible mediators of cancer cachexia? Jpn J Surg. 1996;26:467–75.
88. Keiler U. Pathophysiology of cancer cachexia. Support Care Cancer. 1993;1:290–4.
89. Straton RJ, Dewit O, Crowe R, Jennings G, Viller RN, Elia M. Plasm leptin, energy intake and hunger following total hip replacement surgery. Clin Sci. 1997;93:113–7.
90. Cederholm T, Arter P, Palmviad J. Low circulation leptin level in protein-energy malnourished chronically ill elderly patients. J Intern Med. 1997;242:377–82.
91. Thomas DR. Distinguishing starvation from cachexia. Clin Geriatr Med. 2002;18:883–92.

92. Christou NV, Meakins JL, Gordon J, et al. The delayed hypersensitivity response and host resistance in surgical patients: 20 years later. Ann Surg. 1995;222:534–48.
93. Thomas DR. But is it malnutrition? J Am Med Dir Assoc. 2009;10(5):295–7.
94. Thomas DR. Anorexia: aetiology, epidemiology, and management in the older people. Drugs Aging. 2009;26:557–70.

Chapter 9
Assessment and Management of Wound Colonization and Infection in Pressure Ulcers

Gregory A. Compton

Abstract All chronic wounds are poly-microbial colonized. One aspect pressure ulcer assessment involves determining the degree of bacterial burden and distinguishing colonization from true infection. Heavy bacterial burden may delay healing of a pressure ulcer.

Systemic infection due to pressure ulceration is very uncommon. Bacteremia and sepsis due to a pressure ulcer is rare. Heavy bacterial colonization, often referred to as local infection, is more common in pressure ulcers with necrosis. The presence of heavy necrotic burden, significant exudate, and/or odor is often mistaken for true infection.

This chapter is designed to aid clinicians treating pressure ulcers with critical colonization or systemic infection. It will aid the learner to distinguish between true (systemic) infection and heavy bioburden and discuss the treatments for each condition. Local wound factors that delay healing, including the role of biofilms, will be addressed. Understanding the difference between critical wound bed colonization and true wound related infection is imperative to achieve best outcomes for wound patients.

Keywords Infection • Colonization • Biofilm • Debridement • Wound bed • Chronic wounds

Introduction

The epidemiology of true infection in pressure ulcers has not been extensively studied [1]. The point prevalence of pressure ulcers in long-term care, stage II or higher is between 3 % and 20 % in the USA [2, 3]. This variation is based on the case

G.A. Compton, M.D., C.M.D. (✉)
Geriatric Medicine and Palliative Care, Wound Care Consultant, Hospice Care of South Carolina, 2948 Seabrook Island Road, Johns Island, SC 29455, USA
e-mail: gacompton@comcast.net

D.R. Thomas and G.A. Compton (eds.), *Pressure Ulcers in the Aging Population: A Guide for Clinicians*, Aging Medicine 1, DOI 10.1007/978-1-62703-700-6_9, © Springer Science+Business Media New York 2014

Table 9.1 Infectious complications of pressure ulcers

Failure to heal due to heavy bacterial colonization
Periwound candida infections
Cellulitis
Osteomyelitis (if wound involves contiguous bone)
Necrotizing fasciitis

mix of residents and has not changed significantly over the past two decades. Pressure ulcers are common skin lesions but make up a very small proportion of soft tissue infections.

Pressure ulcers rarely cause cellulitis, deeper SSTI, and osteomyelitis. Skin lesions of all types were the source of bacteremia or fungemia in only 4 % of cases in a recent study [4]. Surgical wound-related bacteremia accounted for another 3 %. Sepsis due to pressure ulcers is rare accounting for less than 4 episodes of bacteremia per 10,000 hospital discharges [5]. A prospective study following 16 nursing home residents for 2,184 days found an infection incidence of 1.4 cases per 1,000 patient-ulcer days [6].

The infectious complications of pressure ulcers are listed in Table 9.1. Chronic wounds with significant necrotic burden were once thought to be a reservoir for nosocomial infection with antibiotic resistant bacteria [7]. More recent studies using standard swab culture in conjunction with bacterium-specific polymerase chain reaction (PCR) techniques reveal that chronic wounds harbor greater bacterial diversity than healthy skin, but overall the flora is not distinct from the normal human microbiome [8, 9]. Chronic wound microbiota arise from skin structures and adjacent orifices. In spite of the diverse colonizing flora in chronic wounds, beta-hemolytic streptococci account for the vast majority of skin and wound-related bacteremia [4].

Skin Biology and Resident Microbial Ecology

The fragile skin of the elderly is predisposed to cellulitis and other forms of skin infection. Typical colonizing skin organisms do not have the ability to degrade keratin and thereby penetrate intact epidermis. They usually gain access by some physical means such as wounds, trauma, excoriation, or surgical incision.

The epidermis is both an active and passive barrier to infection. The structurally intact epidermis is composed of tightly linked epithelial cells covered by a highly cross-linked keratin layer [10, 11]. The stratum corneum, the epidermal top layer, has been described as a "brick and mortar complex." The mortar is composed of intercellular lipids (free fatty acids, wax esters, sterols, and others) that also decrease transepidermal water loss [12]. The skin flora partially hydrolyzes the triglycerides, liberating fatty acids forming the "acid mantle" that is a prohibitive environment for invading microbes as well. The dead keratinocyte bound together by skin lipids is a dry layer that is hostile to bacteria. A summary of the defense mechanisms of intact skin is outlined in Table 9.2.

Table 9.2 Antibacterial defense mechanisms of intact skin

Airflow across skin
Dry skin surface
Intact stratum corneum
Acidic pH of surface
Continuous shedding of surface keratinocytes (squames)
High salt content (residual salt from evaporated sweat)
Antibacterial lipids from sebaceous glands and keratinocytes
Lysozyme produced by keratinocytes, sweat glands and resident staphylococci
Nitrate in sweat activated by cutaneous microbes at low pH
Antimicrobial peptides produced by keratinocytes
From Wilson [86]

Table 9.3 Principle normal skin flora

Organism	Location
Staph saprophyticus	All sites
S. epidermitidis	
Micrococcus spp.	
Staph. aureus	
Aerobic Cornebacterium	Intertriginous areas, including the toe webs
Anaerobic Cornebacterium	Sebaceous and hair follicles
Acinetobacter spp.	Axillae, perineum, and antecubital fossae
Yeast including Pityrosporum spp. and Malassezia furfur	Sebaceous areas of skin (e.g., scalp)

From Hartmann [16] and Blume [87]

The rapid turnover of the keratinocytes and the continuous desquamation of the stratum corneum shed bacteria [13]. Airflow over the skin surface also acts to prevent microbe-containing particles from easily attaching. Additionally, the skin produces a variety of unique defensive molecules called antimicrobial peptides that target microbial membranes [14–16].

Humans are colonized by complex communities of microorganisms that assemble into a beneficial resident microbiota [17]. In the human–microbe interaction, the microbe and host benefit without causing harm to the other. This symbiotic interaction is fundamentally important to human biology. Human skin and mucosa are colonized at birth and there is a lifelong codependent relationship with indigenous microbiota [18]. The common skin flora is listed in Table 9.3.

Wound Flora

Traditionally, wound flora was delineated by culture of the wound bed. It has long been recognized that all open wounds are colonized and the diversity of the microbiome evolves over time [19]. The exact role of various microbes that reside in a chronic wound bed is unknown [20].

Recent techniques in DNA sequencing, using the small subunit (16S) of the ribosomal RNA gene (rRNA), can identify bacteria in a wound sample. Through this precise method all the organisms in a wound tissue sample can be delineated without the inherent problems of the swab or tissue culture methods. This research methodology has shown us that both intact skin and chronic wounds have a much greater microbial diversity that once thought.

A more complete characterization of the microbial diversity of chronic wounds is needed to expand our understanding of how microbiology impacts chronic wound pathology and healing. It is evident when wound healing is delayed, but it is not known exactly how various bacterial colonizers interact. The host response to microbes present in a chronic wound bed depends on their number, the species, and organism virulence factors [21, 22]. Host factors such as microcirculation and nutrition are also important. Slow healing wounds disproportionately affect the frail elderly and diabetics. Future research will aid in understanding the host–wound–microbe interaction and guide specific therapies to speed healing in chronic wounds.

Controversies in the Definition of Wound Infection

The medical literature unfortunately uses the term "infection" interchangeably with heavy colonization. This imprecise lumping of two distinct wound states can lead to inadequate local wound care or overuse of systemic antimicrobials. A point prevalence study found that 6 % of 532 nursing home residents received treatment for infected pressure ulcers [23]. The study shows how a nonspecific definition of infection may lead to overtreatment.

The American Heritage Dictionary of the English Language defines infection as "Invasion by and multiplication of pathogenic microorganisms in a bodily part or tissue, which may produce subsequent tissue injury and progress to overt disease through a variety of cellular or toxic mechanisms" [24]. A widely accepted definition of "infection" in a chronic wound is: those wounds that contain a bacterial cell count of greater than 10^5 colonies per millimeter of tissue [25–27]. The only way to obtain this information is from a quantitate tissue biopsy with culture, a research technique. This definition has no meaning at the bedside and applying it broadly in the management of non-healing wounds is not useful at the bedside [28]. The wound clinician can only use reliable signs, symptoms, and laboratory studies to distinguish the local effects of excessive bacterial burden from systemic infection.

Colonization is defined as the establishment of replicating communities of microorganisms on or within a host [29]. Colonization is considered normal and is not believed to constitute an infection or to inhibit healing [30]. In some circumstances wound colonization by normal microbes has been shown to promote healing.

Heavy or critical colonization is a term that applies to chronic wounds and is a principal cause of delayed healing in pressure ulcers [31]. It is important in the management of chronic wounds to distinguish heavy bioburden that causes a local response from true infection with a systemic response. The labeling of a heavily colonized wound that exhibits delayed healing as "infected" or "locally infected" could result in the unnecessary use of systemic antibiotics that have no wound healing effect and may cause harm [32].

If microbes invade and replicate in viable tissue beyond the wound bed, systemic infection occurs [33]. Suspicion of systemic infection due to a pressure ulcer needs prompt re-evaluation, antimicrobial therapy, debridement if indicated, and/or hospitalization.

Approach to the Pressure Ulcer Patient

In the patient with a pressure ulcer, the clinician must evaluate the patient, the wound bed, and the periwound. Based on a full assessment, treatment of the cause of the wound and local care is initiated. Evaluation and treatment of a patient with a chronic wound is a complex process. The precepts of wound bed preparation are a useful guide to the care process (see Box 9.1) [34, 35].

Assessing the periwound for maceration, inflammatory changes, or infection is the first step in the bedside wound assessment. Next the wound bed is examined. The appearance and type of tissue at the base of the wound will provide information relating to specific local treatment and the presence of complications such as infection. Recognition and documentation of exposed tendons, bone, or hardware is important. Visible bone at the wound base may indicate osteomyelitis and cause delayed healing. The assessment (Chap. 6) and treatment of pressure ulcers (Chap. 7) is covered in detail in other sections of this volume.

Recognizing and Treating Critical Colonization

A well understood model for wound colonization is the burn. Burn injury destroys surface microbes except for Gram-positive organisms located in the depths of the sweat glands or hair follicles. Without prophylactic use of topical antimicrobial

---

Box 9.1 The Wound Bed Preparation Approach to Wound Care

Tier 1
- Treat cause of wound
- Treat medical comorbidities
- Apply local wound care

Tier 2
- Debridement of devitalized tissue
- Minimize bacterial burden
- Maintain wound moisture balance

Table 9.4 Signs and symptoms in true (systemic) pressure ulcer infection

Periwound erythema✓
Periwound induration✓
Local heat*
Otherwise unexplained fever >38 °C, hypotension or tachycardia✓
Otherwise unexplained delirium✓
New wound pain or significant increase in pain✓
Periwound fluctuance or crepitus may signify deep seated infection
Purulent exudate (must distinguish from liquefaction in a necrotic wound)✓
Purpura
Leukocytosis

Items used as criteria in to diagnose systemic infection from pressure ulcers are denoted with checkmarks: according to Practice Guideline by the Infectious Disease Society of America [33]

agents, the burn wound becomes colonized with large numbers of Gram-positive organisms within 48 h. Gram-negative bacteria appear from 3 to 21 days after the injury. Invasive fungal infection is seen later, if at all. This pattern of colonization is seen in pressure ulcers stage III or greater.

Healthy wounds that are progressing go through an orderly, three phase process of inflammation followed by granulation and epithelialization [36]. Pressure ulcers are defined as chronic or slow healing when there is failure of significant improvement in 4–8 weeks [37, 38]. These stalled wounds occur frequently in poor hosts with diabetes or ischemia and are characterized on the cellular level by prolonged inflammation, insufficient deposition of extracellular matrix (ECM), diminished neovascularization, and delayed epithelialization [39, 40].

From the microbes' standpoint a chronic wound is a hostile habitat with unstable and radically changing physical and chemical conditions such as cleansing, debridement, and dressing changes. There are periodic influxes of other competing and incompatible microbes from the patient's environment. The host's immune system and the intrinsic healing processes assault the wound microbiome [41, 42]. These are the reasons why systemic infections in pressure ulcers are so uncommon.

In the chronic wound there is interplay of probiotic and pathogenic microbes that define the balance between colonization and infection [26, 42]. When a wound is not in bacterial balance, it can fail to progress or deteriorate [43]. The bed of a heavily colonized wound may be accompanied by subtle signs of inflammation such as friable granulation tissue or excessive exudate [44] without systemic signs of classic infection [28, 31]. Wound signs of critical bacterial colonization are listed in Table 9.4 [45].

Healthy granulation tissue is pink in color and is an indicator of healing. Unhealthy granulation is pale or has a dark red in color and is friable and bleeds on contact. Excess granulation or hyper-granulation may also be associated with heavy colonization and non-healing wounds. These often respond to cautery with silver nitrate. Chronic wounds may be covered by white or yellow shiny fibrinous tissue, which may be associated with biofilm formation [45]. This tissue is avascular and harbors bacteria. Healing will proceed only when all necrotic tissue, slough, and "film-slough" are removed. The lack of proper wound healing is in part caused by inefficient eradication of pathogens that form biofilms. Biofilms are an emerging concept in critical wound colonization and poor healing.

The Importance of Biofilms in Chronic Wounds

Biofilms are characterized by aggregation of microbes that are no longer planktonic and dwell in a protective carbohydrate matrix. Bacteria producing biofilms have evolved to survive in adverse environments. The matrix allows them to form complex communities and adhere to the wound surface and physically blocks the phagocytic activity of neutrophils [26, 46]. Microbes in biofilms of chronic wounds and bone are resistant to invasion by the host defensive cells and topical or systemic antibiotics [47, 48]. The presence of the biofilm causes a mechanical impediment to wound healing by inhibiting keratinocyte migration [49].

The bacteria in biofilms have a different protein expression pattern from the same organisms when they are in the planktonic form. The organisms in the biofilm also cause a dysregulation of inflammatory proteins by affecting intracellular signaling [50]. The presence of microcolonies in biofilms and the lack of elimination by PMNs are the main causes of inefficient eradication by both antibiotic treatment and activity of the immune system [26]. Small clusters and cell groups are shed more frequently in planktonic form and thereby more likely to invade adjacent viable tissue of the blood stream [51]. The fact that bacteria in biofilms are not in their motile state is one of the reasons why cellulitis and bacteremia are uncommon complications of chronic wounds.

When and How to Culture Pressure Ulcers

Culturing a pressures ulcer, no matter the degree of necrotic burden, is often misleading [46]. The most common technique used to obtain a specimen is superficial swab culture. The results, even when superficial debris is removed from the wound bed and the specimen is promptly delivered to the laboratory, will yield superficial colonizing planktonic bacteria. In most cases a swab culture will be of no clinical value, even in the face of adjacent overt soft tissue infection.

Quantitate tissue biopsy wound culture is the most reliable method to define the degree of bioburden in a chronic wound. The technique involves the removal of devitalized tissue from the wound and sampling viable tissue in the base of the wound. A biopsy tissue sample (often using a 2 or 3 mm punch) and sent to the lab where the sample is weighed. The quantity of each bacterium identified is calculated per gram of tissue. This type of culture is cumbersome and almost never done outside of research studies, because it requires specialized handling in the microbiology lab and is costly. If there is no overt infection present, there is no additional clinical utility of the technique.

The semi-quantitate swab method has been touted as a way to gain valid data without the trauma of a biopsy. The necrotic tissue must be removed from the wound surface, and the viable tissue is swabbed in a back and forth Z-like fashion. The swab is inoculated into a medium and then streaked on to culture plates. Based on the growth on the culture plates, reliable estimates of colony counts can be made by the lab. Not all microbiology labs are set up to do this procedure, and it requires good communication between the practitioner and the lab. This method has also been criticized because of tendency to merely identify surface colonization.

An accepted alternative to the above methods is available, but not widely used. It is sometimes referred to as the Levine method [52]. The wound is cleaned and then a swab is pressed over a 1 cm area with enough pressure to express fluid from within wound tissue. The specimen is sent to the lab in a timely fashion for routine processing. The concept is to sample bacteria, if present, from viable tissue at the wound host interface, not from the wound surface or wound exudate. The results are semi-quantitative.

If an abscess cavity is opened direct sampling of the purulent material with gram stain and routine culture is of clinical value. If surgery is performed for suspected fasciitis, the tissue obtained should be sent for gram stain, aerobic and anaerobic cultures, as well as histology. If bone is curetted or removed, samples should be sent for separate culture and histology.

Another reason that swab wound cultures are not reliable is the presence and structure of the biofilm. It has become increasingly clear that cultures are an ineffective method for characterization of biofilm ecology. Standard wound culture techniques are designed to identify planktonic organisms that grow well in laboratory media. Thus results may reflect the growth of organisms that do not reflect the overall microbiome of a wound [51]. Because of the alginate matrix of biofilms encasing the microorganisms, specimens require special processing to break the carbohydrate bonds and release the encased microbes. This is not done in routine handling of wound culture specimens. There may be a day when routine PCR testing of wound flora is affordable [51, 53].

Identifying True Infection of Chronic Wounds

All chronic wounds are polymicrobial colonized [29]. Heavy bacterial loads may lead to delayed healing. Labeling the wound as infected without evidence of adjacent tissue invasion is misleading.

Infection in viable tissue beyond the wound bed can be diagnosed by a combination of the signs and symptoms listed in Table 9.5. A recent guideline lists criteria

Table 9.5 Wound signs of excessive bioburden	Delay in healing in spite of optimal local intervention and debridement
	Change in appearance of granulation tissue: pale or deep red
	Friable granulation tissue
	Hypergranulation
	Thin fibrinous coating or sheen
	Increase or thickening of exudate
	Deterioration in wound, enlarging, deepening or tunneling
	Wound odor not associated with excess necrotic burden
	See Lazarus et al. [45]

to establish the diagnosis of true wound infection as purulent discharge and four of the following: fever >38 °C; delirium; local warmth; redness, swelling, and increased pain [33]. In general increasing wound pain, surrounding cellulitis, and purulent exudate are the most signs reliable in identifying superficial or deep wound infection [54].

In a patient with a chronic wound presenting with systemic inflammatory response syndrome, pneumonia and urinary tact infections are much more common sources than wound-related infection. It is important to maintain a high index of suspicion for true wound infection particularly with a necrotic wound bed. Wound infection, when it occurs, is initiated from bacterial colonization of the wound base or tracts. Repeated debridement of necrotic tissue from chronic wounds is the best preventative measure. It is only when colonization is combined with other factors such as decreased vascular supply, intrinsic virulence of specific bacteria, and decreased host immunity that true infection occurs [55]. Deep cultures or quantitative biopsies of wound tissue are necessary to determine culpable organisms. But because of biofilms and the polymicrobial nature of wound colonization, the culture data may be misleading. In most instances, it is appropriate to treat true wound infections empirically with systemic antibiotics [56].

It is important to distinguish liquefaction in wounds from purulence. Heavy necrotic wound burden alone can cause both odor and thick exudate. Silver sulfadiazine cream when combined with exudate can produce a thick yellow exudate that can be confused with pus.

Dermatitis from adhesives, candidal infections, and cellulitis all can present on the periwound. Necrotizing fasciitis may first present as changes in surrounding skin. Proper dermatological diagnosis and treatment of adjacent skin findings are part of the wound care clinician's role.

Wound odor is not a reliable sign of infection. Wound odor must be distinguished from dressing odor by removal and proper disposal of the dressing material, cleansing the wound, and then assessing for wound odor. Necrotic wounds often have an unpleasant odor. Anaerobic organisms growing in necrotic tissue create odor by producing volatile fatty acids as an end product of anaerobic metabolism [57]. Topical metronidazole in conjunction with debridement is effective in eliminating wound odor through eradication of anaerobic bacteria.

Inflammation on the Periwound

Periwound erythema has a wide differential, including contact dermatitis, fungal infections, and cellulitis. Satellite lesions may be a clue to a candida infection adjacent to the wound. Diaper dermatitis can occur in incontinent patients and result in maceration and periwound redness. Skin preparations, tactifiers, and dressing adhesives commonly cause periwound contact dermatitis mimicking cellulitis.

Periwound infection can occur from overgrowth of resident fungi, especially in moist or macerated skin [33]. Patients on antimicrobials or corticosteroids are the most susceptible. Such patients may also have trush, denture stomatitis of intertrigo [58]. *Candida albicans* and dermatophytes are the most common organisms. Figure 9.1 is an example of periwound infection due to Candida.

A short course of topical steroids may be necessary to treat surrounding dermatitis. The adverse effects of both systemic and topical steroids on wound healing are well documented. Delayed wound healing due to inhibition of keratinocytes and the local vasoconstrictive effects of the steroids must be considered.

Cellulitis

Cellulitis can occur in the healthy tissue adjacent to a pressure ulcer. The infection is a result of resident wound flora that replicates and invades viable tissues. Cellulitis involves the dermis and subcutaneous tissues. It is sudden in onset and presents as a rapidly spreading erythema, edema, pain, and tenderness. Systemic symptoms occur infrequently and often are mild, including fever, tachycardia, hypotension, and leukocytosis [59]. Cellulitis in the elderly often presents with atypical

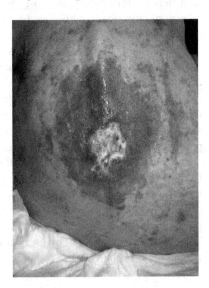

Fig. 9.1 Sacral pressure ulcer complicated by Periwound Candida

symptoms. Fever is uncommon and if present, with or without purulence, a more serious deep-seated infection should be considered.

Less commonly lymphangitic streaks and regional lymphadenopathy occur in cellulitis. Blood cultures are positive in only 4–5 % of cases [60, 61] and do not need to be ordered unless there is evidence systemic toxicity. Cultures of aspirates or punch biopsy specimens have low yields and have no role in routine clinical practice. Swab culture of the pressure ulcer is of no value in predicting the organism involved in adjacent cellulitis.

In cellulitis complicating pressure ulcers, a broad range of microorganisms should be considered as potential pathogens. If this complication develops in a previously institutionalized patient, the known nosocomial pathogens should be considered when deciding on empirical antibiotic coverage.

Necrotizing Fasciitis Complicating Pressure Ulcers

Necrotizing fasciitis is an extremely uncommon but potentially fatal complication of pressure ulcers [62]. The infection rapidly progresses in the skin and deeper structures. It is characterized by necrosis of the skin, subcutaneous tissue, fascia, and at times skeletal muscle. The infection initially spreads along the superficial fascial planes. It starts superficially from skin or mucosa to involve and destroy deeper structures. Fasciitis can cause overwhelming sepsis if not recognized early [63, 64]. Exact categorization of some bacterial infections of the soft tissues may be difficult at presentation [65]. The differences between a superficial skin or soft tissue infection and a classic gas gangrene infection are readily apparent. Initially, the distinction between a superficial and deep infection is difficult [66]. Due to the seriousness of necrotizing infections, a high index of suspicion must be maintained. Fasciitis arising from pressure ulcers are most commonly seen in diabetics and other compromised hosts, and the infections are often polymicrobial.

The exact incidence of fasciitis is unknown but most surgeons see only a few cases per year. There are numerous eponyms given to describe the same condition. Attempts to classify the condition based on location (e.g., Fournier's gangrene), clinical presentation, or bacteriology do not help the bedside clinician since there is little to distinguish between these entities, and their initial management is the same. Broad-spectrum antimicrobial coverage and prompt surgery are indicated.

Osteomyelitis Complicating Pressure Ulcers

Osteomyelitis complicating pressure ulcers is not common and often over treated. Osteomyelitis is predominately bacterial in origin and involves inflammatory destruction of cortical or medullary bone. Bacteria can invade bone directly from a contiguous focus or by hematogenous spread [67]. The Cieny-Mader Staging

System divides osteomyelitis in to four anatomical stages (1) medullary, limited to intramedullary bone as seen in hematogenous cases, (2) superficial, when bone is exposed to necrotic tissue in a wound, (3) localized, full thickness cortical bone involvement, and (4) diffuse [68]. In stage 3 bone cortex can be removed surgically without loss of bone stability. In stage 4, resection would result in loss of bone stability.

The presence of superficial osteomyelitis may cause poor healing in pressure ulcers with or without heavy bioburden, and they often occur together [69]. Exposed bone in a wound bed alone does not establish the diagnosis of osteomyelitis. The best test is combined biopsy and culture of exposed bone [70]. The concept of being able to "probe to the bone" is a clinical technique used in diabetic patients with a foot infection. It involves exploring the wound bed for palpable bone with a sterile blunt metal probe and is often misapplied to pressure ulcer care. Even when used as intended, in diabetic foot ulcers, it has a low positive predictive value. But the technique can be used to reasonably rule out osteomyelitis at the bedside [71]. Positive noninvasive tests such as a plain skeletal X-ray or sedimentation rate greater than 70 mm/h [70, 72] in the proper clinical context raise the probability of osteomyelitis significantly. The best radiographic test is MRI. If prolonged antibiotic treatment is planned, biopsy should be done so to stage the involvement and guide antibiotic therapy. Debridement of involved bone can be done at the time of biopsy. Removal of dead bone and the sessile communities of bacteria in bone-associated biofilm are particularly important in treating chronic osteomyelitis. The involucrum that forms in chronic osteomyelitis has to be excised if healing is to occur [73]. Sinus tracts that develop in apparently healing pressure ulcers should alert the practitioner of underlying chronic osteomyelitis.

Treatment Modalities: Debridement

Sharp debridement is the mainstay of treatment for pressure ulcers with necrosis. All devitalized tissues must be debrided chemically, mechanically, or surgically. At each dressing change the wound bed should be thoroughly cleansed. Any loose slough should be removed and any filmy material should be wiped away with moistened gauze.

It was once thought that returning a stalled chronic wound to an acute wound was needed to reintroduce neutrophils to remove bacteria and activate macrophages so as to promote granulation [74, 75]. But continuous "reactivation" of a wound has its downside. Ideally the inflammatory phase with a predominance of neutrophils needs to be replaced with macrophages that engender angiogenesis and granulation [76].

The choice of debridement technique is based on degree of necrotic burden. Sharp debridement is needed for heavier necrotic loads and can be followed with frequent curettage at the bedside for adherent slough. Enzymatic agents can be used for thinner less adherent slough.

The nonselective papain-urea enzymatic debriding agents have not been available in the USA since 2008. Collagenase (Santyl™) is the only topical debriding agent available in the USA currently. It is selective and will not harm granulation tissue or delay healing [77]. This agent does not penetrate biofilms and has no effect on their eradication [25]. This is also true for commercially available wound cleansers in the absence of mechanical disruption of the biofilm.

Autolytic debridement occurs naturally in a moist wound bed. Dressings that promote autolysis are not known to disrupt biofilms [38]. Maggot Debridement Therapy (MDT) has a number of beneficial effects in chronic wounds with necrotic burden. These include the apparent digestion of established biofilm and suppression of its formation [78].

Treatment Modalities: Topical Antimicrobials

There is a limited role for topical antimicrobial treatment in pressure ulcer care. Many of the recommendations to use topical antimicrobials come from the venous ulcer [79] and diabetic foot ulcer care literature. Potent agents capable of cleansing the skin should never be applied to a wound bed. A good rule of thumb is to never to put anything in the wound that cannot be tolerated comfortably in the conjunctiva [80].

There is limited evidence that topical or systemic antibiotics prevent invasive wound infection. Debridement and the use of topical antimicrobial agents are commonly used together in practice. There is no existing firm evidence to support the routine use of systemic antibiotics to promote healing in venous leg ulcers [81]. There is less evidence for their use in pressure ulcer care.

In spite of the lack of reliable evidence, expert opinion does not recommend discontinuation of any of the commonly used FDA approved topical antimicrobial agents. There is some evidence to support the use of cadexomer iodine [82]. Further research is required before definitive conclusions can be made about the effectiveness of topical preparations such as peroxide-based preparations, ethacridine lactate, mupirocin, and ionic silver products in healing pressure ulceration. There are no trials in support of the use of Dakin's solution at any strength (full strength is a 0.5 % hypochlorite solution). In light of the increasing problem of bacterial resistance, current clinical practice guidelines recommend that antibacterial preparations should only be used in cases of defined infection and not for bacterial colonization [83, 84].

Topical antiseptics and antimicrobials are appropriate treatment in palliative wound care near the end of life. Providone-iodine 10 % solution is used ("painted on") on dry gangrene, necrotic heel, and other pressure ulcers to promote desiccation when healing is not expected at the end of life. Alleviating wound odor can enhance the quality of life of patients. Topical metronidazole 1 % can be effective in eliminating wound odor in necrotic or fumigating wounds when debridement is not indicated [85].

Summary

Cellulitis and other systemic infections complicating pressure ulcers are very uncommon. Nonetheless surveillance for the signs and symptoms of secondary infection must be done with each wound assessment. Noninfectious periwound findings must be distinguished from cellulitis. Critical colonization must be considered when a chronic wound fails to progress. The use of topical antimicrobials including sliver-ion releasing dressings has limited supporting evidence in pressure ulcer care.

Physical examination may indicate the presence of superficial soft-tissue infection, but it is inadequate for determination of the extent of deep-tissue involvement [1]. Wound appearance alone is not useful in the diagnosis of associated osteomyelitis. The presence of bacteria (even as detected by deep-tissue culture) is not sufficient for the diagnosis of true infection. Given that most wound cultures are obtained from the surface of a chronic wound or from wound exudate, the clinical usefulness is limited.

Treatment of chronic, poorly healing pressure ulcers requires a systemic approach addressing extrinsic host factors and intrinsic wound factors. These include all the aspects of wound bed preparation including critical colonization.

References

1. Livesley NJ, Chow AW. Infected pressure ulcers in elderly individuals. Clin Infect Dis. 2002;35:1390–6.
2. Brandeis GH, Ooi WL, Hossain M, Morris JN, Lipsitz LA. The epidemiology and natural history of pressure ulcers in elderly nursing home residents. JAMA. 1990;264:2905–9.
3. Berlowitz DR, Wilking SVB. Pressure ulcers in the nursing home: comprehensive reviews of clinical research, vol. 4. Newbury Park, CA: Sage; 1993. p. 102–30.
4. Pien BC, Sundaram P, Raoof N, Costa S, et al. The clinical and prognostic importance of positive blood cultures in adults. Am J Med. 2010;13:819–28.
5. Bryan CS, Dew CE, Reynolds KL. Bacteremia associated with decubitus ulcers. Arch Intern Med. 2093;1983:143.
6. Nicolle LE, Orr P, Duckworth H, et al. Prospective study of decubitus ulcers in two long term care facilities. Can J Infect Control. 1994;9:35–8.
7. Allman RM. Pressure ulcers among the elderly. N Engl J Med. 1989;320:850.
8. Oates A, Bowling F, Boulton AJM, McBain AJ. Molecular and culture-based assessment of the microbial diversity of diabetic chronic foot wounds and contralateral skin sites. J Clin Microbiol. 2012;50(7):2263–71.
9. Aherro N, Shahi SK, Dwivedi A, Kumar A, et al. Wounds. 2012;24(10):283–8.
10. Fore-Pfliger J. The epidermal skin barrier: implications for the wound care practitioner, part 1. Adv Skin Wound Care. 2004;17:417–25.
11. Fore-Pfliger J. The epidermal skin barrier: implications for the wound care practitioner, part 2. Adv Skin Wound Care. 2004;17:480–8.
12. Fore J. A review of skin and the effects of aging on skin structure and function. Ostomy Wound Manage. 2006;52(9):24–35.
13. Fuchs E. Beauty is skin deep: the fascinating biology of the epidermis and its appendages. Harvey Lect. 2001;94:47–77.
14. Zasloff M. Antimicrobial peptides of multicellular organisms. Nature. 2002;415:389–95.

15. Kazmierczak AK, Szewczyk EM. Bacteria forming a resident flora of the skin as a potential source of opportunistic infections. Pol J Microbiol. 2004;53(4):249–55.
16. Hartmann AA. The influence of various factors on the human resident skin flora. Semin Dermatol. 1990;9(4):305–8.
17. Relman DA, Falkow S. A molecular perspective of microbial pathogenicity in Mandell. In: Mandell G, Douglas R, Bennett's J, editors. Principles and practice of infectious diseases. 7th ed. London: Churchill Livingstone; 2009.
18. Dethlefsen L, McFall-Ngai M, Relman DA. An ecological and evolutionary perspective on human-microbe mutualism and disease. Nature. 2007;449:811–8.
19. Landis S, Ryan S, Woo K, Sibbald RG. Infections in chronic wounds. In: Krasner DL, Rodeheaver GT, Sibbald RG, editors. Chronic wound care: a clinical source book for healthcare professionals. 4th ed. HMP Communications: Malvern, PA; 2007. p. 299–321.
20. Kong HH. Skin microbiome: genomics-based insights into the diversity and role of skin microbes. Trends Mol Med. 2011;17(6):320–8.
21. Howell-Jones RS, Wilson MJ, Hill KE, Howard AJ, Price PE, Thomas DW. A review of the microbiology, antibiotic usage and resistance in chronic skin wounds. J Antimicrob Chemother. 2005;55:143–9.
22. Bowler PG, Duerden BI, Armstrong DG. Wound microbiology and associated approaches to wound management. Clin Microbiol Rev. 2001;14:244–69.
23. Garibaldi RA, Brodine S, Matsumiya S. Infections among patients in nursing homes: policies, prevalence, problems. N Engl J Med. 1981;305:731–5.
24. The American Heritage. Dictionary of the english language. 4th ed. Boston, MA: Houghton Mifflin Company; 2000. Updated in 2009.
25. Rhoads DD, Wolcott RD, Percival SL. Biofilms in wounds: management strategies. J Wound Care. 2008;17(11):502–8.
26. Bjarnsholt T. Why chronic wounds will not heal: a novel hypothesis. Wound Repair Regen. 2008;16(1):2–10.
27. Bendy RH, Nuccio PA, Wolfe E, et al. Relationship of quantitlive wound bacterial counts to healing of decubiti. Effect of topical gentamicin. Antimicrob Agents Chemother. 1964;4:147.
28. White RJ, Cutting KF. Critical colonization–the concept under scrutiny. Ostomy Wound Manage. 2006;52(11):50–6.
29. Dow G, Browne A, Sibbald RG. Infection in chronic wounds: controversies in diagnosis and treatment. Ostomy Wound Manage. 1999;45(8):23–7. 29–40.
30. Bowler PG, Davies BJ. The microbiology of infected and noninfected leg ulcers. Int J Dermatol. 1999;38:573–8.
31. Cooper R. Understanding wound infection. In: Calnie S, editor. European Wound Management Association. Position document: identifying criteria for wound infection. London: Mep Ltd; 2005. p. 2–5.
32. Reddy M, Gill SS, Wu W, Kalkar SR, et al. Does this patient have an infection of a chronic wound? JAMA. 2012;307:605–11.
33. High KP, Bradley SF, Gravenstein S, Mehr DR, et al. Clinical practive guideline for the evaluation of fever and infection in older adult residents of long-term care facilities: 2008 update by the Infectious Disease Society of America. J Am Geriatr Soc. 2009;57:375–95.
34. Panuncialman J, Falanga V. The science of wound bed preparation. Surg Clin N Am. 2009;89:611–26.
35. Sibbald RG, Williamson D, Orstead H, et al. Preparing the wound bed – debridement, bacterial balance and moisture balance. Ostomy Wound Manage. 2000;46(1):14–35.
36. Singer AJ, Clark RA. Cutaneous wound healing. N Engl J Med. 1999;341:738–46.
37. James GA, Swogger E, Wolcott R, et al. Biofilms in chronic wounds. Wound Repair Regen. 2008;16(1):37–44.
38. Black CE, Costerton JW. Current concepts regarding the effect of wound microbial ecology and biofilms on wound healing. Surg Clin N Am. 2010;90:1147–60.
39. Mustoe TA, O'Shaughnessy K, Kloeters O. Chronic wound pathogenesis and current treatment strategies: a unifying hypothesis. Plast Reconstr Surg. 2006;117:35–41.

40. Frank DN, Wysocki A, Specht-Glick DD, Rooney A, et al. Microbial diversity in chronic open wounds. Wound Repair Regen. 2009;17:163–72.

41. Serralta VW, Harrison-Balestra C, Cazzaniga A, Davis SC, Mertz PM. Lifestyles of bacteria in wounds: presence of biofilms? Wounds. 2001;13:29–34.

42. Quatresooz PF, Henry P, Paquet C, Pierard-Franchimont K, Harding G, Pierard E. Deciphering the impaired cytokine cascades in chronic leg ulcers (Review). Int J Mol Med. 2003; 11:411–8.

43. Wysocki AB. Evaluating and managing open skin wounds: colonization versus infection. AACN Clin Issues. 2002;13:382–97.

44. Gardner SE, Frantz RA, Doebbeling BN. The validity of the clinical signs and symptoms used to identify localized chronic wound infection. Wound Repair Regen. 2001;9(3):178–86.

45. Lazarus GS, Cooper DM, Knighton DR. Definitions and guidelines for assessment of wounds and evaluation of healing. Arch Dermatol. 1994;130:489–93.

46. Healy B, Freedman A. ABC of wound healing. Infections. BMJ. 2006;332:838–41.

47. Mertz PM. Feature: cutaneous biofilms: friend or foe. Wounds. 2003;15(5):129–32.

48. Edwards R, Harding KG. Bacteria and wound healing. Curr Opin Infect Dis. 2004;17(2):91–6.

49. Loryman C, Mansbridge J. Inhibition of keratinocyte migration by lipopolysaccharide. Wound Repair Regen. 2008;16(1):45–51.

50. Wolcott RD, Dowd SE. A rapid molecular method for characterizing bacterial bioburden in chronic wounds. J Wound Care. 2008;17(12):513–6.

51. Wolcott RD, Rhoads DD, Dowd SE. Biofilms and chronic wound inflammation. J Wound Care. 2008;17(8):333–41.

52. Levine NS, et al. The quantitate swab culture and smear: a quick simple method for determining the number of viable aerobic bacteria on open wounds. J Trauma. 1976;16(2):89–94.

53. Davies CE, Wilson MJ, Hill KE, Stephens P, Hill CM, Harding KG, Thomas DW. Use of molecular techniques to study microbial diversity in the skin: chronic wounds reevaluated. Wound Repair Regen. 2001;9:332–40.

54. Thomas DR. When is a chronic wound infected? J Am Med Dir Assoc. 2012;13:5–7.

55. Drinka PJ. Swab culture of purulent skin infection to detect infection or colonization with antibiotic resistant bacteria. J Am Med Dir Assoc. 2012;13:75–9.

56. Siddiqui AR. Chronic wound infection: facts and controversies. Clin Dermatol. 2010; 28(5):519–26.

57. Bale S, Tebbie N, Price P. A topical metronidazole gel used to treat malodorous wounds. Br J Nurs. 2004;13(11):S4–11.

58. Hedderwick SA, Wan JY, Bradley SF, Sangeorzan JA, et al. Risk factors for colonization with yeast species in a Veterns Affairs long-term care facility. J Am Geriatr Soc. 1998;46:849–53.

59. Stevens DL, Bisno AL, Chambers HF, Everett ED, et al. Practice guideline for the diagnosis and management of skin and soft-tissue infections. Clin Infect Dis. 2005;41:1373–406.

60. Schwartz MN. Cellulitis. N Engl J Med. 2004;350:904–12.

61. Perl B, Gottehrer NP, Raveh D, Schlesinger Y, et al. Cost-effectiveness of blood cultures for adult patients with cellulitis. Clin Infect Dis. 1999;29:1483–8.

62. Hasham S, Matteucci P, Stanley PRW, Hart NB. Necrotising fasciitis. BMJ. 2005;330:830–3.

63. Hammonson J, Tobar Y, Harkless L. Necrotizing Fasciitis. Clin Podiatr Med Surg. 1996;13: 635–46.

64. Miller LG, Perdreau-Remington F, Rieg G, Mehdi S, et al. Necrotizing fasciitis caused by community-associated methicillin-resistant staphylococcus aureus in Los Angeles. N Engl J Med. 2005;352:1445–53.

65. Seal DV. Necrotizing fasciitis. Curr Opin Infect Dis. 2001;14:127–32.

66. Bisno AL, Cockerill III FR, Bermudez CT. The initial outpatient-physician encounter in Group A streptococcal necrotizing fasciitis. Clin Infect Dis. 2000;31:607–8.

67. Calhoun JH, Brady RA, Shirtliff ME. Osteomyelitis. In: Tan JS, File TM, Salata RA, Tan MJ, editors. Expert guide to infectious diseases. Philadelphia, PA: ACP Press; 2008.

68. Cierny GI, Mader JT, Penninick JJ. A clinical staging system for adult osteomyelitis. Contemp Orthop. 1985;10:17–37.

69. Mader JT, Calhoun JH. Osteomyelitis. In: Mandell GL, Douglas RG, Bennett Jr JE, editors. Principles and practice of infectious dideases. New York, NY: Churchhill Livingston; 1995. p. 1039–51.

70. Butalia S, Palda VA, Sargeant RJ, et al. Does this patient with diabetes have osteomyelitis of the lower extremity? JAMA. 2008;299(7):806–13.

71. Lavery LA, Armstrong DG, Peters EJG, Lipsky BA. Probe-to-bone test for diagnosing diabetic foot osteomyelitis: reliable or relic? Diabetes Care. 2007;30(2):270–4.

72. Lewis Jr VL, Bailey MH, Pulawski G, Kind G, et al. The diagnosis of osteomyelitis in patients with pressure sores. Plast Reconstr Surg. 1988;81(2):229–32.

73. Donlan RM, Costerton JW. Biofilms: survival mechanisms of clinically relevant microorganisms. Clin Microbiol Rev. 2002;15:167–93.

74. Williams RL, Armstrong DG. Wound healing. New modalities for a new millennium. Clin Podiatr Med Surg. 1998;15(1):117–28.

75. Hart J. Inflammation: its role in the healing of chronic wounds. J Wound Care. 2002;11:245–9.

76. Dovi JV, Szpaderska AM, DiPietro LA. Neutraphil function in the healing wound: adding insult to injury? Thromb Haemost. 2004;92:275–80.

77. Brett DW. A historical review of topical enzymatic debridement. Newark, NJ: The McMahon Publishing Group; 2003.

78. Chambers I, Woodrow S, Brown AP, Harris PD, Phillips D, Hall M, Church JCT, Pritchard DI. Degradation of extracellular matrix components by defined proteinases from the greenbottle larva Lucilia sericata used for the clinical debridement of non-healing wounds. Br J Dermatol. 2003;148:14–23.

79. Betts J. Review: evidence for use of systemic antibiotics and topical antiseptics for venous leg ulcers is insufficient. Evid Based Nurs. 2008;11(3):88.

80. Atiyeh BS, Loannovich J, Al-Amm CA, El-Musa KA. Management of acute and chronic wounds: the importance of moist environment in optimal wound healing. Curr Pharm Biotechnol. 2002;3:179–95.

81. O'Meara S, Al-Kurdi D, Ovington LG. Antibiotics and antiseptics for venous leg ulcers. Cochrane Database Syst Rev. 2008;23(1), CD003557.

82. O'Meara SM, Cullum NA, Majid M, et al. Systematic review of antimicrobial agents used for chronic wounds. Br J Surg. 2001;88(1):4–21.

83. Ratliff CR, Bryabt DE, The WOCN Pressure Ulcer Panel. Guideline for prevention and management of pressure ulcers, WOCN clinical practice guideline series. Glenview, IL: Wound Ostomy and Continence Nurses Society; 2003. p. 23.

84. National Pressure Ulcer Advisory Panel and European Pressure Ulcer Advisory Panel. Prevention and treatment of pressure ulcers: clinical practice guideline. Washington, DC: National Pressure Ulcer Advisory Panel; 2009.

85. Paul JC, Pieper BA. Topical metronidazole for the treatment of wound odor: a review of the literature. Ostomy Wound Manage. 2008;54(3):18–27.

86. Wilson M. Microbial inhabitants of humans: their ecology and role in health and disease. New York, NY: Cambridge University Press; 2005. p. 55–8.

87. Blume JE, Levine EG, Heyman WR. Bacterial diseases. In: Bolognia JL, Jorizzo JL, Rapini RP, editors. Dermatology. London: Mosby; 2003. p. 1117.

Chapter 10
Palliative Wound Care and Treatment at End of Life

Kevin Y. Woo, Diane L. Krasner, and R. Gary Sibbald

Abstract The principles of palliative wound and pressure ulcer care should be integrated along the continuum of wound care to address the whole person care needs of older people who often present with chronic debilitating diseases, advanced diseases associated with major organ failure (renal, hepatic, pulmonary or cardiac), profound dementia, complex psychosocial issues, diminished self-care abilities, and challenging wound-related symptoms. This chapter will introduce key concepts for palliative wound and pressure ulcer care that have been developed by the International Interprofessional Wound Care Community and will review the consensus document entitled SCALE: *Skin Changes At Life's End*.

Keywords Palliative wound care • Pain and symptom management • Skin changes at life's end

K.Y. Woo, Ph.D., R.N., F.A.P.W.C.A. (✉)
School of Nursing, Queen's University, 92 Barrie Street, Kingston, ON, Canada K7L 3N6

West Park Health Center, Toronto, ON, Canada
e-mail: kevin.woo@queensu.ca

D.L. Krasner, Ph.D., R.N., C.W.C.N., C.W.S., M.A.P.W.C.A., F.A.A.N.
Wound and Skin Care Consultant, 212 East Market Street, York, PA 17403, USA
e-mail: dlkrasner@aol.com

R.G. Sibbald, B.Sc., M.D., F.R.C.P.C., (M. ed., Derm), M.A.C.P., F.A.A.D., M. ed., M.A.P.W.C.A.
Dermatology Clinic, Unit 23, Suite 210, 1077 North Service Road,
Mississauga, ON, Canada L4Y 1A6
e-mail: rgarysibbald@gmail.com

D.R. Thomas and G.A. Compton (eds.), *Pressure Ulcers in the Aging Population:*   161
A Guide for Clinicians, Aging Medicine 1, DOI 10.1007/978-1-62703-700-6_10,
© Springer Science+Business Media New York 2014

Introduction

Palliative wound and pressure ulcer care is a complex, dynamic, and evolving concept that has gained increased attention over the past decade [1]. In palliative wound and pressure ulcer care, the focus shifts from traditional wound care, where healing and wound closure are the goals, to promoting comfort and dignity, relieving suffering, and improving the quality of life when a palliative wound or pressure ulcer pathway is chosen [2]. As eloquently pointed out by Emmons and Lachman [3], the burden and suffering of people and their circle of care from living with chronic wounds have not been adequately addressed. The scope of palliative wound care should be broadened to encompass the whole person care needs of, particularly, older and frailer people who often present with chronic debilitating diseases, advanced diseases associated with major organ failure (renal, hepatic, pulmonary, or cardiac), profound dementia [4], complex psychosocial issues, diminished self-care abilities, and challenging wound-related symptoms, whether the wound has the potential to heal or not. In other words, the principles of palliative wound and pressure ulcer care should be integrated along the continuum of wound care and its relevance may vary with individual's goals, disease processes, and wound condition (Fig. 10.1). This chapter will introduce key concepts for palliative wound and pressure ulcer care and SCALE: *S*kin *C*hanges *A*t *L*ife's *E*nd that have merged from the International Interprofessional Wound Care Community [5].

The skin is the largest organ of the body and is vulnerable to pressure ulcer development as a result of the deterioration of the body and multiorgan systems failure [6].

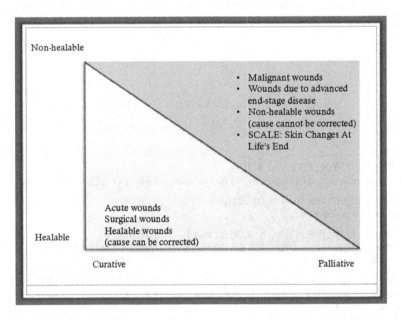

Fig. 10.1 Continuum of Palliative wound care

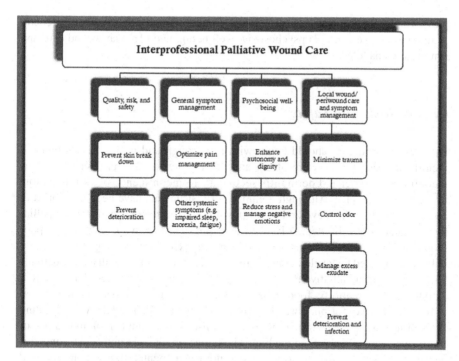

Fig. 10.2 Interprofessional palliative wound care

To maintain hemodynamic stability and normal functioning of vital organs during critical conditions and at life's end, circulation is diverted from the skin, compromising cutaneous perfusion [7, 8]. In fact, hypotension was identified as the strongest predictor of pressure ulcers among critically ill patients with traumatic spinal cord injury [9]. In 2009 an international panel introduced the concept of SCALE: *S*kin *F*ailure *At L*ife's *E*nd in a consensus document based on a modified Delphi process [10]. The National Pressure Ulcer Advisory Panel [7] introduced the term "skin failure" to describe the inevitable damages associated with hypoperfusion of the skin when metabolic demand outstrips supply of oxygen and vital nutrients.

Early signs that herald skin breakdown may include dusky erythema, mottled discoloration, and local temperature change. These signs have been documented in over 50 % of individuals within 2–6 weeks prior to death [10, 11]. In a 2-year audit of a palliative care unit, 26.1 % of 542 individuals were admitted with pressure ulcers and 12.0 % acquired new pressure ulcers during their stay [12]. It is generally accepted that pressure ulcers are largely preventable but not always avoidable due to a number of intrinsic factors that may not be correctable in an individual patient/resident.

Given the complexity of palliative wound care, a systematized and holistic approach integrating interprofessional collaboration is required to optimize patient/resident outcomes [5]. The key components of Interprofessional Palliative Wound Care are outlined in Fig. 10.2 including (1) risk reduction with the key objectives to prevent skin break down and further deterioration of existing ulcers, (2) general symptom management, (3) psychosocial well being, and (4) local wound care and symptom management.

Quality, Risk, and Safety

Palliative wound care should begin with a thorough and holistic assessment to identify the risk for pressure ulcers and other potential skin problems (such as incontinence-associated dermatitis secondary to incontinence or skin tears due to frequent falls) [13]. Although a number of instruments have been developed to assess risk and predict development of pressure ulcers, scales specific to the palliative population are limited. Advanced age, physical inactivity, immobility, poor food and fluid intake, incontinence, and lean body types were among the significant risk factors related to development of pressure ulcers in terminally ill cancer patients [14]. The use of a Palliative Performance Scale that evaluates levels of ambulation, activity, self-care ability, food intake, and consciousness has been demonstrated to be a valid proxy for pressure ulcer risk assessment [15]. The F.R.A.I.L. Healing Probability Assessment Tool [16] has circumscribed a number of indicators of frailty that may affect wound healing. The indicators include immobility; incontinence; poor eating; weight loss; falls; diminished mental status; compromised immunity; poor oxygenation; end-stage renal, liver, or heart disease; and wounds that are complicated by diabetes mellitus, arterial disease, and peripheral vascular disease (PVD) [17].

Palliative care does not preclude active treatment and other supportive strategies to prevent exacerbation of existing wounds. The emergence of new ulcers is equally important. To prevent pressure ulcers, at risk individuals may benefit from therapeutic support surfaces and regular repositioning (frequency determined by the person's condition with some clinicians recommending at least every 4 h) [18–20]. Although best practice recommendations are targeted at pressure redistribution and shear elimination, the plan of care must be customized to promote comfort and meet the needs of the patients/residents including their circle of care. The risk of executing the treatment plan should not outweigh the potential benefits. For instance, repositioning may precipitate vascular collapse or exacerbate shortness of breath. Certain support surfaces may exacerbate dehydration or the potential for aspiration. Individualized plans of care based on individual risk factors and comorbidities are essential.

Among people who develop cachexia, decreased tissue thickness is associated with more pronounced tissue deformation, potentially putting them at high risk for skin breakdown. Poor nutrition could be attributed to factors including impaired absorption, increased metabolic demand, and decreased oral intake as a result of poor appetite, swallowing difficulties, nausea, vomiting, taste alteration, and mucositis. Nutritional supplementation with enriched protein and other micronutrients (zinc, vitamins A, E, and C) should be considered [21, 22]. Meticulous skin care after each incontinent episode together with the use of a mild cleanser and skin protectant may reduce irritation to skin [23, 24]. The role of skin surface temperature and humidity in the formation of pressure ulcers warrants further scrutiny. An increase of 1 °C in skin temperature results in approximately a 13 % increase in tissue metabolic requirements rendering the skin more vulnerable to mechanical damage.

Symptom Management

Pain is consistently reported by patients/residents as one of the worst aspects of living with chronic wounds impacting their quality of life [25]. In a study of 132 patients with pressure ulcers, Dallam and colleagues [26] reported that 59 % experienced some type of pain in an acute care setting with a substantial number of the subjects perceiving pain to be severe. In another study of patients with pressure ulcers, Szor and Bourguignon [27] reported that 42 % of their subjects described pain as continuous even at rest. Proctor et al. [28] performed an analysis based on a minimum dataset involving 3,195 nursing home residents. The result substantiated the significant association between pressure ulcers and daily pain experience (odd ratio = 3.5; 95 % CI = 1.81–6.76). Assessment and measurement of pain assessments should be well documented to facilitate the continuity of patient/resident care and to benchmark the effectiveness of management strategies.

Many methods of pain assessment have been developed, ranging from subjective self-reports to objective behavioral checklists. Pain is a subjective experience. An individual's self-report of pain is the most reliable method to evaluate pain. Other assessment methodologies include physiological indicators, behavioral manifestations, functional assessments, and diagnostic tests. Categorical scales, numerical rating scales, pain thermometers, visual analogue scales, faces scales, and verbal categorical scales are one-dimensional tools commonly used to quantify pain in terms of intensity, quality (characteristics), pain unpleasantness, and pain relief [29]. To obtain a comprehensive assessment of pain, multidimensional measurements are available to evaluate the many facets of pain and its impact on daily functioning, mood, social functioning, and other aspects of quality of life. The key questions to ask about pain can be remembered by *PQRSTU* [30]:

- *P—Provoking and palliating factors*: What makes your pain worse? What makes your pain better (e.g., warm weather, walking, certain types of cleansing solutions or dressings)?
- *Q—Quality of pain*: What does your pain feel like? Descriptors (e.g., burning, electrical shocks, pricking, tingling pins) may help to differentiate the 2 types of pain: nociceptive and neuropathic.
- *R—Regions and radiation*: Where is the pain and does the pain move anywhere (e.g., in and around the wound, the wound region, unrelated)?
- *S—Severity or intensity*: How much does it hurt on a scale of 0–10 with 0 representing no pain and 10 representing pain as bad as it could possibly be?

- *T—Timing or history*: When did the pain start? Is it present all the time? A pain diary may help to map out the temporal pattern of pain (e.g., the pain worsens at night).
- *U—Understanding*: What is important to you for pain relief? How would you like to get better?

As an alternative, studies have shown that the observation of nonverbal indicators encompassing a wide range of vocalized signals and bodily movements may provide a means of assessing pain in patients/residents (e.g., neonates or cognitively impaired) who are not able to verbalize their pain. Clinicians should consider specific tools to evaluate neuropathic pain. There was no one tool that was deemed universal and useful for all individuals; the selection of a specific pain scale must take into account the person's age, language, educational level, sensory impairment, developmental stage, and cognitive status. Once chosen, the same measurement scale should be used for subsequent assessments for ongoing comparison. Changes in pain levels may indicate a need to reassess the choice and timing of analgesics and/or other interventions used in pain management [25] (Table 10.1).

Pharmacotherapy continues to be the mainstay for pain management. Appropriate agents are selected based on severity and specific types of pain. The World Health Organization analgesic ladder proposes that the treatment of mild to moderate nociceptive pain should begin with a nonopioid medication such as acetaminophen and nonsteroidal anti-inflammatory drugs [31]. For controlling more severe and refractory pain, opioid analgesics should be considered. Management of neuropathic pain or associated symptoms (e.g., anxiety and depression) may include the possibility of adding adjuvant treatments. Three classes of medications are recommended as first-line treatments for neuropathic pain: antidepressants with both norepinephrine and serotonin reuptake inhibition (TCAs and selective serotonin and norepinephrine reuptake inhibitors [SSNRIs]), calcium channel ligands (gabapentin and pregabalin), and topical lidocaine (lidocaine patch 5 %). In addition to the severity and pain types, selection of appropriate medications should always take into account the characteristics of the drug (onset, duration, available routes of administration, dosing intervals, side effects) and individual factors (age, coexisting diseases, and other over the counter or herbal medications). For severe pain, it may be necessary to consider oral agents combining long-acting narcotics (oral, patch) as outlined in the World Health Organization Pain Ladder with adjunctive agents for the neuropathic component and short-acting breakthrough agents. In resistant cases, general anesthesia, local neural blockade, spinal analgesia, general anesthesia, or the use of mixed nitrous oxide and oxygen (Entonox) should be considered [25].

As a general rule of thumb, analgesics should be taken at regular intervals until pain is adequately relieved. It may be necessary to consider the use of two or more drugs with complementary mechanisms of action that may provide greater pain relief with less toxicity and lower doses of each drug. For severe pain during dressing change, short acting and potent narcotic analgesics such as sublingual fentanyl (approximately 100 times more potent than morphine) should be considered. In resistant cases, general anesthesia, local neural blockade, spinal analgesia, general anesthesia or the use of mixed nitrous oxide and oxygen (Entonox) should be considered [25].

Table 10.1 Strategies and objectives for pain management

Strategy	Objectives
Education	Web-based learning
	Face to face education:
	Explain mechanism of pain
	Dispel misconceptions about pain
	Address concerns about addiction
	Emphasize the availability of multiple strategies
Pharmacological	Topical:
	Topical ibuprofen (dressing)
	Morphine
	Topical lidocaine
	Systemic
	Nociceptive pain: ASA, NSAIDs, acetaminophen for mild to moderate pain
	Opioids for moderate to intense pain
	Neuropathic pain: SNRI, anticonvulsants
Local wound care	Atraumatic interface (silicone)
	Sequester: remove inflammatory mediators
	Protect periwound skin
	Treat infections
Physical therapies	Heat/cold compress
	Massage
	Exercise
Anxiety reduction	Relaxation
	Imagery
	Distractions
	Education
	Music therapy
	Support groups
Cognitive therapy	Cognitive behavior therapy
	Problem-solving skills
	Positive thinking
Therapeutic alliance	Communication techniques, e.g., reflective listening
	Goal setting
	Align expectations
	Demonstrate sympathy
Empowerment	Allow individual to call "time out"
	Respect individual's choices
	Maximize autonomy: active participation
	Functional-focused therapy

© Woo, 2011

Topical agents or dressings play a role in alleviating wound-related pain. Slow release ibuprofen foam dressings have demonstrated reduction in persistent wound pain between dressing change and temporary pain on dressing removal. The use of topical morphine and lidocaine/prilocaine (EMLA®) may be considered for acute- or procedure-related pain. However, the lack of pharmacokinetic data precludes the routine clinical use of these compounds use at this time. There are many advantages to using local rather than systemic treatment. Any active agent is delivered directly to the affected area, bypassing the systemic circulation, and the dose needed for pain reduction is low with minimal risk of side effects.

Wound-related pain is frequently experienced during dressing changes [32]. Dressing materials may adhere to the fragile wound surface due to the glue like nature of dehydrated or crusted exudate; each time the dressing is removed, potential local trauma may evoke pain. Granulation tissue and capillary loops that grow into the product matrix, especially gauze, can also render dressing removal traumatic. According to a review of dressings and topical agents for secondary intention healing of postsurgical wounds, patients experienced significantly more pain with gauze than other types of dressings including foam, alginate, and hydrocolloid dressings [33]. Nonetheless, gauze continues to be one of the commonly used dressing materials indicating a need to bridge research to practice [34]. Careful selection of dressings with atraumatic and nonadherent interfaces such as silicone has been documented to limit skin damage/trauma with dressing removal and minimize pain at dressing changes.

Next to dressing removal, wound cleansing is also likely to evoke pain during the dressing change [35]. The routine practice of using abrasive materials and gauze to scrub the wound surface is discouraged. Techniques that involve compressing and irrigation may be less traumatic and painful. In the presence of unexpected pain or tenderness, clinicians should consider antimicrobial therapy for wound infection.

Education is a key strategy to empower patients/residents and to improve wound-related pain control. Patients/residents should be informed of various treatment options and be empowered to be active participants in care. Being an active participant involves taking part in the decision-making for the most appropriate treatment, monitoring response to treatment, and communicating concerns to healthcare providers. Common misconceptions about pain management should be addressed.

Fear of addiction and adverse effects had prevented patients/residents from taking regular analgesics. In a pilot study, 5 chronic wound patients described dressing change pain as being more manageable after receiving educational information [36]. Pain-related education is a necessary step in effecting change in pain management by rebuking common misconceptions and myths that may obstruct effective pain management. Cognitive therapy that aims at altering anxiety by modifying attitudes, beliefs, and expectations by exploring the meaning and interpretation of pain concerns has been shown to be successful in the management of pain. This may involve distraction techniques, imagery, relaxation, or altering the significance of the pain to an individual. Patients/residents can learn to envision pain as less threatening and unpleasant through positive imagery by imagining pain disappearing or conjuring a mental picture of a place that evokes feelings and memories of comfort, safety, and relaxation. In addition to pain, clinicians should pay attention to other sources of anxiety that may be associated with stalled wound healing, fear of amputation, body disfigurement, repulsive odor, social isolation, debility, and disruption of daily activities. Relaxation exercises can help to reduce anxiety-related tension in the muscle that contributes to pain [25].

Pruritis

Itch is a common problem in people with chronic wounds. Of 199 people with chronic wounds, Paul, Pieper, and Templin [37] documented that 28.1 % complained of itch. Itch is caused by irritation of the skin most commonly related to dermatitis. People with chronic wounds are exposed to a plethora of potential contact irritants accounting for approximately 80 % of all cases of contact dermatitis [38].

Some of the common irritants including solvents, detergents and soaps, water, and harsh weather conditions are known to remove the skin natural moisturizing factors and interrupt the protective surface lipid bilayers of the stratum corneum. Oral antihistamines, antidepressants, and anticonvulsants have been demonstrated to be effective in relieving itch. Topical steroids should be considered for dermatitis. To achieve a greater anti-itch effect, topical steroid creams can often be kept in the refrigerator or combined with 0.5–1 % of menthol (camphor and phenol are alternatives) to give a cooling effect [38].

Excessive washing and bathing strips away surface lipid and induce dryness that can exacerbate pruritis. People with dermatitis should keep water exposure to a minimum. To replenish skin moisture, humectants or lubricants should be used on a regular basis. Humectant creams are preparations containing urea or lactic acid that contain components of the skin's natural moisturizing factor. Individuals should apply these agents immediately after bathing while the skin is damp. Lubricants are the second type of moisturizer. These products are available in creams or ointments that seal the skin to minimize moisture evaporation. Ointments contain a continuous greasy oil phase, whereas a cream has a continuous water phase with a small amount of suspended oil. A paste adds powder to ointment to give it a firmer consistency like zinc oxide, which may be used to protect periwound skin and resists being washed off easily. A gel (powder in a lattice) increases penetration down hair follicles [38] (Table 10.2).

Psychosocial Well-Being

It is unequivocal that pressure ulcer constitute a significant source of emotional distress to patients/residents and their families [39]. Gorecki and colleagues [40] reviewed 31 studies that investigated quality of life issues in people with pressure ulcers. Some of the emerging themes surrounding having a pressure ulcer include physical restrictions, social isolation, loss of independence, mood disturbance, and financial encumbrance. In a pilot study, 60 % of participants reported high level of stress because of chronic wounds including pressure ulcers [41]. Using a qualitative approach, Lo et al. [42] interviewed 10 patients living with malignant fungating wounds. A recurring theme emerged that articulated the bleak feeling of isolation due to wound-related stigma. Individualized education and appropriate information should be provided to help patients understand the parameters of care.

Table 10.2 Strategies to protect periwound skin

Types	Description	Application	Comments
Silicone	Silicones are polymers that include silicone together with carbon, hydrogen, and oxygen	Apply to periwound skin	Allergy is rare. Certain types of silicone product are tacky facilitating dressing adherence to the skin without any adhesive
Zinc oxide/ Petrolatum	Inorganic compounds that are insoluble in water	Apply a generous quantity to skin	May interfere with activity of ionic silver
Acrylates	Film-forming liquid skin preparation to form a protective interface on skin attachment sites	Spray or wipe on skin sparingly	Allergy is uncommon. Facilitates visualization of periwound skin
Hydrocolloid	A hydrocolloid wafer consists of a backing with carboxymethylcellulose as the filler, water absorptive components such as gelatin and pectin (commercial gelatin desserts) and an adhesive	Window frame the wound margin to prevent recurrent stripping of skin	Allergies have been reported from some colophony-related adhesives (Pentylin H) associated with some hydrocolloid dressings

© Woo & Sibbald, 2009

Local Wound Care

Trauma

The Granulation tissue within a malignant wound is often friable and bleeds easily due to local stimulation of vascular endothelial growth factor (VEG-F), resulting in excess formation of abundant but fragile blood vessels [43]. Reduced fibroblast activity and ongoing thrombosis of larger vessels in infected and malignant wounds may compromise the strength of collagen matrix formation rendering the granulation less resilient to trauma. Even minor trauma from the removal of wound dressings that adhere to wound surface could provoke bleeding.

Repeated application and removal of adhesive tapes and dressings pull the skin surface from the epithelial cells and this can precipitate skin damage by stripping away the stratum corneum. In severe cases, contact irritant and allergic dermatitis results in local erythema, edema, and blistering on the wound margins [43, 44]. Enzyme-rich exudate may spill onto the periwound skin causing maceration and tissue erosion with a subsequent increased risk of trauma and pain. To minimize trauma induced by adhesives, a number of sealants, barriers, and protectants such as wipes, sprays, gels, and liquid roll-ons are useful on the periwound skin.

Odor

Unpleasant odor and putrid discharge are associated with increased bacterial burden, particularly involving anaerobic and certain gram-negative (e.g., pseudomonas) organisms. Metabolic by-products that produce this odor include: volatile fatty acids, (propionic, butyric, valeric, isobutyric, and isovaleric acids), volatile sulfur compounds, putrescine, and cadaverine [13]. To eradicate wound odor, metronidazole as an anti-inflammatory and anti-infective agent against anaerobes has been demonstrated to be efficacious [45]. Topical application of metronidazole is readily available as gel and cream. Alternatively, gauze can be soaked with intravenous metronidazole solution to use as a compress or tablets can be ground into powder and sprinkled onto wound surface [46]. Some individuals derive the greatest benefit if the metronidazole is administered orally.

Activated charcoal dressing has been used to control odor with some success. To ensure optimal performance of charcoal dressing, edges should be sealed and the contact layer should be kept dry. If topical treatment is not successful or practical, kitty litter beneath the bed may act as an effective odor-reducing technique.

Exudate

Excessive moisture creates an ideal wound environment for bacteria to proliferate especially when the host defense is compromised. Moisture is usually contraindicated in non-healable wounds; hydrating gels and moisture-retentive dressings (hydrocolloids) should usually be avoided if the wound is non-healable [13]. To contain and remove excess exudate from the wound, a plethora of absorbent dressings have been developed. Major categories of dressings include foams, alginates, and hydrofibers. When drainage volume exceeds the fluid handling capacity of a dressing, enzyme-rich and caustic exudate may spill over to wound margins causing maceration or tissue erosion (loss of part of the epidermis but maintaining an epidermal base) and pain [47]. Irritant dermatitis is not uncommon from the damage of wound effluent; topical steroids continue to be the mainstay therapy.

The moist and warm environment is also ideal for proliferation of fungi and yeast including Candida. Individuals with coexisting conditions that affect the immune system (such as diabetes mellitus, kidney disease, and hepatitis C) or receiving immunosuppressive drugs (e.g., steroids) or chemotherapy are more susceptible for fungal infection. In addition, antibiotic use may disrupt the normal ecology of skin flora permitting the overgrowth of fungi. Besides the typical raised red lesions with satellite lesions extending around the wound margin, the patient may complain of burning and itching. As a treatment option, Candida can be effectively treated with Nystatin, a polyene antifungal agent. For the treatment of infection related to dermatophytes or tinea, Terbinafine (Lamisil), an allylamine, has been shown to be the most effective. Clotrimazole cream (an azole) is only effective against 70–80 % of infections related to dermatophytes or yeasts but it also possesses anti-inflammatory and minor antibacterial properties.

SCALE: Skin Changes at Life's End

In 2008 an expert panel was established to formulate a consensus statement on Skin Changes At Life's End (SCALE) [10]. The panel consists of 18 internationally recognized key opinion leaders including clinicians, caregivers, medical researchers, legal experts, academicians, a medical writer, and leaders of professional organizations. The panel discussed the nature of SCALE, including the proposed concepts of the Kennedy Terminal Ulcer (KTU) and skin failure along with other end of life skin changes. The final consensus document and statements were edited and reviewed by the panel after the meeting. The document and statements were initially externally reviewed by 49 international distinguished reviewers. A modified Delphi process was used to determine the final statements and 52 international distinguished reviewers reached consensus on the final statements [48–50].

The skin is the body's largest organ and like any other organ is subject to a loss of integrity. It has an increased risk for injury due to both internal and external insults. The panel concluded that our current comprehension of skin changes that can occur at life's end is limited; that the SCALE process is insidious and difficult to prospectively determine; additional research and expert consensus is necessary; and contrary to popular myth, not all pressure ulcers are avoidable.

Specific areas requiring research and consensus include (1) the identification of critical etiological and pathophysiological factors involved in SCALE, (2) clinical and diagnostic criteria for describing conditions identified with SCALE, and (3) recommendations for evidence-informed pathways of care.

The statements from this consensus document (Fig. 10.3) are designed to facilitate the implementation of knowledge-transfer-into-practice techniques for quality patient outcomes. This implementation process should include interprofessional teams (clinicians, lay people, and policy makers) concerned with the care of individuals at life's end to adequately address the medical, social, legal, and financial ramifications of SCALE (Fig. 10.3).

The Ten SCALE Consensus Statements

Statement 1: Physiologic changes that occur as a result of the dying process may affect the skin and soft tissues and may manifest as observable (objective) changes in skin color, turgor, or integrity, or as subjective symptoms such as localized pain. These changes can be unavoidable and may occur with the application of appropriate interventions that meet or exceed the standard of care.

Statement 2: The plan of care and patient response should be clearly documented and reflected in the entire medical record. Charting by exception is an appropriate method of documentation.

Statement 3: Patient-centered concerns should be addressed including pain and activities of daily living.

Statement 4: Skin changes at life's end are a reflection of compromised skin (reduced soft tissue perfusion, decreased tolerance to external insults, and impaired removal of metabolic wastes).

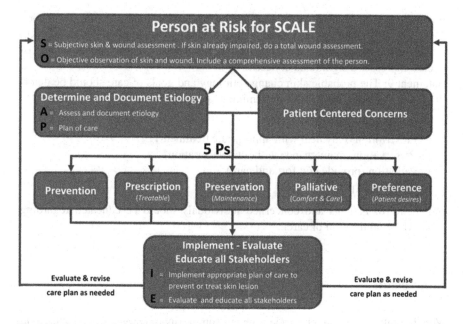

Fig. 10.3 Implementing SCALE: The SOAPIE mnemonic with the 5P enabler

Statement 5: Expectations around the patient's end of life goals and concerns should be communicated among the members of the interprofessional team and the patient's circle of care. The discussion should include the potential for SCALE including other skin changes, skin breakdown, and pressure ulcers.

Statement 6: Risk factors symptoms and signs associated with SCALE have not been fully elucidated, but may include:

- Weakness and progressive limitation of mobility
- Suboptimal nutrition including loss of appetite, weight loss, cachexia and wasting, low serum albumin/pre-albumin, and low hemoglobin as well as dehydration
- Diminished tissue perfusion, impaired skin oxygenation, decreased local skin temperature, mottled discoloration, and skin necrosis
- Loss of skin integrity from any of a number of factors including equipment or devices, incontinence, chemical irritants, chronic exposure to body fluids, skin tears, pressure, shear, friction, and infections
- Impaired immune function

Statement 7: A total skin assessment should be performed regularly and document all areas of concern consistent with the wishes and condition of the patient. Pay special attention to bony prominences and skin areas with underlying cartilage. Areas of special concern include the sacrum, coccyx, ischial tuberosities, trochanters, scapulae, occiput, heels, digits, nose, and ears. Describe the skin or wound abnormality exactly as assessed.

Statement 8: Consultation with a qualified healthcare professional is recommended for any skin changes associated with increased pain, signs of infection, skin breakdown (when the goal may be healing), and whenever the patient's circle of care expresses a significant concern.

Statement 9: The probable skin change etiology and goals of care should be determined. Consider the 5 Ps for determining appropriate intervention strategies:

- Prevention
- Prescription (may heal with appropriate treatment)
- Preservation (maintenance without deterioration)
- Palliation (provide comfort and care)
- Preference (patient desires)

Statement 10: Patients and concerned individuals should be educated regarding SCALE and the plan of care.

Conclusion

With the shifting demographics and growing complexity of chronic wounds, the principles of palliative wound care are becoming more relevant in clinical practice. Starting with an assessment of the whole person, it is important to maintain high quality of care, manage general symptoms, address psychosocial concerns, and implement strategies that minimize the unpleasant impact of living with a chronic wound.

References

1. Tippett A. An introduction to palliative chronic wound care. Ostomy Wound Manage. 2012;58(5):6.
2. Alvarez OM, Meehan M, Ennis W, Thomas DR, Ferris FD, Kennedy KL, et al. Chronic wounds: palliative management for the frail population. Wounds. 2002;14(10):13–8.
3. Emmons KR, Lachman VD. Palliative wound care: a concept analysis. J Wound Ostomy Continence Nurs. 2010;37(6):639–44. quiz 645–6.
4. O'Brien T, Welsh J, Dunn FG. ABC of palliative care. Non-malignant conditions. BMJ. 1998;316(7127):286–9.
5. Krasner DL, Rodeheaver G, Sibbald RG, Woo KY. International interprofessional wound caring. In: Krasner DL, Rodeheaver G, Sibbald RG, Woo KY, editors. Chronic would care 5: a clinical source book for healthcare professionals, vol. 1. HMP Communications, LLP: Malvern, PA; 2012. p. 3–24.
6. Manzano F, Navarro MJ, Roldan D, Moral MA, Leyva I, Guerrero C, et al. Pressure ulcer incidence and risk factors in ventilated intensive care patients. J Crit Care. 2010;25(3):469–76.
7. Langemo D. General principles and approaches to wound prevention and care at end of life: an overview. Ostomy Wound Manage. 2012;58(5):24–6. 30 passim.
8. Langemo DK, Black J. National pressure ulcer advisory P. Pressure ulcers in individuals receiving palliative care: a National Pressure Ulcer Advisory Panel white paper. Adv Skin Wound Care. 2010;23(2):59–72.

9. Wilczweski P, Grimm D, Gianakis A, Gill B, Sarver W, McNett M. Risk factors associated with pressure ulcer development in critically ill traumatic spinal cord injury patients. J Trauma Nurs. 2012;19(1):5–10.

10. Sibbald RG, Krasner DL, Lutz J. SCALE: skin changes at life's end: final consensus statement: October 1, 2009. Adv Skin Wound Care. 2010;23(5):225–36. quz 237–238.

11. Sibbald RG, Krasner DL, Woo KY. Pressure ulcer staging revisited: superficial skin changes & deep pressure ulcer framework(c). Adv Skin Wound Care. 2011;24(12):571–80. quiz 581–2.

12. Galvin J. An audit of pressure ulcer incidence in a palliative care setting. Int J Palliat Nurs. 2002;8(5):214–21.

13. Woo KY, Sibbald RG. Local wound care for malignant and palliative wounds. Adv Skin Wound Care. 2010;23(9):417–28. quiz 429–30.

14. Henoch I, Gustafsson M. Pressure ulcers in palliative care: development of a hospice pressure ulcer risk assessment scale. Int J Palliat Nurs. 2003;9(11):474–84.

15. Maida V, Ennis M, Kuziemsky C, Corban J. Wounds and survival in cancer patients. Eur J Cancer. 2009;45(18):3237–44.

16. F.R.A.I.L. Healing Probability Assessment Tool. 1999. http://www.frailcare.org/images/Palliative%20Wound%20Care.pdf.

17. Black JM, Edsberg LE, Baharestani MM, Langemo D, Goldberg M, McNichol L, et al. Pressure ulcers: avoidable or unavoidable? Results of the National Pressure Ulcer Advisory Panel Consensus Conference. Ostomy Wound Manage. 2011;57(2):24–37.

18. Vanderwee K, Grypdonck MHF, De Bacquer D, Defloor T. Effectiveness of turning with unequal time intervals on the incidence of pressure ulcer lesions. J Adv Nurs. 2007;57(1):59–68.

19. Krapfl LA, Gray M. Does regular repositioning prevent pressure ulcers? J Wound Ostomy Continence Nurs. 2008;35(6):571–7.

20. McInnes E, Bell-Syer SEM, Dumville JC, Legood R, Cullum NA. Support surfaces for pressure ulcer prevention. Cochrane Database Syst Rev. 2008;13(4), CD001735.

21. Dorner B, Posthauer ME, Thomas D, National Pressure Ulcer Advisory Panel. The role of nutrition in pressure ulcer prevention and treatment: National Pressure Ulcer Advisory Panel white paper. Adv Skin Wound Care. 2009;22(5):212–21.

22. Iizaka S, Okuwa M, Sugama J, Sanada H. The impact of malnutrition and nutrition-related factors on the development and severity of pressure ulcers in older patients receiving home care. Clin Nutr. 2010;29(1):47–53.

23. Beeckman D, Schoonhoven L, Verhaeghe S, Heyneman A, Defloor T. Prevention and treatment of incontinence-associated dermatitis: literature review. J Adv Nurs. 2009;65(6):1141–54.

24. Hodgkinson B, Nay R, Wilson J. A systematic review of topical skin care in aged care facilities. J Clin Nurs. 2007;16(1):129–36.

25. Woo KY, Krasner DL, Sibbald RG. Pain in people with chronic wounds: clinical strategies for decreasing pain and improving quality of life. In: Krasner DL, Rodeheaver G, Sibbald RG, Woo KY, editors. Chronic wound care 5: a clinical source book for healthcare professionals, vol. 1. Malvern, PA: HMP Communications, LLC; 2012. p. 85–96.

26. Dallam L, Smyth C, Jackson BS, Krinsky R, O'Dell C, Rooney J, et al. Pressure ulcer pain: assessment and quantification. J Wound Ostomy Continence Nurs. 1995;22(5):211–5. discussion 217–8.

27. Szor JK, Bourguignon C. Description of pressure ulcer pain at rest and at dressing change. J Wound Ostomy Continence Nurs. 1999;26(3):115–20.

28. Proctor WR, Hirdes JP. Pain and cognitive status among nursing home residents in Canada. Pain Res Manag. 2001;6(3):119–25.

29. Woo KY, Sibbald RG. The improvement of wound-associated pain and healing trajectory with a comprehensive foot and leg ulcer care model. J Wound Ostomy Continence Nurs. 2009;36(2):184–91. quiz 192–3.

30. Registered Nurses Association of Ontario. Assessment and management of pain. Toronto, ON: RegisteredNurses Association of Ontario; 2002.

31. Coutts P, Woo KY, Bourque S. Treating patients with painful chronic wounds. Nurs Stand. 2008;23(10):42–6.

32. Woo KY. Exploring the effects of pain and stress on wound healing. Adv Skin Wound Care. 2012;25(1):38–44. quiz 45–6.

33. Woo KY. The use of antimicrobial dressings in chronic wounds: NERDS and STONEES principles. Surg Technol Int. 2010;20:73–82.

34. Probst S, Arber A, Faithfull S. Malignant fungating wounds: a survey of nurses' clinical practice in Switzerland. Eur J Oncol Nurs. 2009;13(4):295–8.

35. Woo KY. Meeting the challenges of wound-associated pain: anticipatory pain, anxiety, stress, and wound healing. Ostomy Wound Manage. 2008;54(9):10–2.

36. Gibson MC, Keast D, Woodbury MG, Black J, Goettl L, Campbell K, et al. Educational intervention in the management of acute procedure-related wound pain: a pilot study. J Wound Care. 2004;13(5):187–90.

37. Paul JC, Pieper B, Templin TN. Itch: association with chronic venous disease, pain, and quality of life. J Wound Ostomy Continence Nurs. 2011;38(1):46–54.

38. Woo KY, Sibbald RG. The ABCs of skin care for wound care clinicians: dermatitis and eczema. Adv Skin Wound Care. 2009;22(5):230–6. quiz 237–8.

39. Langemo DK, Melland H, Hanson D, Olson B, Hunter S. The lived experience of having a pressure ulcer: a qualitative analysis. Adv Skin Wound Care. 2000;13(5):225–35.

40. Gorecki C, Brown JM, Nelson EA, Briggs M, Schoonhoven L, Dealey C, et al. Impact of pressure ulcers on quality of life in older patients: a systematic review. J Am Geriatr Soc. 2009;57(7):1175–83.

41. Upton D, Solowiej K, Hender C, Woo KY. Stress and pain associated with dressing change in patients with chronic wounds. J Wound Care. 2012;21(2):53–4. 56, 58 assm.

42. Lo SF, Hu WY, Hayter M, Chang SC, Hsu MY, Wu LY. Experiences of living with a malignant fungating wound: a qualitative study. J Clin Nurs. 2008;17(20):2699–708.

43. Woo KY, Harding K, Price P, Sibbald G. Minimising wound-related pain at dressing change: evidence-informed practice. Int Wound J. 2008;5(2):144–57.

44. Woo K, Sibbald G, Fogh K, Glynn C, Krasner D, Leaper D, et al. Assessment and management of persistent (chronic) and total wound pain. Int Wound J. 2008;5(2):205–15.

45. Paul JC, Pieper BA. Topical metronidazole for the treatment of wound odor: a review of the literature. Ostomy Wound Manage. 2008;54(3):18–27. quiz 28–9.

46. Nicks BA, Ayello EA, Woo K, Nitzki-George D, Sibbald RG. Acute wound management: revisiting the approach to assessment, irrigation, and closure considerations. Int J Emerg Med. 2010;3(4):399–407.

47. Cutting KF, White RJ. Maceration of the skin and wound bed. 1: its nature and causes. J Wound Care. 2002;11(7):275–8.

48. Skin Changes At Life's End Expert Panel. SCALE: skin changes at life's end. WOUNDS. 2009;21(12):329–36.

49. Krasner DL. Five FAQs about SCALE. Long term living Magazine 2010 Feb 26–27.

50. Sibbald RG, Krasner DL, Lutz J. Skin changes at life's end: part 1. Director. 2011;19(4):32–8.

Chapter 11
Quality of Care

Barbara M. Bates-Jensen and Janet Cheng

Abstract Pressure ulcer prevention and care is an indicator of quality care across all healthcare settings. Evaluating pressure ulcer quality of care is complicated by multiple quality indicators developed by multiple organizations which are applied in different care settings. Regulations related to pressure ulcer care in different care settings creates further complexity. While a wealth of pressure ulcer clinical practice guidelines exist, evidence of implementation of practice guidelines with sustainability is lacking. This chapter explores pressure ulcer quality of care. We review outcome and process measures related to pressure ulcer prevention, present current pressure ulcer regulations and quality indicators, and recommend specific strategies for implementing pressure ulcer prevention programs all of which are essential for improving pressure ulcer quality of care.

Keywords Pressure ulcer quality • Quality indicators • Pressure ulcer regulations • Implementation of pressure ulcer programs

Quality of care is an increasingly important concept as the USA focuses on cost containment in health care among its aging population. One area where the emphasis on improving the quality of care is evident in all healthcare settings is pressure ulcer prevention and care. Pressure ulcers are a highly complex, multifactorial, and costly global health problem common in all healthcare settings. The Joint Commission estimates that 2.5 million patients in US acute care hospitals are treated for pressure ulcers each year [1] and this number is likely to increase as the

B.M. Bates-Jensen, R.N., Ph.D. (✉)
Associate Professor, School of Nursing & David Geffen School of Medicine,
University of California, Los Angeles, USA
e-mail: bbatesjensen@sonnet.ucla.edu

J. Cheng, R.N., M.S.N., M.P.H.
School of Nursing, University of California, Los Angeles, USA

D.R. Thomas and G.A. Compton (eds.), *Pressure Ulcers in the Aging Population:*
A Guide for Clinicians, Aging Medicine 1, DOI 10.1007/978-1-62703-700-6_11,
© Springer Science+Business Media New York 2014

population ages. Unlike facility-specific conditions (such as surgical site infection or ventilator-associated pneumonia), pressure ulcers present across all care settings and patients, especially among geriatric populations.

Pressure ulcers are costly. Annual costs were estimated at $10.5–$17.8 billion for 2010. The cost for managing a single full-thickness pressure ulcer is as much as $70,000 [1]. One study reports the average hospital-associated costs for managing one full-thickness stage IV ulcer and related complications for one hospital admission at $129,248 and costs for managing a community-acquired stage IV ulcer over an average of four hospital admissions at $124,327 [2]. The Centers for Medicare and Medicaid Services (CMS) reports the cost of treating a pressure ulcer in acute care (as a secondary diagnosis) is $43,180.00 per hospital stay [3]. Contributing cost factors include increased length of stay due to pressure ulcer complications such as pain, infection, high tech support surfaces, and decreased functional ability [4]. The Agency for Healthcare Research and Quality (AHRQ) reported that pressure ulcer-related hospitalizations ranged from 13 to 14 days and cost $16,755–$20,430 compared to the average stay of 5 days and costs approximately $10,000 [5]. Healthcare utilization and costs of caring for persons with SCI who experience the complication of a severe (stage III/IV) pressure ulcer are high (in excess of $100k annually) [6]. Clearly there are considerable financial repercussions related to pressure ulcers. With so much at stake economically, it is no wonder that so much emphasis is being placed on the healthcare services clinicians provide related to pressure ulcer prevention care. Most importantly, how does one define quality as it relates to pressure ulcers? How can it be meaningfully quantified and how can clinicians incorporate quality pressure ulcer prevention care into the existing healthcare infrastructure?

This chapter will review outcome and process measures related to pressure ulcer prevention, pressure ulcer regulations and quality indicators, and specific strategies for implementing pressure ulcer prevention programs all of which are essential for improving quality of care for pressure ulcers.

Why Pressure Ulcers and Why Now?

Pressure ulcers are caused by multiple factors and require coordinated care delivered by multiple disciplines. As such, pressure ulcers have been considered a marker of quality within organizations. Pressure ulcers have long been a concern in nursing homes (NHs). In NHs, pressure ulcers are associated with morbidity, mortality, and other quality of care problems [7–11]. Estimates of the prevalence of pressure ulcers among NH residents range from 2 to 29 %, and incidence estimates are similar with higher rates reported in clinical studies and lower rates derived from data-based studies [9, 11–15]. Furthermore, pressure ulcer incidence increases over time with longer NH residency associated with increased pressure ulcer incidence [14, 15]. The major pressure ulcer care processes have been identified in practice guidelines [16–21] and in quality indicators [1, 22, 23]. Yet, pressure ulcers remain one of the most frequently cited deficiencies in NHs and pressure ulcers continue to be identified as a significant problem by the Government Accounting Office (GAO) and other federal agencies [2, 4, 24–27]. Furthermore, NHs with high rates of pressure ulcers are likely to also have other quality of care problems [7–9, 11]. Hence, pressure ulcer practice in NHs is highly regulated with pressure ulcer development one of three sentinel events that prompts external regulators to further assess quality of care in the nursing home and this has spawned multiple efforts directed at improving the quality of pressure ulcer care in NHs.

Pressure ulcers are not only a problem in NHs. In 2006, President Bush signed the Tax Relief and Health Care Act, which authorized CMS to establish and implement a physician quality reporting system, shifting from a fee-for-service to a pay-for-performance system [28]. Fee-for-service reimbursement pays physicians based on the number of services they perform; hence, the more services that physicians bill, the more they are paid. The pay-for-performance system attempts to tie reimbursement to patient outcomes, such that physicians are paid when their patients improve clinically, independent of the number of procedures performed. The difference between the two is that emphasis is placed on the value of healthcare services in the latter, rather than the volume of services in the former. Paramount to pay-for-performance is the determination of value in a way that is clinically relevant and practical for patients and clinicians. In an effort to encourage quality measure reporting, the Medicare Improvements for Patients and Providers Act of 2008 authorized a 2 % bonus for those who successfully *reported* quality measures, increasing the bonus to 4 % in 2011 [28].

President Obama signed in 2010 the Health Information Technology for Economic and Clinical Health (HITECH) Act. This mandate provides over $20 billion dollars to incentivize clinicians and hospitals to adopt health information technology (HIT). The Medicare Electronic Health Record Incentive Program pays up to a $44,000 bonus to each eligible provider who adopts and "meaningfully uses" an electronic medical record. Physicians who report their data are to be compensated by taking away money from the physicians who don't report, beginning in 2015. In 2015, non-reporting physicians will lose 1 % of their Medicare revenue, in 2016, they will see a 2 % deduction, and in 2017, a 3 % deduction [28].

The Patient Protection and Affordable Care Act signed into law in 2010 aims to curb overall costs of health care. Similar to the Tax Relief and Health Care Act of 2006, the Affordable Care Act focuses Medicare reimbursements on quality of care [29]. The law imposes penalties on 25 % of hospitals whose rate of hospital-acquired conditions are highest, resulting in a projected cost savings of $3.2 billion over 10 years [30]. Since pressure ulcers are considered a hospital-acquired condition, tighter regulations are being implemented that affect care reimbursements, spurring the interest in measuring quality of care.

Outcome and Process Measures

In the context of healthcare quality, pressure ulcer quality of care is primarily measured by examining prevalence and incidence data. Evaluation of hospital length of stay, cost factors, and mortality may also be used as measures of pressure

---

Box 11.1 Example of Prevalence Calculation for Prevalence of Patients Receiving a Risk Assessment on Admission

$$\begin{array}{l}\textit{Number / percentage of patients} \\ \textit{who received a pressure ulcer} \\ \textit{risk assessment upon admission}\end{array} = \frac{\begin{array}{l}\textit{Number of patients who have} \\ \textit{a pressure ulcer risk assessment} \\ \textit{completed during the admission process}\end{array}}{\textit{Number of patients admitted to the facility}}$$

Box 11.2 Example of Prevalence Calculation for Prevalence of Residents at Risk for Pressure Ulcers

$$\begin{array}{l}\textit{Number of residents who are} \\ \textit{at risk for a pressure ulcer}\end{array} = \frac{\begin{array}{l}\textit{Number of residents who have an} \\ \textit{at risk score on a risk assessment tool}\end{array}}{\begin{array}{l}\textit{Number of residents who have a} \\ \textit{completed risk assessment tool}\end{array}}$$

Box 11.3 Example of Incidence Calculation for Yearly Incidence of Hospital Acquired Stage III or IV Pressure Ulcers

$$\begin{array}{l}\textit{Incidence of stage III or IV} \\ \textit{pressure ulcers in 2011}\end{array} = \frac{\begin{array}{l}\textit{Number of patients who develop} \\ \textit{a stage III or IV while in the hospital}\end{array}}{\begin{array}{l}\textit{Number of patients admitted to the hospital} \\ \textit{from Jan 1 to Dec 31, 2011}\end{array}}$$

---

ulcer quality. Prevalence is defined as the proportion of a population found to have a condition, where the condition is the numerator and population is the denominator. Boxes 11.1 and 11.2 present two examples of calculations for the prevalence of patients who are at risk for pressure ulcers. Incidence measures the number of occurrences within the specified population over a length of time. Box 11.3 presents an example of the calculation for incidence of stage III and IV pressure ulcers.

Both prevalence and incidence are valuable in determining quality of care related to pressure ulcers. For example, if nursing home A has an incidence of 10 % in the last 3 months and implemented a quality improvement targeted at early identification, it can evaluate its effectiveness by comparing pressure ulcer incidence before the intervention at baseline and after the intervention. For example, Tippet used pressure ulcer incidence for the outcome measure of prevention efforts in a NH [31]. Pre-initiative average incidence data for this 151-bed facility was 5.19 % (168 ulcers over 3,234 person-months). Post-initiative average incidence data 4 years out was 0.73 % (47 ulcers over 6,446 person-months). The initiative involved training programs, implementation of care protocols, use of support surfaces and wound and skin products.

Prevalence may also be used as a measure of the effectiveness of pressure ulcer prevention programs, though this measure includes those patients who have a pressure ulcer already. Interpretation of effectiveness may need to take into account the *change* in prevalence rate, not necessarily overall prevalence rate. Prevalence studies are often conducted for a 1-day period, often termed point prevalence, which when conducted in acute care may inadvertently capture patients with longer lengths of stay. Patients with longer hospital stays may have higher acuity and thus greater risk of developing pressure ulcers. If prevalence includes evaluation of facility-acquired pressure ulcers, it provides a direct outcome measure similar to incidence.

Milne and colleagues used prevalence data to measure improvement in pressure ulcer care in the long-term acute care hospital (LTACH) setting [32]. They identified the need for quality improvement in pressure ulcer care, but found no data for LTACHs for use in benchmarking their facility data. The facility created a wound care team, developed a data collection form that included pressure ulcer assessment, risk, treatment, and care planning, and provided staff education. After the quality improvement initiative, monthly prevalence rates of pressure ulcers decreased by 37 %, and the mean facility-acquired pressure ulcer prevalence rates fell to 4.2 % from 41 % [32].

Another possible measure of quality in acute care is hospital length of stay. Length of hospital stay increases when pressure ulcers develop. Hospital stays principally for pressure ulcers are reported as slightly longer than hospital stays for those with a secondary pressure ulcer diagnosis (14.1 days versus 12.7 days) [5]. The length of stay for hospitalizations principally for pressure ulcers is reported as nearly three times longer than hospitalizations with no diagnosis of pressure ulcers (14.1 days versus 5.0 days). Data from the national Medicare Patient Safety Monitoring System database for hospitalized patients in 2006 and 2007 determined that: national hospital-acquired pressure ulcer (HAPU) incidence was 4.5 %, but significant variation between states existed, with higher incidence rates in the Northeast and Missouri [33]. HAPU development was significantly associated with higher in-hospital mortality (11.2 %), mortality 30 days after discharge (15.3 %), and longer hospital stays (11.6 ± 10.1 days for those with HAPU versus 4.9 ± 5.2 days for those without) [33].

Financial factors can also affect quality related to pressure ulcers. In a longitudinal study of US NHs between 1999 and 2005, a $10 a day increase in Medicaid reimbursement rates was associated with a 2.1 % decline in pressure ulcer incidence, even after taking the implementation of Medicaid case-mix reimbursement policies into account (reimbursement is positively correlated to patient acuity, the higher the population acuity, the higher the reimbursement amount) [34].

Process Versus Outcome Measures

For the purposes of comparing quality of health care, understanding the difference between process and outcome measures is important [35]. Process measures are more sensitive to quality of care because they are a *direct* measure of the care provided, whereas outcome measures *indirectly* measure care quality by measuring the supposed end product of care delivery. For example, a process measure related to pressure ulcer prevention is that all patients have a risk assessment conducted within 24 h of admission to the organization. This measures the action of the care providers, conducting the risk assessment, as opposed to the end product of the action, the outcome of pressure ulcer incidence. Process measures are most valuable if linked to an outcome measure; however, both process and outcome measures must be taken into account when considering quality of care. As an example, Zingmond et al. [36] demonstrated that higher quality of care as measured by meeting certain care processes was associated with improved functional status (the outcome measure) using routinely collected Medicare and Medicaid claims data. Care processes refer to the care provided to the patient if the patient was eligible for the criteria: for instance, patients who were at risk for atrial fibrillation or flutter would have received quality care if they received anticoagulation or antiplatelet therapy. If process and outcome data are collected successively, this data may be used to monitor the effect of interventions or changes in the healthcare system over time. This is similar to how CMS claims data has been used to evaluate quality of care [36]. Table 11.1 presents examples of process and outcome measures related to pressure ulcer screening, prevention, and treatment.

Outcome measures are affected by differences in patient type, data collection, quality of care, and chance. For example, pressure ulcer risk is quite different for critically ill adults compared to persons with spinal cord injury or nursing home residents, thus pressure ulcer incidence (the outcome measure) is different among the three populations. The most appropriate outcome measures to evaluate the effectiveness of pressure ulcer prevention programs are incidence and prevalence rates. When a prevention program is successful, the organization's incidence of pressure ulcer development should decrease or remain at a low level. Incidence and prevalence data should be risk adjusted by using risk-stratification techniques when gathering data. Risk stratification identifies individual risk factors that affect a person's probably for an outcome (in this case, pressure ulcers). For example, individual risk factors might be age, mobility, nutritional status, and comorbidities. Using risk stratification allows comparison of data with other healthcare facilities for benchmarking and adequate evaluation of prevention programs as case-mix of the organization varies over time. For patients who already have a pressure ulcer, an outcome for demonstrating successful pressure ulcer prevention is no further areas of skin breakdown. Again, risk-stratification techniques should be used so that data can be compared with other facilities and so that severity of pressure ulcers can be evaluated accurately.

Table 11.1 Examples of process and outcome measures for pressure ulcer care

	Process measures	Outcome measures
Prevention screening	Percent patients with risk assessment at 12 h	Percent of patients with PUs identified on admission (POA) within
	Percent patients with skin assessment	Percent of low risk patients who develop a PU
	Percent patients with mobility screening	
Prevention interventions for at-risk population	Percent patients with support surface within 6 h	Percent of high risk patients who develop PU
	Percent patients with nutritional assessment	Incidence
	Percent patients with mobility/repositioning plan	
Treatment	Percent with weekly wound assessment	Percent patients healed (by stage, st 2 in 60 days; full thickness in 12 weeks)
	Percent with minimum four wound characteristics documented (stage, size, location, appearance)	Time to healing
	Percent with necrosis who have debridement within X period of time	50 % wound size decrease by 4 weeks
		Percent who have PU which is new/worsened

Quality Indicators

Efforts to improve pressure ulcer quality of care have resulted in development of quality indicators for monitoring care processes in addition to monitoring of outcomes [22, 23, 25, 27, 37–43]. Quality indicators have been developed by multiple organizations for all healthcare settings. Understanding the quality indicators used in all healthcare settings is essential for improvement efforts and continuity of care. This is particularly true as more attention is focused on transitioning patients between care settings. Advancement of health information technology has spawned the electronic medical record, making it more feasible to gather and report data on quality along the health care continuum. Implementation of value-based purchasing is underway to transform the US health care infrastructure into an efficient, high quality, and economical healthcare system where patient information and quality data are transmitted seamlessly between care settings. In this section, quality indicators across all healthcare settings are first discussed and then setting specific indicators.

Quality Indicators Across All Health Care Settings

While multiple organizations have developed quality indicators and measures related to pressure ulcers, it is important to note that these quality measures across organizations and healthcare settings are not comparable, which makes evaluating the indicators and the meaning tied to each indicator difficult and complicated.

National Quality Forum

The National Quality Forum (NQF) is a private, nonprofit organization comprised of members from all sectors of the healthcare system whose mission is to improve the quality of the American healthcare system [37]. Endorsement of a healthcare performance measure by NQF, which involves a formal Consensus Development Process and evidence-based reviews, virtually guarantees the measure will become a gold standard in the healthcare system. Major healthcare payers use NQF-endorsed measures to determine reimbursement fees. A national quality measure system allows not only for comparison among facilities across regions but also across the continuum of care, as patients transition from an acute care setting to NH or home health. At this time, there are no quality measures endorsed by NQF related to pressure ulcers.

In addition to endorsement of quality measures, NQF also endorses a set of adverse events deemed serious reportable events (SREs), which refers to "...an event must be unambiguous, largely preventable, and serious, as well as adverse, indicative of a problem in a healthcare setting's safety systems, or important for public credibility or public accountability.... SREs that are entirely preventable and those that are largely preventable should be publicly reported" [38]. Twenty-nine SREs are listed under the seven areas of surgical/invasive procedures, product/device, patient protection, care management, environmental, radiological, and potential criminal events. The definition of an SRE associated with pressure ulcers is "any stage III, stage IV, and unstageable pressure ulcers acquired after admission/presentation to a healthcare setting" [39]. Pressure ulcers fall under care management SREs, among SREs such as patient death or serious injury related to falls, medication errors, unsafe administration of blood products, and failure to follow up or communicate test results [38]. The presence of pressure ulcers as a SRE denotes its importance as an outcome quality measure in health care.

The Joint Commission National Patient Safety Goals

The Joint Commission developed the National Patient Safety Goals (NPSGs) in 2002 to provide federal guidance to healthcare facilities on increasing patient safety and benchmarks [40]. A panel of health professionals, including nurses, physicians, pharmacists, risk managers, and others comprise the Patient Safety Advisory Group, which advises The Joint Commission on patient safety issues relevant to all healthcare settings. Currently, Goal 14 is the only goal that focuses on pressure ulcers: "Prevent healthcare-associated pressure ulcers (decubitus ulcers)" [41]. Because the Joint Commission accredits the majority of healthcare facilities, the National Patient Safety Goals are also used to benchmark quality. While goal 14 is currently only listed under guidelines for LTACHs, the goal has previously been applied to all health facilities.

The Assessing Care of Vulnerable Elders Quality Indicators

The Assessing Care of Vulnerable Elders (ACOVE) quality indicator set consists of explicit if–then rules (based on expert opinion and evidence) that, if adhered to, measure whether care provided meets a specified quality standard [22, 42, 43]. Now in its third rendition, ACOVE-3 includes 13 QIs related to pressure ulcers [43]. In the ACOVE project, care processes empirically related to positive outcomes or recommended in practice guidelines were converted into indicators and validated by expert consensus methodology [44]. The ACOVE quality indicators provide a baseline for measures that may discriminate between quality and substandard care.

The ACOVE indicators cover pressure ulcer measures in risk assessment, preventive intervention, pressure ulcer assessment, and pressure ulcer management appropriate for any healthcare setting [22]. The three risk assessment measures require that a pressure ulcer risk assessment using a standardized scale should be performed upon admission and at regular intervals (48 h for hospitals, weekly then quarterly for NHs, and weekly then biweekly for home health) if the patient is found to be at risk for pressure ulcers. Preventive interventions are targeted to patients at risk for pressure ulcers; interventions should include pressure reduction and/or repositioning strategies, and nutritional assessment and support if the patient is also at risk for malnutrition. For patients who already have a pressure ulcer, the pressure ulcer assessment dictates that the pressure ulcer documentation should include location, depth/stage, size, and wound bed and any pressure ulcer pain should be assessed and treated. The pressure ulcer management indicators provide guidance on treating pressure ulcers based on stage, wound bed characteristics, and post-treatment time. Table 11.2 shows the ACOVE indicators.

Quality Indicators in Acute Care Settings

In acute care settings, three main organizations provide quality indicators and measures: the National Database of Nursing Quality Indicators (NDNQI), the Collaborative Alliance for Nursing Outcomes (CALNOC), and the CMS. CALNOC and NDNQI both target pressure ulcers as a nursing-sensitive or nursing-specific quality measure. The CMS targets HAPU in a general, more punitive fashion (i.e., lack of reimbursement for stage III or IV HAPUs) and public reporting of HAPU rates.

The National Database of Nursing Quality Indicators

The NDNQI is a national project established by the American Nurses Association in 1998 to monitor quality indicators in hospitalized patients that are nursing sensitive.

Table 11.2 ACOVE pressure ulcer quality indicators for vulnerable elders (VE) [42]

Indicator	IF	THEN
Risk assessment		
	1. IF a VE who is admitted to a hospital is unable to reposition himself or herself or has limited ability to do so	THEN risk assessment for PUs using a standardized scale should be performed upon admission, and if the patient is found to be at risk, the assessment should be repeated at least every 48 h thereafter
	2. IF a VE is admitted to a skilled nursing facility	THEN risk assessment for PUs using a standardized scale should be performed upon admission, every week during the first 4 weeks and every 3 months thereafter
	3. IF a VE is admitted to a home healthcare organization	THEN risk assessment for PUs using a standardized scale should be performed upon admission, and if the patient is found to be at risk, then weekly for 4 weeks and every other week thereafter
Preventive intervention		
	4. IF a VE is identified as at risk for PU development or presents with a PU	THEN preventive interventions should be instituted that address pressure reduction (or management of tissue loads) and repositioning needs
	5. IF a VE who is at risk for PU development or has a PU also demonstrates malnutrition	THEN a nutritional assessment to identify nutritional deficiencies and nutrition support should be provided
PU assessment		
	6. IF a VE presents with a PU	THEN the PU should be assessed for the following wound characteristics. Location Depth and stage Size Wound bed (e.g., necrotic tissue, exudates, wound edges for undermining and tunneling, presence or absence of granulation and epithelialization)
	7. IF a VE has a PU	THEN he or she should be assessed for PU pain daily in the hospital and at each outpatient visit, and the pain should be treated, if present
PU management		
	8. IF a VE presents with a full-thickness PU covered with necrotic debris or eschar (unless dry eschar presents on the heel)	THEN debridement interventions using sharp, mechanical, enzymatic, biosurgery, or autolytic procedures should be instituted within 24 h
	9. IF a VE presents with a PU that is clean or free of necrotic tissue	THEN wound cleansing with normal saline or a noncytotoxic cleanser should be instituted at each dressing change

(continued)

Table 11.2 (continued)

Indicator	IF	THEN
	10. IF a VE presents with a clean full-thickness or partial thickness PU	THEN a moisture-retentive topical dressing such as thin-film dressings, hydrocolloids, hydrogels, foams, or alginates should be provided for treatment and not dry gauze in any form
	11. IF a VE with a full-thickness stage III or IV PU presents with systemic signs and symptoms of infection, such as elevated temperature, elevated white blood count, and confusion and agitation, and it is likely the sepsis is due to the wound	THEN the PU should be debrided to eliminate necrotic debris within 24 h, and a tissue biopsy, needle aspiration, or quantitative swab after debridement should be obtained for bacterial culture and appropriate systemic antibiotics initiated
	12. IF a VE presents with a clean full-thickness stage III or IV PU at 2–4 weeks post-treatment with no improvement in PU status (e.g., decrease in surface area or depth or according to standardized wound healing tool score)	THEN the appropriateness of the treatment plan and presence of complications should be reassessed
	13. IF a VE presents with a partial-thickness stage II PU at 1–2 weeks post-treatment with no improvement in PU status	THEN the appropriateness of the treatment plan and presence of complications should be reassessed
Related QIs for PUs		
Mobilization of hospital Patient (Hosp #7)	7. IF a VE who is ambulatory as an outpatient is hospitalized for longer than 48 h and is not receiving intensive or palliative care	THEN there should be a plan to increase mobility within 48 h of admission
Mobilization of postoperative patient (Hosp #27)	POSTOPERATIVE CARE Mobilization 27. IF a VE who was ambulatory as an outpatient has major surgery and is not in intensive care	THEN ambulation should be performed by postoperative day 2

In 2000, the NDNQI added HAPUs as one of the patient safety and quality of care indicators to monitor in participant hospitals. Hospital sites in 2011 include 1,721 hospitals in 50 states. Participating institutions collect data by medical record abstraction and direct skin assessments and enter it into a secure Web site [45]. Hospitals pay fees to participate and have access to unit-level performance comparison reports to state, national, and regional percentile distributions. All indicator data are reported quarterly at the nursing unit level and reflect the structure, process, and outcomes of nursing care. Participating hospitals use the NDNQI data as quality measures, outcomes of quality improvement efforts, and benchmark performance to other participating facilities. The NDNQI also provides online education on pressure ulcers [44, 46].

The Collaborative Alliance for Nursing Outcomes

Similar to NDNQI, The CALNOC is a nonprofit organization that accumulates nursing-sensitive indicators into a national registry database that provides patient outcomes to guide healthcare professionals [47]. Indicators include unit data (type of unit), structural measures (ratio, staff mix, RN characteristics, unit admissions/transfers/discharges), process measures, and outcome measures (HAPUs by stage). Registered nurses enter data and participating institutions have access to benchmarking. Participating CALNOC hospitals have reduced their HAPU rates from 10 to 2.8 % [47]. CALNOC meets Regulatory Compliance and Accreditation requirements—CALNOC is a recognized registry for the Centers for Medicare and Medicaid Services and Joint Commission. In addition, CALNOC has been approved for Magnet Qualification. Awarded by the American Nurses Credentialing Center, Magnet designation started in 1990 as a means of recognizing hospitals that offer excellent nursing care. Since then, only 258 of the nation's 7,569 hospitals have been designated as Magnet hospitals [48]. One of the qualifications for magnet status is that nurses are engaged with quality improvement practices and quality outcomes [48]. Hospitals that participate in CALNOC or NDNQI use their participation as evidence of the requirement.

The Centers for Medicaid and Medicare Services

The 2005 Deficit Reduction Act required that Health and Human Services identify health conditions that (1) were high cost, high volume, or both; (2) resulted in higher payment when presented as a secondary diagnosis; and (3) could reasonably have been prevented through implementation of evidence-based guidelines [49] in the acute care setting. The current hospital-acquired conditions (HACs) incorporate 11 categories, including HAPUs that are stage III or IV. Any care provided to treat a HAC is not reimbursable by Medicare unless the HAC was documented as present on admission. In the case of pressure ulcers, care provided for patients who present to the acute care setting without a pressure ulcer documented on admission or were not admitted with pressure ulcer as the admitting diagnosis and are treated for a stage III or IV pressure ulcer will not be reimbursable. A hospital's HAPU rates are reportable to CMS, who then makes the data available on consumer websites for public knowledge.

Quality Indicators for NHs

The Minimum Data Set (MDS) is part of the federally mandated process for clinical assessment of all residents admitted in Medicare or Medicaid-certified NHs. The entire process, called the Resident Assessment Instrument (RAI), provides a comprehensive assessment of each resident's functional capabilities and helps NH facility staff identify health problems. The RAI–MDS has been adopted by other countries for use in long-term care facilities to standardize assessment data and improve quality of care-based quality indicators. The MDS was not originally designed as a quality measurement instrument, but researchers have used data from the MDS to develop quality indicators [23, 50]. MDS-derived quality indicators have been tested and provide a basis for quality improvement efforts in long-term care. MDS quality indicator data is reported on public Web sites for all Medicare-certified NHs in the USA [51] Quality indicators are calculated according to the presence or absence of a particular indicator for an individual. The data for all individuals in a facility are summed providing a facility level measure of the quality indicator. Some indicators are calculated based on prevalence (e.g., percent of residents bedfast) and others are calculated based on incidence (e.g., percent of short-stay residents with pressure ulcers that are new). Quality indicators related to pressure ulcers include the percent of short-stay residents with pressure ulcers that are new or worsened and percent of long-stay high-risk residents with pressure ulcers [52]. Using MDS data to compute indicators of care quality for use in quality improvement programs has been problematic. Stevenson and Mor [53] evaluated quality indicators by using the CMS identified target NHs (pressure ulcer rates greater than 20 % or restraint rates greater than 11 % in study period) and analyzing the target NH facility characteristics, performance on other quality indicators (pain, low risk for pressure ulcer, high risk for pressure ulcer, weight loss, restraints, UTI, indwelling catheters, incontinence, activity of daily living decline, deficiencies on prior performance) and whether status as targeted NHs would have differed in previous years. While one in four NHs was targeted in the US, the geographical spread throughout the US was skewed. Targeted NHs were not necessarily poor performers on other quality indicators, suggesting that had other indicators been selected as targets by the CMS, different NHs would have been targeted. Finally, changes over time in NH target status did not address NH performance changes over time [53]. Thus, poor scores on a single quality indicator if used to target improvement activities for a facility can mask that the facility can perform well on other quality indicators while performing poorly on the target indicator [53]. Further, performance of individual facilities on a specific quality indicator may change with time. This complicates the interpretation of the MDS-derived quality indicators.

Several studies of MDS quality indicators related to pressure ulcer care provide examples of the complexity associated with the MDS-derived quality indicators. Bates-Jensen and colleagues [54] compared NHs that scored in the highest and lowest quartile for the MDS bedfast quality indicator. Based on interviews and hourly direct observations, the proportion of time that bedfast patients were found in bed in higher prevalence bedfast NHs was significantly higher, as was observed activity and reported mobility assistance, than the same measures for bedfast patients in lower prevalence bedfast NHs, though the RAI–MDS bedfast indicator was underreported across all NH facilities. They concluded that while the MDS bedfast quality indicator discriminated facilities in which residents spent greater time confined to bed, it failed to identify differences in activity and mobility as those NHs with higher bedfast quality indicator scored provided more activity and mobility assistance.

The same research group found that NHs with lower rates on incontinence quality indicators (prevalence of incontinence and prevalence of incontinence without toileting plan) had significantly higher documentation for evaluation of incontinence history and for toileting assistance by staff [55]. There was no difference in frequency of scheduled toileting assistance for incontinent residents rated as receiving assistance compared to those rated as not receiving assistance, indicating no association between care process and MDS incontinence quality indicators [55]. The studies evaluating the MDS-derived quality indicators have all evaluated the MDS 2.0. With the advent of the MDS 3.0, MDS-derived quality indicators may be easier to understand and new quality indicators may be developed.

While not quality indicators themselves, the skin assessment data on the MDS provides data on pressure ulcer care in NHs. The current version, MDS 3.0, collects data that include pressure ulcer risk assessment, presence of pressure ulcers on admission, number of new, healed, and unhealed pressure ulcers, and classification of each pressure ulcer including the categories of suspected deep tissue injury and unstageable [45, 56].

Quality Indicators for Long-Term Acute Care Hospitals

For LTACHs, the CMS has provided the Long-Term Care Hospital Continuity Assessment Record & Evaluation (CARE) Data Set to collect pressure ulcer quality measures [57]. The dataset gathers information on medical complexity and status (medical diagnoses, comorbid conditions, major treatments during stay, medications, skin integrity, and physiologic factors), functional status (impairments including bladder and bowel, swallowing, vision, hearing, weight-bearing status, respiratory status, self-care, mobility, medication management, and IADLs), cognitive status (memory/recall, delirium, confusion, behavioral symptoms, including depression, and presence of pain), and social support (structural barriers in the home, living situation, caregiver availability, need for assistance, and discharge complications).

How Can Consumers Use Quality Indicators?

Resources are available to help consumers understand quality improvement efforts. The CMS has provided an online database [58] that can guide consumers in choosing hospitals, NHs, home health agencies, and even medical equipment suppliers and healthcare plans. The tool breaks down the numbers such that consumers can easily interpret comparison charts among their results. For example, using Nursing Home Compare [59], a consumer can look at the percent of short-stay NH residents with pressure ulcers that are new or worsened and compare the facility's percentage to state and national averages. A reminder under each heading informs the consumer whether a high or low number is better, allowing the consumer to quickly compare results rather than learning how ratios are determined. Hospital Compare [60] gathers similar pressure ulcer data, quantifying the incidence of pressure ulcers per 1,000 patient discharges for each hospital against the national average (for example, 0.241 pressure ulcers per 1,000 patient discharges against the national incidence of 0.136 pressure ulcers per 1,000 patient discharges). Again, consumers just need to know in this case that lower numbers are better.

Regulations and Quality Indicators: What Drives What?

The driving force behind regulations is reimbursement for medical care and public and patient safety, which is different from the forces behind development of quality indicators. The two are often confused; there is a distinct difference between quality indicators and regulations. Regulations have evolved over time and are often the result of extreme events. Regulations develop because of financial concerns and ethical care issues often related to safety. Quality indicators develop from scientific evidence over time. While quality indicators are developed using a different model than regulations, regulations often use quality indicator data as performance measures to evaluate compliance with particular care processes.

Each healthcare setting sets forth regulations to monitor and report pressure ulcer-related events. The increasing shift of value over volume in healthcare services has spurred compliance to setting-specific regulations to receive reimbursement. These regulations are prime motivators that have driven the development of quality indicators to monitor quality of care. General regulations in acute care, LTACHs, and NHs are discussed. The following are several settings and their regulations.

Acute Care Hospitals

The CMS oversees the regulations that dictate healthcare reimbursement by Medicare. Those regulations related to pressure ulcers include performing a risk assessment on each patient at admission including but not limited to skin, nutrition, and activity level; documentation of existing ulcers at admission and treatments utilized; and prevention strategies for patients without pressure ulcers on admission. Regulations also dictate that facilities will not be reimbursed for treatment of stage III or IV pressure ulcers if the pressure ulcer developed during that admission [61].

The Deficit Reduction Act of 2005 mandated that any treatment provided for HACs not present on admission would not be reimbursed. The healthcare provider must be able to prove that the HAC was present on admission through medical records or in the case of pressure ulcers, that the pressure ulcer was the patient's primary diagnosis. Should the pressure ulcer be billed as a secondary diagnosis, there must be proof that the pressure ulcer was unavoidable. There are no clear regulations for determining when a pressure ulcer is avoidable in the acute care setting. However, in February 2010, the National Pressure Ulcer Advisory Panel (NPUAP) hosted a conference to establish consensus on whether there are individuals in whom pressure ulcer development may be unavoidable and whether a difference exists between end-of-life skin changes and pressure ulcers [62]. Unavoidable pressure ulcers are determined after the fact and refer to those pressure ulcers that develop among patients where pressure cannot be relieved, nutrition cannot be delivered, or those persons who are hemodynamically unstable [62].

Long-Term Acute Care Hospitals

A long-term acute care hospital (LTACH) refers to "a hospital [which] must have a provider agreement with Medicare and must have an average Medicare inpatient length of stay of greater than 25 days" [63]. Since no standardized datasets were being used in LTACHs, healthcare facilities that bridge the gap in the care continuum between acute care and NHs, the CMS developed the Long-Term Care Hospital Continuity Assessment Record & Evaluation (LTACH CARE) Data Set to collect data for pressure ulcers among these facilities [63], based on the MDS 3.0 and CARE tool (Continuity Assessment Record & Evaluation). The LTACH CARE dataset is the first standardized dataset used in the LTACH setting and includes measures on pressure ulcer documentation, selected factors related to pressure ulcers, and patient demographic information [64]. Pressure ulcers (i.e., the percent of patients with one or more stage II–IV pressure ulcers that are new or have worsened), are one of the three initial measures reported to the CMS that began in October 2012, with Section M focusing on skin conditions. Unlike NHs, LTACHs must complete an admission assessment within 3 days of admission (NHs have 14 days to complete an initial assessment) and complete the LTACH CARE dataset within 5 additional days [65] for all patients, regardless of payer. The CMS has incorporated NQF-endorsed measures in the initial reporting system for LTACHs (with more measures to be added in 2014) and this emphasizes the CMS's initiative to improve health care quality and pressure ulcer care quality across all settings.

Nursing Homes

Federal regulations by the CMS dictate that NHs "must ensure that—(1) A resident who enters the facility without pressure ulcers does not develop pressure ulcers unless the individual's clinical condition demonstrates that they were unavoidable; and (2) A resident having pressure ulcers receives necessary treatment and services to promote healing, prevent infection and prevent new sores from developing" [62, 65]. Pressure ulcers are further categorized into avoidable and unavoidable for the NH setting [65]:

- "Avoidable" = the NH staff failed to do one or more of the following: assess clinical condition, conduct pressure ulcer risk assessment, implement prevention strategies, monitor and evaluate the impact of the interventions; or revise the interventions as appropriate.
- "Unavoidable" = the resident developed a pressure ulcer even though the NH staff assessed the clinical condition, conducted a pressure ulcer risk assessment; defined and implemented prevention interventions; monitored and evaluated the impact of the interventions; and revised as appropriate [65].

For any NH to be reimbursed by the CMS, they must complete the Resident Assessment Instrument (RAI) process within 14 days of admission, annually and when there is a significant change in status [66, 67]. The CMS mandates that this assessment must include the MDS, a set of core measures that must be included within each assessment. As noted earlier, currently in version 3.0, the MDS requires more specific data related to pressure ulcers.

F-tag 314 refers to the federal regulation that determines compliance with pressure ulcer prevention and treatment [65, 67]. F-tag 314 explains the intent of the law, defines terms, and provides instructions on determining compliance. Surveyors who visit the NH use the protocol outlined in F-tag 314 to determine NH facility compliance, where compliance to the regulation means that that the standard is met. Noncompliance may lead to additional investigation of other potential noncompliance within the NH.

Can We Measure Quality of Pressure Ulcer Care by Evaluating Quality Indicators? Do Quality Indicators Reflect Care Quality?

Quality of care may not be directly measured using quality indicators. Process measures are better more direct measures of quality of care as they provide data on actual care delivery. There is not necessarily a direct relationship between care delivery or process measures and quality indicators. This is most noticeable in using the MDS-derived quality indicators in NHs. For example, Rapp and colleagues [68] found that NHs with low prevalence of pressure ulcers did not self report more guideline-recommended interventions compared to those with high prevalence of pressure ulcers. When using direct observation as compared to self-report data or medical record data, the questionable relationship between quality indicators and care delivery is more pronounced.

Bates-Jensen and colleagues studied NHs in the highest and lowest quartile for the MDS pressure ulcer quality indicator to evaluate if facilities with lower pressure ulcer quality indicator scores provided better pressure ulcer care [69]. Care processes were measured from medical record data, direct observation, and use of wireless movement monitors to quantify repositioning activity. They found no differences between high and low pressure ulcer quality indicator NHs for most pressure ulcer care processes with the exception of more frequent use of pressure reducing support surfaces in the high pressure ulcer quality indicator NHs. Of interest, repositioning for residents unable to self-reposition was not routinely performed at 2-hour intervals based on the movement monitor data despite medical record documentation that indicated 2-hour repositioning was occurring for nearly all residents. They concluded the MDS pressure ulcer quality indicator was not an accurate measure of the quality of pressure ulcer care delivery [69]. These findings are similar for other related quality indicators. NHs identified as performing in the upper quartile of the MDS bedfast quality indicator had a higher proportion of bedfast residents and more residents at risk for physical decline, direct observation verified this finding. No differences were shown between NHs with high MDS bedfast quality indicator scores and those NHs with low MDS bedfast quality indicator scores. Significant differences between the two groups of NHs existed based on direct observation of time residents spent in bed. In addition residents who required moderate to complete assistance for transfer or bed mobility were 4.4 times more likely to be observed in bed more than 50 % of the time; those who could not stand and bear weight were 5.4 times more likely to be found in bed more than 50 % of the time compared to those who could. Residents in high bedfast homes who required physical assistance or were totally dependent were 3.5 times more likely to be found in bed compared to their counterparts in lower performing NHs [54].

Can We Improve Quality of Pressure Ulcer Care?

While there are number of quality improvement organizations as described previously, the CMS contracts with regional and state quality improvement organizations (QIOs) to review medical care and implement improvements to quality of care for all Medicare beneficiaries across health care settings [70]. QIOs have been instrumental in evaluating the quality of care related to pressure ulcers especially in the NH setting. In fact, improving pressure ulcer care has been part of the past ten statements of work (the language for the CMS QIO contracts) [70]. In most cases, a collaborative approach is used where organizational leaders and direct care staff learn from each other as they progress through quality improvement plan–do–study–act processes and then progress is measured by evaluating pressure ulcer outcomes such as prevalence and incidence. Several investigators have used similar approaches with success. Horn and colleagues [71] conducted an observational study of 11 NHs that implemented a standardized certified nurse assistant (CNAs) documentation tool that incorporated best-practice information found that the high risk pressure ulcer quality measure (a prevalence measure that includes admissions with pressure ulcers and pressure ulcers that develop after admission) decreased

33 % from baseline, while the incidence of pressure ulcers decreased from 12.1 to 4.6 % after tool implementation. The success of the Horn and colleagues study demonstrates the effect of and need for standardized documentation and communication across all NHs that is easily collected by front line staff (e.g., CNAs) and easily interpreted by management to implement change processes [71].

Several investigators have looked at pressure ulcer outcome measures after quality improvement programs [72–76]. Rantz and colleagues evaluated Medicaid-certified facilities in Missouri deemed "at risk" for quality that voluntarily enrolled in a quality improvement program which included staff education, clinical site visits, guidance on evidence-based guidelines, and assessment tools [73]. Rates of pressure ulcer prevalence and pressure ulcer prevalence among high risk residents improved by 21 % and 26 %, respectively, after implementation of the quality improvement program. Limitations of this study included self-selection of NHs into the quality improvement program, based on prevalence data, which does not control for case-mix or variation over time. This limitation is similar for many of the QIO or collaborative-based intervention studies as in most cases the NHs self-select into the program.

Some investigators have looked at use of technology as a method of improving pressure ulcer quality. Baier and colleagues [74] evaluated NHs using a Web-based tool (Setting Targets Achieving Results-STAR) that tracks and provides feedback on six quality measures; the tool collects longitudinal data, provides information to help select annual quality indicator performance targets, and tracks improvement over time. NHs using the STAR tool were grouped into ambitious and less ambitious categories based on percent of improvement over time on the pressure ulcer quality measure. On average, NHs with ambitious targets were 9 times more likely to improve on the pressure ulcer quality measure than those with less ambitious targets [74]. Similarly Sharkey and colleagues [75] evaluated NHs in Washington DC that implemented an On-Time quality indicator tool, which provides clinical decision making tools, strategies for tool use, and guided facilitation for frontline NH staff. NHs were categorized into three levels of implementation for analysis. Those NHs with high levels of implementation (and better outcomes) were associated with greater team participation in workgroup calls (especially from top leadership), presence of an internal champion, and team willingness to trial and redesign process improvements [75].

Other investigators have examined the relationships between quality and staffing. Temkin-Greener and colleagues [76] explored the relationship between NHs work environment and risk of pressure ulcers and incontinence. Residents in NHs who had higher staff cohesion (the extent to which staff are perceived to have common goals, values, and strong group identity) had significantly lower odds of pressure ulcers and incontinence. There was no association between consistent assignments or prevalence of formally organized teams with pressure ulcers and incontinence. Interestingly, a 1 percent higher prevalence of self-managed teams resulted in a 2.3 % decrease in the odds of having a pressure ulcer, leveling off at 12 %, though team dynamics did not affect incontinence [76].

In most cases, multipronged and multidisciplinary pressure ulcer prevention approaches have also led to improvements in pressure ulcer prevalence and incidence rates in acute care and LTACHs as well as NHs [77, 78]. Most studies evaluating pressure ulcer prevention interventions evaluate recurring components of pressure ulcer prevention programs including pressure redistribution (repositioning and use of support surfaces), nutritional assessment and support, incontinence management, skin hygiene, inspection, and assessment [77, 78]. These programs are implemented using a wide variety of approaches [79–101] including: clinical performance monitoring and feedback [79–83, 85, 90, 92, 98], skin care champions [80, 83, 84, 86, 89, 90, 93–95], educational support materials [83–88, 90, 92, 93, 95–97] (including stickers [82, 83, 85, 89], turn clocks [79] pocket guides [83, 85, 88], newsletters [84, 85, 95], posters [85, 88], theme songs [79, 80, 83], and penlights [98]), protocol development [80, 82, 83, 86, 88, 90, 94, 99, 100], risk assessment [79, 81–83, 86, 88, 89, 91, 95, 96, 100, 101], staff education [79–82, 84–91, 93–101], bed support surfaces [83, 86, 88, 90, 91, 95, 96, 100, 101], and use of skin teams [80, 83, 84, 86, 89, 90, 93, 95]. Outcomes reported in these studies include both prevalence and incidence. Very few studies measured care processes [92–95, 97] which may further delineate why an intervention is successful. The difficulties with most of these studies are no comparison groups, few process measurements, and no measure of sustainability of programs with continued improvement in pressure ulcer quality indicators but they do provide persuasive evidence that pressure ulcer care can be improved.

Quality Indicators and Clinical Practice Guidelines

"Quality indicators are not the same as practice guidelines; care not meeting the standards set by quality indicators almost certainly represents poor-quality care. Practice guidelines, in contrast, strive to define optimal care in the context of complex medical decision-making. Furthermore, this comprehensive set of quality indicators is designed to measure care at the level of the health system, health plan, or medical group."—Wenger et al. [43]

What is the difference between guidelines and quality indicators? As Wenger et al. [43] suggest, guidelines are evidence-based *best* practice, which is constantly being updated as more research becomes available. Quality indicators, on the other hand, comprise the baseline, or the *minimum*, standard of care. For example, to prevent pressure ulcers, patients should be repositioned at routine intervals to offset the friction and load on any one body part. If a nursing home resident is bedridden and is turned every 3 hours by staff, that resident is receiving the *minimum* standard of care for pressure ulcer prevention. However, if the resident is turned every hour (perhaps an eager nursing student is present that day), this not only meets the standard of scheduled repositioning but also exceeds it since the resident is being turned more than what is considered the minimal standard. Thus, an unmet quality indicator is a failure to provide standard care compared to an unmet clinical practice guideline, which is a failure to provide best care.

Multiple clinical practice guidelines for pressure ulcers exist and they can be overwhelming in terms of the number of recommendations typically included in each guideline. Table 11.3 presents selected organizations pressure ulcer clinical

Table 11.3 Selected pressure ulcer clinical practice guidelines

Organization (National Guideline Clearinghouse reference #)	Guideline	Outcomes
NPUAP EPUAP (2009) (NGC 8204)	Evaluation/Treatment/Management Classification of pressure ulcers Assessment and monitoring of healing Assessment of the individual Pressure ulcer assessment Methods for monitoring healing Providing adequate nutritional support Pain assessment and management Education of individuals, family, and healthcare providers in pain management Support surfaces and positioning for treatment of pressure ulcers Positioning while in bed and in a chair Interventions for critically ill individuals, spinal cord-injured individuals, bariatric individuals Wound cleansing Debridement Dressings (e.g., hydrocolloid, transparent film, hydrogel, alginate) Assessment and treatment of infection Biophysical agents in pressure ulcer management (e.g., electrical stimulation, electromagnetic agents, phototherapy, acoustic energy, hydrotherapy) Biological dressings (insufficient evidence to recommend) Growth factors (insufficient evidence to recommend) Surgery for pressure ulcers Pressure ulcer management in individuals receiving palliative car, including patient and risk assessment, pressure redistribution, nutrition and hydration Control of wound odor	Incidence and prevalence of pressure ulcers Hospital lengths of stay, readmission rates, and hospital charges Infections Morbidity and mortality

(continued)

Table 11.3 (continued)

Organization (National Guideline Clearinghouse reference #)	Guideline	Outcomes
NPUAP, EPUAP (2009) (NGC 8145)	Risk assessment Establishing a risk assessment policy Educating staff in risk assessment Documentation of risk assessment Use of structured approach to risk assessment (e.g., use of Braden and other standard scales) Consideration of factors involved in pressure ulcer development: Nutritional indicators Factors affecting perfusion and oxygenation Skin moisture Advanced age Skin assessment Friction and shear risks (Subscale Braden Scale) Sensory perception (Subscale Braden Scale) General health status Development of pressure ulcer prevention plan Prevention Ensuring comprehensive skin assessment policy is in place Educating staff in skin assessment Performing regular skin assessments, noting areas of heat, edema, induration Skin care, including use of emollients and avoidance of massage, friction, and excessive moisture Nutrition for pressure ulcer prevention Nutritional screening and assessment Providing nutritional support Offering high-protein mixed oral nutritional supplements and/or tube feeding Administering oral nutritional supplements (ONS) and/or tube feeding (TF) Repositioning for the prevention of pressure ulcers Technique in bed and in seated positions Frequency of repositioning Documentation of repositioning Education and training of all involved in care	Incidence and prevalence of pressure ulcers Hospital lengths of stay, readmission rates, and hospital charges Infections Morbidity and mortality

	Use of support surfaces	Incidence and prevalence of pressure ulcers
	Appropriateness and functionality of the support surfaces	Efficacy of intervention for preventing the development of pressure ulcers, and facilitating wound healing
	Use of high-specification foam mattresses	Validity of tools used to assess patients at risk and pressure ulcer healing
	Alternating-pressure active support overlays and replacement mattresses	Morbidity
	Heel and elbow protection devices	Cost
	Pressure-redistributing seat cushion	
	Natural sheepskin pads	
	Special considerations for patients in the operating room	
	Risk assessment of individuals undergoing surgery	
	Using pressure-redistributing mattresses on the operating table	
	Positioning of the patient	
WOCN (2010) (NGC 7973)	Paying attention to pressure redistribution prior to and after surgery	
	Evaluation/Risk assessment	
	Assessment of individual risk for developing pressure ulcers using risk assessment tools	
	Assessment of other intrinsic/extrinsic risk factors	
	Assessment of skin	
	Assessment of nutritional status	
	Assessment for history of prior ulcer and/or presence of current ulcer, previous treatments, or surgical interventions	
	Assessment for potential complications associated with pressure ulcers	
	Prevention/Management/Treatment	
	Measures to minimize shear-related injury	
	Measures to redistribute pressure	
	Use of skin protectant	
	Nutritional management	
	Use of a low-air loss or air-fluidized surface	
	Bowel/bladder management program	
	Implement strategies to optimize healing	
	Wound management	
	Use of antibiotics (e.g., topical, systemic)	
	Debridement of devitalized tissue	
	Adjunctive therapies as indicated	
	Evaluation of need for operative repair	
	Evaluation and management of pain	
	Patient/caregiver education	

(continued)

Table 11.3 (continued)

Organization (National Guideline Clearinghouse reference #)	Guideline	Outcomes
ICSI (2012) (NGC 8962)	Evaluation/Prevention/Risk assessment Assessment and daily reevaluation of all patients for the risk of pressure ulcer development (use of Braden Scale or Braden Q scale) Documentation of the risk assessment Prevention plan and documentation Initiation of pressure ulcer prevention plan (minimizing/eliminating friction, minimizing pressure, support surfaces, managing moisture, maintaining adequate nutrition/hydration) Educating patients and caregivers Skin inspection and documentation Management/Treatment Comprehensive assessment including wound evaluation and documentation Review of history and physical, with emphasis on pressure ulcer Wound description/staging Review of etiology of pressure Assessment of nutritional status Monitoring the wound for signs of infection Assessment of psychosocial needs Pressure ulcer treatment Establishing the treatment goal Moist wound healing Cleansing the wound Choosing appropriate topical wound care products Wound debridement Consideration of adjunct therapy (including negative pressure wound therapy, electrical stimulation) Pain management Management of nutrition (specific nutrient goals, vitamin and mineral supplement) Surgical consultation Patient and staff education Discharge plan or transfer of care Documentation of all items in patient's medical record	Prevalence of pressure ulcers in healthcare facilities Effectiveness of treatment http://www.icsi.org/pressure_ulcer_treatment_protocol_ulcer_treatment_protocol_review_and_comment_/pressure_ulcer_treatment_protocol__.html

Guideline	Recommendations	Measures
AAWC (2010) (NGC 8120)	**Evaluation/Risk assessment/Screening** Initial and continuous pressure ulcer risk assessment using valid, reliable scales (including Braden scale) Nutritional assessment with a validated measure Document medical and surgical history Assessment of psychosocial conditions and quality of life Environmental assessment Physical examination including wound assessment Diagnostic tests **Prevention/Rehabilitation** Skin inspection and maintenance Hydration and nutrition plan of care Rehabilitative and restorative programs Positioning standards of care to manage pressure ulcers Off-loading equipment including chairs, intensive care, and operating rooms Interdisciplinary team approach Education **Management/Treatment** Remove/alleviate all causes of pressure ulcer damage Debride, cleanse, and dress the wound Advanced or adjuvant interventions Surgical interventions Documentation of response Palliative care	Risk-adjusted pressure ulcer prevalence and incidence Risk-adjusted pressure ulcer healing time, pain, odor, and infections Risk-adjusted percent of pressure ulcers healed by 4–20 weeks of care Risk-adjusted pressure ulcer recurrence Patient and professional satisfaction with pressure ulcer care and outcomes Cost effectiveness of healing (e.g., per pressure ulcer healed) Cost-effectiveness of prevention (e.g., per 100 pressure ulcer-free days)
AMDA (2008) (NGC 6410)	**Recognition/Assessment** Examination of the patient's skin thoroughly to identify pressure ulcers Assessment for risk factors for developing pressure ulcers such as comorbid conditions, drugs that may affect ulcer healing, history of pressure ulcers, impaired or decreased mobility, and others using risk assessment instruments (e.g., the Braden Scale for Predicting Pressure Sores, the Norton Score) Assessment of the patients overall physical and psychosocial health and characterization (staging) of the pressure ulcer	Prevalence and incidence of pressure ulcers in long-term care settings Reliability and validity of risk assessment tools for pressure ulcers Efficacy of intervention measures Time to healing

(continued)

Table 11.3 (continued)

Organization (National Guideline Clearinghouse reference #)	Guideline	Outcomes
	Identification of physiologic, functional, and psychosocial factors that can affect ulcer treatment and healing	
	Identification of priorities in managing the ulcer and the patient including identification and treatment of causative factors and modifiable comorbid conditions, optimal nutritional support, prevention and management of infection of the ulcer, and others	
	Treatment/Prevention	
	Establishment of a realistic, individualized interdisciplinary care plan	
	Provision of general support for the patient including hydration, nutrition, pain management, and psychosocial support	
	Management of pressure by proper positioning, turning and transferring techniques; using appropriate positioning devices, support surfaces, and offloading devices; maintaining the lowest possible head elevation	
	Management of infection using topical antibiotics (e.g., bacitracin–polymyxin) if indicated or silver dressing	
	Debridement of necrotic tissue from the ulcer (autolytic, enzymatic, mechanical, surgical)	
	Covering and protecting the ulcer and surrounding skin using appropriate ulcer care products and dressings	
	Management of comorbid conditions (e.g., anemia, chronic obstructive pulmonary disease, diabetes, heart failure, peripheral vascular disease) that may contribute to pressure ulcer risk	
	Monitoring	
	Monitoring and documentation of the patient's progress and ulcer healing	
	Recognition and management of ulcer complications such as increasing necrosis, infection, cellulitis	
	Reassessment of treatment and change in approaches if indicated; consideration of surgery and adjunctive therapies (e.g., negative pressure wound therapy)	
	Monitoring of the facility's management of pressure ulcers using specific indicators	
HIGN (2008) (NGC 6346)	Assessment of pressure ulcers	Prevalence of new pressure ulcers
	Risk assessment	Prevalence of nonhealing pressure ulcers
	Braden Risk Score	
	Stage I pressure ulcers in patients with darkly pigmented skin	

Prevention strategies	
Braden Risk Score	
Management of pressure ulcers	
Risk assessment documentation	
Care issues and interventions: mobilization, skin care, moisture, positioning, use of devices, nutrition, friction and shear	
Assessment of skin tears	
Risk assessment	
Three group risk assessment tool	
Payne-Martin classification system	
Prevention	
Safe environment	
Staff/caregiver education	
Protect from self-injury and skin injury during routine care	
Management/Treatment of skin tears	
Assess size of wound	
Cleaning wounds	
Application and removal of dressings	
Use of skin sealants, protective ointments, liquid barriers	Prevalence of skin tears
	Prevalence of nonhealing skin tears

NPUAP National Pressure Ulcer Advisory Panel, European Pressure Ulcer Advisory Panel. Pressure ulcer prevention recommendations. In: Prevention and treatment of pressure ulcers: clinical practice guideline. Washington (DC): National Pressure Ulcer Advisory Panel; 2009

WOCN Wound, Ostomy, and Continence Nurses Society. Guideline for prevention and management of pressure ulcers. Mount Laurel (NJ): Wound, Ostomy, and Continence Nurses Society (WOCN); 2010 Jun 1. 96 p (WOCN clinical practice guideline; no. 2)

ICSI Institute for Clinical Systems Improvement. Pressure ulcer prevention and treatment protocol. Health care protocol. Bloomington (MN): Institute for Clinical Systems Improvement (ICSI); 2012 Jan. 88

AAWC Association for the Advancement of Wound Care. Association for the Advancement of Wound Care guideline of pressure ulcer guidelines. Malvern (PA): Association for the Advancement of Wound Care (AAWC); 2010. 14 p

AMDA American Medical Directors Association. Pressure ulcers in the long-term care setting. Columbia (MD): American Medical Directors Association (AMDA); 2008. 44 p

HIGN Hartford Institute for Geriatric Nursing. http://www.hartfordign.org from Ayello EA, Sibbald RG. Preventing pressure ulcers and skin tears. In: Capezuti E, Zwicker D, Mezey M, Fulmer T, editor(s). Evidence-based geriatric nursing protocols for best practice. 3rd ed. New York (NY): Springer Publishing Company; 2008 Jan. pp. 403–29

practice guidelines for comparison. In general, pressure ulcer prevention clinical practice guidelines all involve attention to risk assessment, skin assessment, management of tissue loads with repositioning and use of pressure redistribution support surfaces, nutrition assessment, and incontinence management. Much of pressure ulcer prevention is routine care that is delivered at frequent intervals 24 hours a day, 7 days a week in the context of other care delivery. Yet, even as the care is routine, it is also necessary to individual pressure ulcer prevention to the individual risk factors for a particular patient. A successful pressure ulcer prevention program is multidisciplinary and multifaceted.

The pressure ulcer quality indicators previously discussed are instrumental for monitoring care delivery, reporting, and reimbursement purposes. However, documentation and implementation are separate issues. For quality indicators to be meaningful, they must be put into practice. In addition to tying quality indicators to reimbursement, quality indicators must be written in such a way that is feasible in terms of time and cost for health care providers to implement.

Suggestions for Improving Practice

One of the obstacles in preventing pressure ulcers is implementing and maintaining a prevention program within an organization [102]. Facilities often fail to show an improvement in pressure ulcer outcomes such as incidence because attention has not been focused on the process of implementing and maintaining new interventions in an organization. Successful pressure ulcer prevention requires a comprehensive multipronged approach for implementation. A single implementation strategy is not a successful approach. Use of multiple implementation strategies is more likely to succeed and those discussed below have demonstrated success across health care settings.

An interdisciplinary approach is fundamental in pressure ulcer prevention [102]. One of the commonalities prevalent in recent successful quality improvement efforts in acute care and NHs is multidisciplinary collaboration. Stakeholders that may be included in the pressure ulcer team are: wound care specialists, nurses, nutritionists or dieticians, physical therapists, social workers, and physicians or primary care providers from a variety of disciplines (e.g., vascular surgery, plastic surgery, geriatricians, nurse practitioners). The cross-disciplinary care can allow for a resident to receive debridement from a certified wound specialist or plastic surgeon, diet, and nutritional status evaluation by a nutritionist, wheelchair support surface pressure mapping and mobility conditioning by a physical therapist, and pain management by a primary care provider. Through the coordinated efforts of the multidisciplinary team, effective and efficient care can be successfully achieved. This can be accomplished with skin care rounds. Use of a multidisciplinary team that meets/rounds on at-risk patients weekly is a strategy that has worked in all health care settings as the key clinicians have an opportunity to provide input into the care plan for individual patients. Yet, when a multidisciplinary team is involved, there are opportunities for failed communication. Thus, those pressure ulcer prevention programs that have demonstrated success incorporate methods of improving communication among the health care team as part of the implementation plan. Implementation of a standardized means of communication such as SBAR (situation, background, assessment, and recommendation) for acute care can facilitate continuity of care. Using standardized communication ensures that there is little misunderstanding on the severity or meaning of words used. This standardized communication can ensure that each member of the healthcare team has a current understanding of the patient's condition and is aware of the priority goals of care. A critical part of this communication vehicle is use of standard tools for reporting activities. For example, if a NH uses the Braden Scale for Predicting Pressure Sores as the pressure ulcer risk assessment tool, then all clinicians including direct care staff should be familiar with the tool. Use of the same standard tools facilitates accurate communication about the patient's pressure ulcer risk status, prevention strategies in use, and response to prevention.

Research has shown improved pressure ulcer prevention outcomes for programs that bundle a standardized set of care practices and create an acronym for the bundled care practices [83, 85, 87, 90, 102–105]. Similar to the bundles created for prevention of ventilator-associated pneumonia (VAP) or surgical site infection (SSI) in the acute care setting, the NO ULCERS and SKIN bundles have been established as a means to prevent the inadvertent omission of any steps in pressure ulcer care. The NO ULCERS bundle, created by the New Jersey Hospital Association is an acronym for Nutrition and fluid status, Observation of skin, Up and walking or turn and position, Lift (don't drag) skin, Clean skin and continence care, Elevate heels, Risk assessment, and Support surfaces for pressure redistribution [104]. Similarly, the SKIN (Surface selection, Keep turning, Incontinence management, and Nutrition) bundle acts as an alternative tool kit for standardizing pressure ulcer prevention and management [83, 85, 102, 104]. Such bundles serve as a reminder of what procedures of pressure ulcer care are most important and provide clinicians with a consistent set of interventions that can be referenced for improved communication. The acronyms assist in communication and motivation, examples of other acronyms include SOS—save our skin; PUPP—pressure ulcer prevention program. Bundles work because they have built in redundancy; if one aspect of care is missed when the next care practice is delivered, the missed care is caught and corrected. One of the distinct advantages of bundles is that it allows multiple disciplines to communicate effectively regarding the status of care already received and care that has yet to be performed. Thus, the bundle can clarify when and where to make referrals and ease the continuity of care between disciplines and effectively direct front line staff such as CNAs.

Incorporating routine audits of behaviors with prompt feedback on performance to clinicians is an essential component of most successful implementation strategies. Providing feedback on performance communicates the status of the implementation of the new program and demonstrates where improvement is needed. Providing feedback from data-based audits is most successful when the feedback is timely and focused and unit based. For example, feedback should be provided on a unit or individual level as compared to on an organization as whole.

The audit procedure to collect data on clinician behavior needs to be quick and easily conducted or there is a risk of the audit becoming so burdensome and time consuming that it is not performed. This leads to lack of feedback data to clinicians and the disappearance of the program. Audit data provides the information that can be used to further improve the program. Thus, implementation is a continual process that is data-driven based on frequent use of audit and feedback approaches. Small experiments to improve the program can be conducted through quality improvement cycles of plan–do–study–act [102]. This is the premise that drives the collaborative approach to improving pressure ulcer care.

Another process that is effective in implementing pressure ulcer prevention programs is use of a unit-based skin champion, a clinician that is focused on improving the skin care of patients on a particular unit. But involvement of clinicians and direct care providers is not enough. Leadership of the organization must be actively supportive of the program. The influence that top administration can make on motivating direct care providers in implementing the program cannot be overstated. Ongoing support, commitment, and recognition from all levels of leadership in the organization is critical to success.

Many investigators have found use of visual cues such as turning clocks, stickers on medical records, arm bands on patients at risk, pocket sized reference cards for nurses, or newsletters updating staff on progress. These cues provide a nonverbal method of quickly communicating patient status to all who work in the organization or provide a quick reference for nurses and direct care providers at the bedside.

While these recommendations do not include all strategies for implementing a pressure ulcer prevention program, they provide some guidance on what has worked in organizations. One of the difficulties in evaluating implementation of pressure ulcer prevention programs is that there is limited data on sustainability of such programs. There is little data available to know what strategies are successful in different types of organizations or with long-term sustainability of a program or even *if* a program can be institutionalized such that it is maintained. These strategies assume that the organization has a person who is knowledgeable about pressure ulcers. In some areas, access to a knowledgeable wound care clinician is not available. In these cases, use of telehealth may be helpful in implementing a pressure ulcer prevention program.

Quality of Life

While quality of care is important, it is also important to take into account the related concept, quality of life. Quality-adjusted life years (QALY) is a measure of disease burden, including both the quality and the quantity of life lived [105]. It is used in assessing the value for money of a medical intervention. The QALY model requires utility independent, risk neutral, and constant proportional tradeoff behavior [105]. Limited data exist to help us examine this. QALY is a measurement that takes into account length of survival and the quality of that survival (based on public ranking of the health condition), with low quality. The QALY is useful to compare quality of life between individuals in the same population or for the same individual provided different treatment options.

Pham and colleagues [106] compared current pressure ulcer prevention practice in 613 LTACHs in Canada with four quality improvement strategies and evaluated lifetime risk of stage II–IV pressure ulcers, QALYs, and lifetime costs. The four strategies included (1) pressure redistribution support surfaces for all residents, (2) oral nutritional supplements for high risk residents with recent weight loss, (3) skin emollients for high-risk residents with dry skin, and (4) foam cleansing for high-risk residents requiring incontinence care. Strategies on average cost $11.66 per resident and they reduced lifetime risk. The associated numbers needed to treat for each strategy were 45, 333, 158, and 63, respectively. The probability that each quality improvement strategy is cost effective increases as decision makers increase their willingness-to-pay for more QALYs. Strategy 1 and 4 slightly improved QALYs and reduced mean lifetime cost by $115 and $179 per resident, respectively. The authors report that clinical and economic evidence supports pressure redistribution support surfaces (strategy 1) for all long-term care residents [106]. Additional studies evaluating QALYs are not available related to pressure ulcer care, yet these data are valuable for making informed decisions about pressure ulcer prevention.

Pressure ulcers are complex multifaceted costly clinical conditions that require sustained coordinated approaches for successful outcomes. This is true for all healthcare settings. Quality of pressure ulcer care is monitored in each health care setting using quality indicators developed from multiple organizations. The issue of quality of pressure ulcer care is complicated by numerous regulations and multiple clinical practice guidelines. In this chapter we have reviewed outcome and process measures related to pressure ulcer prevention, pressure ulcer regulations and quality indicators across healthcare settings, and specific strategies for implementing pressure ulcer prevention programs all of which are essential for improving quality of care for pressure ulcers.

References

1. Strategies for preventing pressure ulcers. Jt Comm Perspect Patient Saf. 2008; 8(1):5–7(3). Available from: http://www.jcrinc.com/Pressure-Ulcers-stage-III-IV-decubitis-ulcers/. Accessed 23 Mar 2013.
2. Centers for Medicare & Medicaid Services. Proposed fiscal year 2009 payment, policy changes for inpatient stays in general acute care hospitals. Available from: http://www.cms. hhs.gov/apps/media/press/factsheet.asp. Accessed 4 Aug 2010.
3. Brem H, Maggi J, Nierman D, Rolnitzky L, Bell D, Rennert R, Golinko M, Yan A, Lyder C, Vladeck B. High cost of stage IV pressure ulcers. Am J Surg. 2010;200(4):473–7.
4. Centers for Medicare & Medicaid Services. Medicare program; proposed changes to the hospital inpatient prospective payment systems and fiscal year 2009 rates; proposed changes to disclosure of physician ownership in hospitals and physician self-referral rules; proposed collection of information regarding financial relationships between hospitals and physicians: proposed rule. Federal register. 2008;73(84):23550. Available from: http://edocket.access. gpo.gov/2008/pdf/08-1135.pdf. Accessed 4 Aug 2010.

5. Russo C, Steiner C, Specter W. Hospitalizations related to pressure ulcers among adults 18 years and older, 2006. Healthcare Cost and Utilization Project. 2008. Available from: http://www.hcup-us.ahrq.gov/reports/statbriefs/sb64.pdf. Accessd 4 Aug 2010.

6. Stroupe K, Manheim LM, Evans CT, Guihan M, Ho C, Li K, Cowper-Ripley D, Hogan TP, St. Andre JR, Huo Z, Smith B. Cost of treating pressure ulcers for persons with spinal cord injury. Top Spinal Cord Inj Rehab. 2011;16(4):62–73.

7. Berlowitz DR, Brandeis GH, Morris JN, et al. Deriving a risk-adjustment model for pressure ulcer development using the minimum data set. J Am Geriatr Soc. 2001;49:866–71.

8. Allman RM. Pressure ulcer prevalence, incidence, risk factors, and impact. Clin Geriatr Med. 1997;13:421–36.

9. Allman RM. Pressure ulcers: using what we know to improve quality of care. J Am Geriatr Soc. 2001;49:996–7.

10. Xakellis Jr GC. Quality assurance programs for pressure ulcers. Clin Geriatr Med. 1997;13:599–606.

11. Berlowitz DR, Bezerra HQ, Brandeis GH, Kader B, Anderson JJ. Are we improving the quality of nursing home care: the case of pressure ulcers. J Am Geriatr Soc. 2000;48(1):59–62.

12. Bergstrom N, Braden B. A prospective study of pressure sore risk among institutionalized elderly. J Am Geriatr Soc. 1992;40(8):747–58.

13. National Pressure Ulcer Advisory Panel, Pieper B, editors. Pressure ulcers: prevalence, incidence and implications for the future. Reston, MA: NPUAP; 2012.

14. Brandeis GH, Morris JN, Nash DJ, Lipsitz LA. The epidemiology and natural history of pressure ulcers in elderly nursing home residents. JAMA. 1990;264(22):2905–9.

15. Berlowitz DR, Brandeis GH, Anderson J, Du W, Brand H. Effect of pressure ulcers on the survival of long-term care residents. J Gerontol A Biol Sci Med Sci. 1997;52(2):M106–10.

16. Wound, Ostomy, and Continence Nurses Society (WOCN). Guideline for prevention and management of pressure ulcers. Mount Laurel, NJ: Wound, Ostomy, and Continence Nurses Society (WOCN); 2010. p. 96. WOCN clinical practice guideline; no. 2.

17. Institute for Clinical Systems Improvement (ICSI). Pressure ulcer prevention and treatment protocol. Health care protocol. Bloomington, MN: Institute for Clinical Systems Improvement (ICSI); 2012. p. 88.

18. Association for the Advancement of Wound Care (AAWC). Association for the advancement of wound care guideline of pressure ulcer guidelines. Malvern, PA: Association for the Advancement of Wound Care (AAWC); 2010. p. 14.

19. American Medical Directors Association (AMDA). Pressure ulcers in the long-term care setting. Columbia, MD: American Medical Directors Association (AMDA); 2008. p. 44.

20. European Pressure Ulcer Advisory Panel and National Pressure Ulcer Advisory Panel. Prevention and treatment of pressure ulcers. Washington, DC: National Pressure Ulcer Advisory Panel; 2009.

21. Whitney J, Phillips L, Aslam R, Barbul A, Gottrup F, Gould L, Robson MC, Rodeheaver G, Thomas D, Stotts N. Guidelines for the treatment of pressure ulcers. Wound Repair Regen. 2006;14(6):663–79. doi:10.1111/j.1524-475X.2006.00175.x. Article first published online: 2 Jan 2007.

22. Bates-Jensen BM, MacLean CH. Quality indicators for the care of pressure ulcers in vulnerable elders. J Am Geriatr Soc. 2007;55:S409–16. doi:10.1111/j.1532-5415.2007.01349.x.

23. Zimmerman DR, Karon SL, Arling G, et al. Development and testing of nursing home quality indicators. Health Care Financ Rev. 1995;16(4):107–27.

24. Report to the Special Committee on Aging, U.S. Senate, California Nursing homes care problems persist despite federal and state oversight. GAO/HEHS-98-202. Washington, DC: United States General Accounting Office: 1998.

25. Harrington C, Carrillo H. The regulation and enforcement of federal nursing home standards, 1991–1997. Med Care Res Rev. 1999;56(4):471–94.

26. Harrington C, Zimmerman D, Karon SL, Robinson J, Beutel P. Nursing home staffing and its relationship to deficiencies. J Gerontol B Psychol Sci Soc Sci. 2000;55(5):S278–87.

27. Park-Lee E, Caffrey C. Pressure ulcer among nursing home residents: United States, 2004. U.S. Department of Health and Human Services, Centers for Disease Control and Prevention, National Center for Health Statistics, NCHS Data Brief, No. 14, February 2009.

28. Fife C. The changing face of wound care: measuring quality. Today's wound clinic. 2012. pp. 10–14. Available from: http://www.todayswoundclinic.com/files/TWC_October2012_Fife2.pdf

29. Schaum KD. 25 years of Medicare reimbursement changes for wound care. Adv Skin Wound Care. 2012;25(2):96.

30. Centers for Medicare and Medicaid. Affordable care act update: implementing medicare cost savings. 2010. Available from: http://www.cms.gov/apps/docs/aca-update-implementing-medicare-costs-savings.pdf. Accessed 24 May 2013.

31. Tippet AW. Reducing the incidence of pressure ulcers in nursing home residents: a prospective 6-year evaluation. Ostomy Wound Manage. 2009;55(11):52–8.

32. Milne CT, Trigilia D, Houle TL, Delong S, Rosenblum D. Reducing pressure ulcer prevalence rates in the long-term acute care setting. Ostomy Wound Manage. 2009;55(4):50–9.

33. Lyder CH, Wang Y, Metersky M, et al. Hospital-acquired pressure ulcers: results from the national Medicare Patient Safety Monitoring System study. J Am Geriatr Soc. 2012;60(9):1603–8.

34. Mor V, Gruneir A, Feng Z, Grabowski DC, Intrator O, Zinn J. The effect of state policies on nursing home resident outcomes. J Am Geriatr Soc. 2011;59(1):3–9.

35. Mant J. Process versus outcome measures in the assessment of quality of health care. Int J Qual Health Care. 2001;13(6):475–480. Available from: http://intqhc.oxfordjournals.org/content/13/6/475.full.pdf

36. Zingmond DS, Ettner SL, Wilber KH, Wenger NS. Association of claims-based quality of care measures with outcomes among community-dwelling vulnerable elders. Med Care. 2011;49(6):553–9.

37. National Quality Forum. NQF: home. Last updated 2013. Available from: http://www.qualityforum.org/Home.aspx. Accessed 25 May 2013.

38. National Quality Forum. Serious reportable events in healthcare 2011. 2011. Available from: http://www.qualityforum.org/WorkArea/linkit.aspx?LinkIdentifier=id&ItemID=69573. Accessed 25 May 2013.

39. National Quality Forum. NQF: serious reportable events. Available from: http://www.qualityforum.org/Topics/SREs/List_of_SREs.aspx. Accessed 25 May 2013.

40. The Joint Commission. National patient safety goals. 2013. Available from: http://www.jointcommission.org/standards_information/npsgs.aspx. Accessed 24 May 2013.

41. The Joint Commission. 2013 National patient safety goals slide presentation. 2013. Available from: http://www.jointcommission.org/assets/1/18/2013_NPSG_Presentation_FINAL_021513.ppt. Accessed 8 May 2013.

42. Askari M, Wierenga PC, Eslami S, Medlock S, De Rooij SE, Abu-Hanna A. Studies pertaining to the ACOVE quality criteria: a systematic review. Int J Qual Health Care. 2012;24(1):80–7. Epub 2011 Dec 2.

43. Wenger NS, Roth CP, Shekelle P, The ACOVE Investigators. Introduction to the assessing care of vulnerable elders-3 quality indicator measurement set. J Am Geriatr Soc. 2007;55:S247–52. doi:10.1111/j.1532-5415.2007.01328.x.

44. Bates-Jensen BM. Pressure ulcers: pathophysiology, detection, and prevention. In: Sussman C, Bates-Jensen BM, editors. Wound care: a collaborative practice manual for health care practitioners. 4th ed. Baltimore, MD: Lippincott Williams & Wilkins; 2012.

45. Centers for Medicare and Medicaid. MDS 3.0 RAI manual. Updated May 8, 2013. Available from: http://www.cms.gov/Medicare/Quality-Initiatives-Patient-Assessment-Instruments/NursingHomeQualityInits/MDS30RAIManual.html. Accessed 25 May 2013.

46. National Database of Nursing Quality Indicators (NDNQI). Available from: http://nursingworld.org/MainMenuCategories/ThePracticeofProfessionalNursing/PatientSafetyQuality/Research-Measurement/The-National-Database/NDNQIBrochure.pdf. Accessed 25 May 2013.

47. Collaborative Alliance for Nursing Outcomes. CALNOC – collaborative alliance for nursing outcomes. Available from: http://www.calnoc.org/. Accessed 25 May 2013.
48. American Nurses Credentialing Center (ANCC). Magnet recognition program overview. Available from: http://www.nursecredentialing.org/Magnet/ProgramOverview
49. Centers for Medicare and Medicaid. Hospital-acquired conditions. Available from: http://www.cms.gov/Medicare/Medicare-Fee-for-Service-Payment/HospitalAcqCond/Hospital-Acquired_Conditions.html. Accessed 24 May 2013.
50. Hutchinson AM, Milke DL, Maisey S, et al. The resident assessment instrument-minimum data set 2.0 quality indicators: a systematic review. BMC Health Serv Res. 2010;10:166.
51. Centers for Medicare and Medicaid. Nursing home compare. Available from: http://www.medicare.gov/NursingHomeCompare/search.aspx. Accessed 25 May 2013.
52. Centers for Medicare and Medicaid Services. Nursing home quality initiatives: quality measures. Last updated April 12, 2013. Available from: http://www.cms.gov/Medicare/Quality-Initiatives-Patient-Assessment-Instruments/NursingHomeQualityInits/NHQIQualityMeasures.html. Accessed 24 May 2013.
53. Stevenson DG, Mor V. Targeting nursing homes under the Quality Improvement Organization program's 9th statement of work. J Am Geriatr Soc. 2009;57(9):1678–84.
54. Bates-Jensen BM, Alessi C, Cadogan M, et al. The Minimum Data Set bedfast quality indicator: Is it accurate and does it reflect differences in care processes related to time in bed and mobility decline? Journal of the American Geriatrics Society. Apr 2003;51(4):S71-S71.
55. Schnelle JF, Cadogan MP, Yoshii J, Al-Samarrai NR, Osterweil D, Bates-Jensen B, Simmons S. The minimum data Set urinary incontinence quality indicators: do they reflect differences in care processes related to incontinence? Med Care. 2003;41(8):909–22.
56. Levine JM, Roberson S, Ayello EA. Essentials of MDS 3.0 section M: skin conditions. Adv Skin Wound Care. 2010;23(6):273–84. quiz 285–276.
57. Centers for Medicare and Medicaid. Long-term care hospital quality reporting program guidance. Last updated March 1, 2012. Available from: http://www.cms.gov/Medicare/Quality-Initiatives-Patient-Assessment-Instruments/LTCH-Quality-Reporting/Downloads/LTCH-Quality-Reporting-QGP-Guidance.pdf. Accessed 24 May 2013.
58. Centers for Medicare and Medicaid. Quality care finder. Available from: http://www.medicare.gov/quality-care-finder/. Accessed 25 May 2013.
59. Centers for Medicare and Medicaid. Nursing home compare. Available from: http://www.medicare.gov/nursinghomecompare/. Accessed 25 May 2013.
60. Centers for Medicare and Medicaid. Hospital compare. Available from: http://www.medicare.gov/hospitalcompare/. Accessed 25 May 2013.
61. Clancy CM. CMS's hospital-acquired condition lists link hospital payment, patient safety. Am J Med Qual. 2009;24(2):166–8.
62. Black JM, Edsberg LE, Baharestani MM, et al. Pressure ulcers: avoidable or unavoidable? Results of the National Pressure Ulcer Advisory Panel Consensus Conference. Ostomy Wound Manage. 2011;57(2):24–37.
63. Centers for Medicare and Medicaid. Post-Acute care payment reform demonstration: final report. Available from: http://www.cms.gov/Research-Statistics-Data-and-Systems/Statistics-Trends-and-Reports/Reports/Downloads/PAC-PRD_FinalRpt_Vol2of4.pdf. Accessed 25 May 2013.
64. Centers for Medicare and Medicaid. Federal Register. Volume 77(102). 2012. Available from: http://www.gpo.gov/fdsys/pkg/FR-2012-08-31/pdf/2012-19079.pdf. Accessed 25 May 2013.
65. Centers for Medicare and Medicaid. Guidance to surveyors for long term care facilities. Available from: http://www.cms.gov/Regulations-and-Guidance/Guidance/Manuals/downloads/som107ap_pp_guidelines_ltcf.pdf. Accessed 24 May 2013.
66. Lyder CH, Ayello EA. Pressure ulcer care and public policy: exploring the past to inform the future. Adv Skin Wound Care. 2012;25(2):72–6.
67. Thomas DR. The new F-tag 314: prevention and management of pressure ulcers. J Am Med Dir Assoc. 2006;7(8):523–31.

68. Rapp MP, Nelson F, Slomka J, Persson D, Cron SG, Bergstrom N. Practices and outcomes: pressure ulcer management in nursing facilities. Nurs Adm Q. 2010;34(2):E1–e11.
69. Bates-Jensen BM, Cadogan M, Osterweil D, et al. The minimum data set pressure ulcer indicator: does it reflect differences in care processes related to pressure ulcer prevention and treatment in nursing homes? J Am Geriatr Soc. 2003;51(9):1203–12.
70. Centers for Medicare and Medicaid. Quality improvement organizations. Available from: http://www.cms.gov/Medicare/Quality-Initiatives-Patient-Assessment-Instruments/QualityImprovementOrgs/index.html?redirect=/qualityimprovementorgs. Accessed 25 May 2013.
71. Horn SD, Sharkey SS, Hudak S, et al. Beyond CMS quality measure adjustments: identifying key resident and nursing home facility factors associated with quality measures. J Am Med Dir Assoc. 2010;11(7):500–5.
72. Rantz MJ, Cheshire D, Flesner M, et al. Helping nursing homes "at risk" for quality problems: a statewide evaluation. Geriatr Nurs. 2009;30(4):238–49.
73. Rantz MJ, Zwygart-Stauffacher M, Hicks L, et al. Randomized multilevel intervention to improve outcomes of residents in nursing homes in need of improvement. J Am Med Dir Assoc. 2012;13(1):60–8.
74. Baier R, Butterfield K, Patry G, Harris Y, Gravenstein S. Identifying star performers: the relationship between ambitious targets and nursing home quality improvement. J Am Geriatr Soc. 2009;57(8):1498–503.
75. Sharkey S, Hudak S, Horn SD, Barrett R, Spector W, Limcangco R. Exploratory study of nursing home factors associated with successful implementation of clinical decision support tools for pressure ulcer prevention. Adv Skin Wound Care. 2013;26(2):83–92. quiz p.93-84.
76. Temkin-Greener H, Cai S, Zheng NT, Zhao H, Mukamel DB. Nursing home work environment and the risk of pressure ulcers and incontinence. Health Serv Res. 2012;47(3 Pt 1):1179–200.
77. Soban LM, Hempel S, Munjas BA, Miles J, Rubenstein LV. Preventing pressure ulcers in hospitals: a systematic review of nurse-focused quality improvement interventions. Jt Comm J Qual Patient Saf. 2011;37(6):245–52.
78. Niederhauser A, VanDeusen LC, Parker V, Ayello EA, Zulkowski K, Berlowitz D. Comprehensive programs for preventing pressure ulcers: a review of the literature. Adv Skin Wound Care. 2012;25(4):167–88. quiz 189–190.
79. Baldelli P, Paciella M. Creation and implementation of a pressure ulcer prevention bundle improves patient outcomes. Am J Med Qual. 2008;23(2):136–42.
80. Bales I, Padwojski A. Reaching for the moon: achieving zero pressure ulcer prevalence. J Wound Care. 2009;18(4):137–44.
81. Catania K, Huang C, James P, Madison M, Moran M, Ohr M. Wound wise: PUPPI: the Pressure Ulcer Prevention Protocol Interventions. Am J Nurs. 2007;107(4):44–52. quiz 53.
82. Chicano SG, Drolshagen C. Reducing hospital-acquired pressure ulcers. J Wound Ostomy Continence Nurs. 2009;36(1):45–50.
83. Courtney BA, Ruppman JB, Cooper HM. Save our skin: initiative cuts pressure ulcer incidence in half. Nurs Manage. 2006;37(4):36, 38, 40 passim.
84. Dibsie LG. Implementing evidence-based practice to prevent skin breakdown. Crit Care Nurs Q. 2008;31(2):140–9.
85. Gibbons W, Shanks HT, Kleinhelter P, Jones P. Eliminating facility-acquired pressure ulcers at Ascension Health. Jt Comm J Qual Patient Saf. 2006;32(9):488–96.
86. Hopkins B, Hanlon M, Yauk S, Sykes S, Rose T, Cleary A. Reducing nosocomial pressure ulcers in an acute care facility. J Nurs Care Qual. 2000;14(3):28–36.
87. LeMaster KM. Reducing incidence and prevalence of hospital-acquired pressure ulcers at Genesis Medical Center. Jt Comm J Qual Patient Saf. 2007;33(10):611–6. 585.
88. Sacharok C, Drew J. Use of a total quality management model to reduce pressure ulcer prevalence in the acute care setting. J Wound Ostomy Continence Nurs. 1998;25(2):88–92.
89. Stoelting J, McKenna L, Taggart E, Mottar R, Jeffers BR, Wendler MC. Prevention of nosocomial pressure ulcers: a process improvement project. J Wound Ostomy Continence Nurs. 2007;34(4):382–8.

90. Young J, Ernsting M, Kehoe A, Holmes K. Results of a clinician-led evidence-based task force initiative relating to pressure ulcer risk assessment and prevention. J Wound Ostomy Continence Nurs. 2010;37(5):495–503.
91. Young ZF, Evans A, Davis J. Nosocomial pressure ulcer prevention: a successful project. J Nurs Adm. 2003;33(7–8):380–3.
92. Baier RR, Gifford DR, Lyder CH, et al. Quality improvement for pressure ulcer care in the nursing home setting: the Northeast Pressure Ulcer Project. J Am Med Dir Assoc. 2003;4(6):291–301.
93. McKeeney L. Improving pressure ulcer prevention in nursing care homes. Br J Community Nurs. 2008;13(9):S15–6. S18, S20.
94. De Laat EH, Schoonhoven L, Pickkers P, Verbeek AL, Van Achterberg T. Implementation of a new policy results in a decrease of pressure ulcer frequency. Int J Qual Health Care. 2006;18(2):107–12.
95. Elliott R, McKinley S, Fox V. Quality improvement program to reduce the prevalence of pressure ulcers in an intensive care unit. Am J Crit Care. 2008;17(4):328–34. quiz 335; discussion 336–327.
96. Hiser B, Rochette J, Philbin S, Lowerhouse N, Terburgh C, Pietsch C. Implementing a pressure ulcer prevention program and enhancing the role of the CWOCN: impact on outcomes. Ostomy Wound Manage. 2006;52(2):48–59.
97. Abel RL, Warren K, Bean G, et al. Quality improvement in nursing homes in Texas: results from a pressure ulcer prevention project. J Am Med Dir Assoc. 2005;6(3):181–8.
98. Rosen J, Mittal V, Degenholtz H, et al. Ability, incentives, and management feedback: organizational change to reduce pressure ulcers in a nursing home. J Am Med Dir Assoc. 2006;7(3):141–6.
99. Gunningberg L, Stotts NA. Tracking quality over time: what do pressure ulcer data show? Int J Qual Health Care. 2008;20(4):246–53.
100. Stausberg J, Lehmann N, Kroger K, Maier I, Schneider H, Niebel W. Increasing pressure ulcer rates and changes in delivery of care: a retrospective analysis at a University Clinic. J Clin Nurs. 2010;19(11–12):1504–9.
101. Elliott J. Strategies to improve the prevention of pressure ulcers. Nurs Older People. 2010;22(9):31–6.
102. Berlowitz D, VanDeusen Lukas C, Parker V, Niederhauser A, Silver J, Logan C, Ayello E, Zulkowski K. Preventing pressure ulcers in hospitals. Quality improvement implementation toolkit. Agency for Healthcare Research and Quality. 2011. Available from: http://www.ahrq.gov/research/ltc/pressureulcertoolkit/. Accessed 29 Apr 2011.
103. Armstrong DG, Ayello EA, Capitulo KL, Fowler E, Krasner DL, Levine JM, Sibbald RG, Smith APS. New opportunities to improve pressure ulcer prevention and treatment: implications of the CMS inpatient hospital care present on admission (POA) indicators/hospital-acquired conditions (HAC) policy. J Wound Ostomy Continence Nurs. 2008;35(5):485–92.
104. Ayello E, Lyder C. Protecting patients from harm: preventing pressure ulcers in hospital patients. Nursing. 2007;37:36–40.
105. McClimans L, Browne JP. Quality of life is a process not an outcome. Theor Med Bioeth. 2012;33(4):279–92. doi:10.1007/s11017-012-9227-z.
106. Pham B, Stern A, Chen W, et al. Preventing pressure ulcers in long-term care: a cost-effectiveness analysis. Arch Intern Med. 2011;171(20):1839–47.

Chapter 12
Legal Aspects of Pressure Ulcer Care

Gregory A. Compton

Abstract Pressure ulcers are serious reportable events that occur in all healthcare settings. Their overall prevalence has not declined dramatically in the past two decades in spite of efforts by multiple government and nongovernmental entities. They account for 45 % of all nursing home litigation in the USA and are a significant proportion of suits filed in other care settings. Tort law as applied to medicine and nursing is designed to deter misconduct and compensate those harmed.

Pressure ulcers are easily recognized, discrete injuries that occur in elderly, frail, and chronically ill people. The individuals affected dwell in complex systems of care and often encounter providers from multiple disciplines. The development of a pressure ulcer that occurs within a system of care not as the result of the action or omission of a single provider is not negligence per se.

To prevail in a malpractice action a plaintiff must show the existence of a doctor–patient relationship, a duty owed to the patient, a breach of the standard of care, and harm. In addition, the alleged harm must be the proximate cause of the injury that prompted the action. Medical experts are needed to offer opinions as to the standard of care particular to the case. Death claims are common in pressure ulcer litigation (approximately 30 %). Malpractice claims can be defended by contesting liability for the undesired outcome, on the amount of alleged damages or both. Many claims are settled pre-suit and most do not go to trial.

Most wound care professionals agree that some pressure ulcers are unavoidable. Identifying patients at risk and applying focused preventative strategies are the duty of the providers in a care system. Developing a reasoned plan of care and effectively applying devices to prevent injury are also part of that duty.

Evidence-based clinical practice guidelines may add value to the care process. Good quality evidence for effective prevention and treatment is lacking. Therefore

G.A. Compton, M.D., C.M.D. (✉)
Geriatric Medicine and Palliative Care, Wound Care Consultant, Hospice Care
of South Carolina, 2948 Seabrook Island Road, Johns Island, SC 29455, USA
e-mail: gacompton@comcast.net

D.R. Thomas and G.A. Compton (eds.), *Pressure Ulcers in the Aging Population:*
A Guide for Clinicians, Aging Medicine 1, DOI 10.1007/978-1-62703-700-6_12,
© Springer Science+Business Media New York 2014

providing a firm basis for the applicable standard of care is difficult and most often left to expert opinion. In addition to practice guidelines, state practice acts and facility policy and procedures may be used as evidence.

The legal route to dispute resolution is a lengthy and arduous process. Anger, fear, and guilt often drive plaintiffs to initiate a case. Defendants are the second victims when a case is filed. Open two-way communication between patients and providers is the proper approach in any clinical situation. It is also the best malpractice avoidance tool yet devised.

Keywords Pressure ulcers • Malpractice • Tort • Legal • Elderly • Standard of care • Expert testimony • Experts • Nursing • Prevention • Wound care • Nursing homes • Hospitals

Tort Law Explained

The chapter covers aspects of pressure ulcer care that has the potential to devolve into civil litigation. A civil suit is brought as a result of a dispute citizens have with each other. The discussion will be further limited to negligent torts since most medical malpractice suits are of that type. A tort is an alleged noncriminal civil wrong for which damages are sought and is distinguished from breach of contract and property disputes. Malpractice is negligence on the part of a professional. Tort law as applied to medicine, nursing, and other healthcare disciplines is intended to deter misconduct and compensate those harmed. It has several other goals including meting out justice, enhancing safety, and providing an outlet to air grievances. Most researchers agree that the current medical malpractice tort system is inefficient and does not meet the stated goals [1]. After 200 years of American jurisprudence and waves of tort reform, most medical professionals view medical malpractice as excessively adversarial, shaming, and unfair [2, 3].

Medical Professional Malpractice as a Cause of Action

Medical malpractice is defined as a failure to "exercise the degree of care and skill that a physician or surgeon of the same medical specialty would use under similar circumstances" [4]. In tort, claiming injury is not enough. The plaintiff must show the following four legal conditions for negligence (1) the defendant(s) owed a duty of care, (2) the defendant(s) failed to conform to the required standard of care, (3) the failure was the proximate cause of the injury, and (4) that the plaintiff suffered harm that is monetary, physical, or emotional damages or death. The standard of proof is the preponderance of evidence. This is sometimes stated as "more likely than not" or greater than a 50 % likelihood. The standard of proof is direct cause (interchangeable with proximate cause), a cause that directly produces the event without any intervening cause. The injury must be reasonably anticipated by the wrongful act. The language in each state's statutes varies, but in essence will involve one of the two following questions. Was the practitioner's breach a substantive element in causing the injury? Would the injury have occurred without the alleged negligence?

Standard of Care

A negligent tort is committed by the failure to observe the standard of care. The standard of care is defined as the degree of care that a reasonable, prudent, or competent provider of similar specialty would exercise under similar circumstances. It is a measure of duty determined by a given set of circumstances, meaning a particular patient, with a specific condition at a defined time and place [5]. It is not general guidance. In addition, the standard of care may involve the practitioner's attention to risks and benefits of an action (or withholding aspects of care). It also assumes appreciation of the potential dangers and pitfalls of the clinical decision. Nowhere in the legal definition is there an explicit duty to communicate with the patient regarding the medical decision. Patient and family communication is within the domain of medical ethics (patient autonomy) [6].

Experts are required, on both sides, to opine as to the standard of care in almost all cases of alleged medical negligence. Many cases require experts from multiple disciplines, one from each type of practitioner who is accused of wrongful behavior.

Role of Experts in Malpractice Litigation

Physician and other professional experts are generally misunderstood by their peers. Courts need credible expert information and opinion to evaluate information that they are not fully competent to understand. Medical malpractice cases rely heavily on expert opinion and testimony because of the specialized nature of the facts. An expert, at time of trial, must be qualified by the court to testify. If disqualified, the expert's testimony may not be heard by the jury.

Balanced experts that do merit reviews for the plaintiff's attorneys can limit frivolous malpractice cases. The plaintiff's bar, for the most part, does not want to waste resources on meritless cases and value expert opinion. Experts who evaluate plaintiff cases and find no merit provide a valuable service by stopping cases before they start. This function is not appreciated by their peers.

In many states, a document or affidavit, often called a certificate of merit, has to be filed with the court in order to proceed. Generally the certificate, signed by an expert, must state that the defendant(s) owed a duty, breached that duty, and there was actual harm. The requirements to file a case vary greatly state to state. Tort reform in many states has narrowed the requirements for experts. Examples include disqualifying retired individuals and limiting the amount of professional time spent on legal matters.

Most medical and nursing professional societies have some form of statement or guidance for member's performance as expert witnesses. The American College of Physicians, the largest Internal Medicine professional association in the USA, encourages members to participate in the legal process "as a component of their professional activities in order to meet the need for medical testimony" [7]. The Council of Medical Specialty Societies has produced a Statement on Qualification and Guidelines for the Physician Expert Witness [8]. It promulgates set of qualifications and recommended behaviors for experts. The American College of Physicians and the American College of Surgeons [9, 10], among others, have adopted these for their members. Nowhere does it discourage physicians to serve as expert witnesses. The guidelines do warn that behaviors and opinions offered are subject to the normal peer review process.

Medical Errors

Alain Enthoven, in his excellent and still timely treatise *Health Plan*, lists seven misconceptions of the recipients of healthcare services [11]. He explodes the myths in detail. They apply to physicians and other healthcare professionals and are listed below:

1. The doctor should be able to know what condition the patient has, be able to answer patient questions precisely, and prescribe the right treatment. If the doctor doesn't, that is incompetence or even malpractice."
2. For every medical condition there is a "best" treatment. It is up to the doctor to know about the treatment and use it. Anything else is unnecessary surgery, waste, fraud, or underservice.
3. Medicine is an exact science. Unlike 50 or 100 years ago, there is now a firm scientific base for what the doctor does. Standard treatments are supported by scientific proof of efficacy.
4. Medical care consists of standard products that can be described precisely and measured meaningfully in standard units such as "inpatient days," "outpatient visits," or "doctor office visits."
5. Much of health care is a matter of life and death or serious pain or disability.
6. More medical care is better than less medical care.
7. People have no control over the timing of their need for medical care. Whatever care is needed is needed right away.

These common misconceptions give context to the concept of perceived medical errors. All bad outcomes are not the result of an error nor do all errors result in harm. Many patients have unrealistic expectations. Even with the best-known care some patients will have complications or die [12].

There are many unknowns in pressure ulcer care [13]. In spite of development and implementation of new technologies for prevention and treatment, the prevalence of

Table 12.1 Important outstanding questions in pressure ulcer care

What are the most important risk factors?
Is the current staging system adequate?
What is the best way to prevent pressure ulcers?
How do providers choose among the myriad of treatment options?
What should be the competencies of the front line wound care professionals?
What should be the competencies of the domain experts called for consultation?

pressure ulcers has not declined significantly in the last 10 years [14, 15]. This is in spite of a growing literature discussing systematic changes to reduce error and improve outcomes in health care in general [16]. Some important unknowns are outlined in Table 12.1. Many of these questions are part of the current research agenda.

Pressure Ulcers and Medical Complexity

Pressure ulcers are defined as localized tissue injury involving interplay of multiple external forces, such as pressure, shear, and friction [17]. Pressure is the perpendicular force that is applied to skin, distorting and compressing the underlying soft tissues and muscle over a bony prominence. Shear stress is diagonal displacement of tissues. Any pressure injury that is accompanied by shear or friction will result in enhanced tissue damage. This is a simple definition. But the mechanisms of development of pressure ulcers belie that simplicity. Many intrinsic, patient-specific factors contribute to the development of pressure ulcers and are ignored in a simple pressure-shear only model [18].

The pressure ulcer is a disease state and is considered a Geriatric Syndrome [19]. The geriatric syndrome is an evolving concept that describes multifactorial health conditions that occur in vulnerable individuals due to the accumulated impairments in multiple systems [20]. Pressure ulcers occur in frail compromised individuals, particularly when there is a precipitous decline in their condition. More than 100 risk factors have been identified for their development.

There are new models emerging to understand which patients develop pressure ulcers and why. One of these models is the association between the evolving syndrome of frailty and pressure ulcers [21]. The burden of disease in a society changes and evolves with advancement in science. One of the barriers to success in decreasing the worldwide pressure ulcer prevalence is that our systems of care are designed to manage diseases of the past and a growing elderly population [22].

One of the roles of the defense attorney is to teach the jury. The lawyer, in concert with an expert, must explain the complex nature of the disease state to a lay audience in terms they understand. Each pressure ulcer case is different with multiple risks and multiple inputs leading to the end result. How well this is done often drives the outcome in litigation.

Patient Safety and Preventable Harm

The concepts of patient safety and medical malpractice are linked. Patient safety as a concept continues to evolve and is an important component of care quality. The Institute of Medicine (IOM) launched "The Quality of Healthcare in America" project in 1998 with the goal of developing strategies that would result in what they deemed "threshold improvements" in healthcare quality over 10 years. The first publication of that project was "To Err is Human: Building a Safer Health System in 1999" [23]. The publication received wide attention in the medical and public press. It sparked debate and was followed by other credible patient safety works [24, 25].

The terms harm, adverse event, and injury should not be used interchangeably. Injury had a legal connotation and suggests negligence when there may be none. The Canadian Disclosure Guidelines define harm as "an outcome that negatively affects a patient's health and/or quality of life" and an adverse event as "an event which results in unintended harm to a patient and is related to care" provided and is unrelated to the underlying medical conditions [26]. There is no consensus on the best metrics to quantify specific types of harm or global harm in a health care system [27].

In 2001 Ken Kizer of the National Quality Forum (NQF) coined the term "Never-Event" [28]. It referred to egregious errors that should never occur such as wrong side surgery. The list was introduced in 2002 and expanded in 2006 to include 27 items. While some items on the list are true never events and can be considered negligence per se, most are not. The term itself is unfortunate and inclusion of "Stage 3 or 4 pressure ulcers acquired after admission to a healthcare facility" is misleading. A better term, also used in NQF reports, is a "serious reportable event." The definition states that the adverse event is unambiguous, is serious, and is usually preventable [29]. Reportable in this context means the occurrence should be internally tracked as an institutional quality metric.

No one will disagree with including "preventing pressure ulcers" as a high priority national patient safety goal. But the nuances must be understood. It should be stressed that neither the NQF nor the Joint Commission is stating that all pressure ulcers are preventable. Further, the NQF definition includes added a specification that excludes progression from Stage 2 to 3 if Stage 2 was recognized on admission.

There is widespread misunderstanding that the Centers for Medicare and Medicaid Services (CMS) views pressure ulcers as "never events" in hospitals. Pressure ulcers are considered "hospital-acquired conditions" (HAC) and are considered "reasonably preventable" if not present on admission [30]. The new CMS designations are designed to limit DRG payments to hospitals for facility-acquired pressure ulcers and other hospital-acquired complications. A HAC is should not be interpreted as an admission of fault. In fact at a recent National Pressure Ulcer Advisory Panel Consensus Conference 100 % of the expert panelists agreed that not all pressure ulcers are preventable [31].

CMS has recognized that, in long-term care settings, pressure ulcers can be unavoidable. This is codified in Tag F314 in the Survey Procedures for Long-Term Care Facilities that lists the methodology to determine if the pressure ulcer was unavoidable [32]. In short a facility must (1) evaluate the resident's clinical condition and risk factors; (2) define and implement interventions that are consistent with the resident's risks and goals; and (3) monitor and evaluate the impact of the intervention or revise the interventions as appropriate in order to call a pressure ulcer unavoidable. It is notable that the surveyors' job is to assess compliance with federal regulations, not make medical determinations as to the standard of care [33].

In 2003 the IOM placed "Frailty associated with old age-preventing falls and pressure ulcers, maximizing function, and developing advanced care plans" in its top 20 priority areas for national action [25]. An updated NQF-endorsed list of Safe Practices for Better Healthcare was published in 2003 and updated in 2009. Safe Practice 27 is Pressure Ulcer Prevention [34]. Pressure Ulcer care and prevention, particularly in the frail elderly, has been high on the policy agenda for 10 years. There is not yet wide consensus on what system changes need to be made to reach these goals [31, 35, 36].

Wound Care Clinical Practice Guidelines and Regulations

There are many extant wound-related Clinical Practice Guidelines. They are useful to understand the best available evidence and the opinions of the writers at the time they are published. Guidelines should never be held out as a definition of the standard of care. Warren Warwick quoted in the New Yorker says of Guidelines, they are a "record of the past they should come with an expiration date" [37]. This is true of the original AHCPR (now AHRQ) Clinical Practice Guidelines Numbers 3 and 15: Pressure Ulcers in Adults: Prediction and Prevention (1992) and Treatment of Pressure Ulcers (1993). While groundbreaking and used extensively to teach wound care principles at the time, these documents have been supplanted by newer research. To quote the preface of these guidelines they are "systematically developed statements to assist practitioner and patient decisions" [38, 39]. Table 12.2 is a current list of useful Practice Guidelines.

The National Guideline Clearinghouse (NGC) is a public resource for evidence-based clinical practice guidelines (found at http://www.guidelines.gov/). There have been few crosswalk comparison of the various pressure ulcer guidelines. There has been some "guideline syntheses" where pressure ulcer recommendations from different associations are compared. A systematic side-by-side comparison of the major guidelines has not been done and content for many has not been validated [41].

The Medical Record as Legal Document

The principal reason to have a complete and accurate record is a vehicle of communication among providers of care. Additionally a clear, accurate, and contemporaneous medical record is the best defense in a lawsuit. Charting by exception is

Table 12.2 Listing of pressure ulcer clinical practice guidelines by major professional societies in the USA, Europe, and Canada

Guideline name and source	Year published NGC #
Pressure ulcers in the long-term care setting. American Medical Directors Association	1996; revised 2008 NGC:006410
Guideline for prevention and management of pressure ulcers. Wound, Ostomy, and Continence Nurses Society—Professional Association	2003 (updated 2010 Jun 1). NGC:007973
Pressure ulcer treatment recommendations. In: Prevention and treatment of pressure ulcers: clinical practice guideline. European Pressure Ulcer Advisory Panel	2009 NGC:008204
Pressure ulcer prevention recommendations. In: Prevention and treatment of pressure ulcers: clinical practice guideline. National Pressure Ulcer Advisory Panel and the European Pressure Ulcer Advisory Panel	2009 NGC:008145
(1) Risk assessment and prevention of pressure ulcers. (2) Risk assessment & prevention of pressure ulcers 2011 supplement. Registered Nurses' Association of Ontario	2002; revised 2005; addendum released 2011 NGC:008720
Association for the Advancement of Wound Care guideline of pressure ulcer guidelines. Association for the Advancement of Wound Care	2010 NGC:008120
Preventing pressure ulcers and skin tears. In: Evidence-based geriatric nursing protocols for best practice. Hartford Institute for Geriatric Nursing	2003; revised 2008 NGC:006346
Guidelines for the Prevention of Pressure Ulcers. Wound Healing Society	2008 [40]

acceptable. Late entries in the record, while better than no entry can be questioned. The late entry should be made as soon as practicable. Accidental charting on the wrong day or time does occur, but can be used to call the entire chart into question.

Wound care documentation is a special case requiring many data elements. Best practice includes length, width, depth, amount, and type of exudate; a description of the wound bed; and the periwound with each sequential assessment. Weekly assessment of each wound is an accepted standard. Photos of wounds are an adjunct and should not be used in place of above. Whether to take photos and place in the record is controversial. Written consent is needed for photos. See Chap. 4 for more detail on wound documentation.

A full head-to-toe assessment is advised on transition to a new care setting or transfer to another unit. A detailed and well-documented skin assessment is a part of that evaluation. If multiple providers are involved, their examinations should comport. The initial head to toe assessment on transfer allows a provided to show that a lesion was present on admission as promoted by CMS.

The monitoring and documentation of skin status at regular intervals in at-risk individuals prior to breakdown is a best practice. While formal documentation is not required under the standard of care, its presence in the record shows diligence and attention to details.

Incident reports and facility statistics are not usually discoverable, but can be put into evidence if it supports a provider's care of the patient. In the nursing home, state survey data is a matter of public record, including resident-specific complaint surveys. If the plaintiff brings nursing home surveys into evidence, the trier of fact needs to be reminded that the case is about a specific patient at a specific time under a unique set of circumstances. Results of surveys are to be used by facilities to monitor compliance with federal regulations and improve overall care processes and are irrelevant in particular.

The Evidence in Pressure Ulcer Care

This chapter will not recapitulate the best practice recommendations for prevention and treatment of pressure ulcers outlined in other chapters. Experts and others who offer opinions about the quality of care rendered in a particular case need to have a firm basis for that opinion. The term evidence-based medicine gets at using randomized controlled trials (RTC) to inform medical decision making and guidelines. Experts that opine in pleadings and at trial should use the best available evidence from the medical literature as the basis of their opinions. They should only fall back on expert opinion when support from the literature does not exist.

One example of available evidence is the state of understanding of topical treatment for pressure ulcers. Saline wet-to-moist dressings, by maintaining a moist wound bed was once the gold standard in topical wound care. Its use is still within the standard of care in spite of the availability of a multitude of advanced wound products and devices. In a recent systematic review by Reddy and colleagues they showed that no particular treatment for pressure ulcers is clearly superior [13]. In another systematic review, hydrocolloid wound dressings were superior to saline dressings in six trials [42]. Otherwise there are few rigorous RCTs comparing treatments in the wound literature. Many of the newer more costly treatment options can be costly and complicated and few have a solid evidence base.

Leape and others leaders in health safety recommend a balanced approach between implementing evidenced-based safety practices versus those that make sense but lack literature support [43]. Innovation in patient care cannot wait for RCTs prior to thoughtful introduction and use. But newer therapies should not used to define the standard of care in legal proceedings.

A pressure ulcer as a cause of contribution to death is an uncommon even. If the ulcer does not heal, most frail individuals die with the ulcer rather than because of it. In the period 1990–2001 the national multiple cause of death database was mined for pressure ulcer-related deaths. The National Center for Health Statistics defines the underlying cause of death as "the disease or injury that initiated the train of events leading to death or the circumstances of the accident or violence, which produced the fatal injury." It was found that pressure ulcers were linked to 114,380 of a total of 27,572,153 recorded deaths in the USA [44]. Pressure ulcer-related deaths, assuming accuracy of death certificate data, account for 0.04 % of the total deaths for that period. Pressure ulcers are an uncommon cause of death.

Communication and Setting Goals

Open two-way communication between patients and providers is the proper approach in any clinical situation. It is also the best malpractice avoidance tool yet devised. Rapport with patients and their families is essential in the clinical encounter. If a pressure ulcer develops, full disclosure of its presence and explanation of the plan of care is essential. Continue to educate the patient and family so to assure adherence and understand goals of care. Education also allows patients or their surrogate to have realistic expectations which may forestall litigation.

There is growing body of literature on care transitions [45]. A proper clinical "hand off" is an essential part of the care when a patient moves to another level of care. Transitional care is defined as "a set of actions designed to ensure the coordination and continuity of health care as patients transfer between different locations or different levels of care within the same location" [46]. As with other health conditions, detailed information regarding the location, stage, measurements, and treatments in progress for the pressure ulcer(s) should be transmitted to the next provider. This should be in writing and be part of the verbal nursing report.

The Ask–Tell–Ask approach to data gathering is a successful paradigm in palliative medicine and works in pressure ulcer care as well. Once informed of the skin status, ask about the patient's perspective on prognosis. This conversation will set the stage for a discussion about goals of pressure ulcer care. Complete healing is often not possible. The time line to closure may exceed 2 years in stage IV pressure ulcers in the elderly [47]. Patients and caregivers need to know what the practitioner knows.

Summary

A pressure ulcer is complex disease entity with multiple etiologies that almost always occurs in compromised patients. Decreasing the prevalence of pressure ulcers continues to challenge practitioners in all care settings. The rates of facility acquired pressure ulcers are considered a quality indicator [48]. They are associated with considerable morbidity and substantial costs. The development of a pressure ulcer is a frequent cause for action in medical malpractice cases.

Many malpractice cases begin with a search for answers to explain an unexpected bad outcome. The legal route to dispute resolution is a lengthy and arduous process. Pressure ulcer lesions have a very distressing appearance to family caregivers. Anger, fear, and guilt often drive plaintiffs to initiate a case when there is lack of understanding of the why and how of a bad, unexpected clinical outcome [49]. Physicians need to take the lead early in the process. It is unfair to the generalist bedside nurse to carry all the burden of explaining complex issues to patients and families. Effective clinical communion and conflict resolution at the bedside is a learned skill [Personal communication J. Richard Compton, M.D.]. If a bedside provider does not feel they are the proper person to answer the patient's query, the concern needs to be acknowledged and prompt referral to the proper authority.

Wound care practitioners need to know the pressure ulcer prevention and treatment guidelines and apply them as appropriate. Detailed documentation serves the patient and is the best defense. Compassionate communication with at-risk patients and families is the physician's ethical obligation and will forestall legal action. Anticipatory guidance promotes understanding of the complexity of the frail, at risk patient. It works better than saying you are sorry and can prevent "second victims" [50].

References

1. Sloan FA, Chepe LM. Medical malpractice. Cambridge, MA: MIT Press; 2008. p. 1.
2. Mehlman MJ. The shame of medical malpractice. J Leg Med. 2006;27:17–32.
3. Annas GJ. Doctors, patients, and lawyers—two cenruries of health law. N Engl J Med. 2012;367:445–50.
4. Garner BA. Black's law dictionary. 7th ed. New York, NY: West; 1999. p. 971.
5. Smith H. A model for validating an expert's opinion in medical negligence cases. J Leg Med. 2005;26:207–31. p. 208.
6. Beauchamp TL, Childress JF. Principle of biomedical ethics. 4th ed. Oxford: Oxford University Press; 1994. p. 120.
7. Position Paper. Guidelines for physician expert witness. Ann Intern Med. 1990; (10):789.
8. Statement on Qualification and Guidelines for the Physician Expert Witness. Council of Medical Specialty Societies. 1989. http://www.cmss.org/DefaultTwoColumn.aspx?id=79. Accessed 7 Jul 2012.
9. Statement on the physician expert witness by the American College of Surgeons. Bulletin of the American College of Surgeons vol. 85, No. 6, Page 24. 2000. http://www.facs.org/fellows_info/statements/st-8.html
10. Jerrold L. The role of the expert witness. Surg Clin North Am. 2007;87(4):889–901. vii–viii.
11. Enthoven AC. Health plan: the practical solution to the soaring cost of medical care. Washington, DC: Addison-Wesley & Beard Books; 1980. p. 2–8. Reprinted 2002.
12. Pronovost PJ, Colantuoni E. Measuring preventable harm helping science keep pace with policy. JAMA. 2009;301:1273–5.
13. Reddy M, Gill SS, Kalkar SR, et al. Treatment of pressure ulcers: a systematic review. JAMA. 2008;300:2647–62.
14. National Pressure Ulcer Advisory Panel, Cuddington J, Ayello EA, Sussman C, editors. Pressure ulcers in America: prevalence, incidence, and implications for the future. Reston, VA: NPUAP; 2001.
15. VanGilder C, Amlung S, Harrison P. Results of the 2008–2009 International Pressure Ulcer Prevalence Survey and a 3-year acute care, unit specific analysis. Ostomy Wound Manage. 2009;55(11):39–45.
16. Leape LL. Error in Medicine. JAMA. 1994;272:1851–7.
17. Black J, Baharestani MM, Cuddigan J, National Pressure Ulcer Advisory Panel, et al. National pressure ulcer advisory panel's updated pressure ulcer staging system. Adv Skin Wound Care. 2007;20:269–74.
18. Thomas DR. Does pressure cause pressure ulcers? An inquiry into the etiology of pressure ulcers. J Am Med Dir Assoc. 2010;11:397–405.
19. Inouye SK, Studenski S, Tinetti ME, Kuchel GA. Geriatric syndromes: clinical, research, and policy implications of a core geriatric concept. J Am Geriatr Soc. 2007;55:780–91.

20. Tinetti ME, Inouye SK, Gill TM, et al. Shared risk factors for falls, incontinence, and functional dependence. Unifing the approach to geriatric syndromes. JAMA. 1995;273:1348–53.
21. Campbell KE. A new model to identify shared risk factors for pressure ulcers and frailty in older adults. Rehabil Nurs. 2009;34:242–7.
22. Jones DS, Podolsky SH, Greene JA. The burden of disease and the changing task of medicine. N Engl J Med. 2012;366:2333–8.
23. Kohn LT, Corrigan JM, Donaldson MS, editors. To err is human: building a safer health system. Washington, DC: National Academies Press; 1999. p. xi.
24. Aspden P, Corrigan JM, Wolcott J, Erickson SM, editors. Patient safety: achieving a new standard for care. Washington, DC: National Academies Press; 2004.
25. Priority areas for national action: transforming health care quality. Washington, DC: National Academies Press; 2003.
26. Disclosure Working Group. Canadian disclosure guidelines. Edmonton, AB: Canadian Patient Safety Institute; 2008.
27. Parry G, Cline A, Goldmann D. Deciphering harm measurement. JAMA. 2012;307(20):2155–6.
28. National Quality Forum. Serious reportable adverse events in health care: update 2006. Washington, DC; 2006.
29. AHRQ: never events. http//www.psnet.ahrq.gov/primer.aspx?priomerID=3. Accessed 15 Jul 2012.
30. Hospital Acquired Conditions. Centers for Medicare and Medicaid Services Web site. https://www.cms.gov/HospitalAcqCond/. Accessed 28 Aug 2012.
31. Black JM, Edsberg LE, Bahaharestani MM, The National Pressure Advisory Panal, et al. Pressure ucers: avoidable or unavoidable? The results of the national pressure ulcer advisory panel consensus conference. Ostomy Wound Manage. 2011;57(2):24–37.
32. Centers for Medicare and Medicaid Services Tag F314. http://www.cms.gov/Regulations-and-Guidance/Guidance/Manuals/downloads/som107ap_pp_guidelines_ltcf.pdf. Accessed 22 Aug 2012.
33. Fife CE, Yankowsky KW, Ayello EA, Capitulo KL, et al. Legal issues in the care of pressure ulcer patients: key concepts for healthcare providers-a consensus paper from the International Expert Wound Care Advisory Panel. Adv Skin Wound Care. 2010;23(11):493–507.
34. National Quality Forum (NQF). safe practices for better healthcare—2009 update: a consensus report. Washington, DC: NQF; 2009.
35. Ayello EA, Lyder CH. A new era of pressure ulcer accountability in acute care. Adv Skin Wound Care. 2008;21:134–40.
36. Sibbald RG, Krasner DL, Woo KY. Pressure ulcer staging revisited: superficial skin changes and deep tissue pressure ulcer framework. Adv Skin Wound Care. 2011;24(12):571–80.
37. Gawande A. The bell curve: what happen when patients find out how good their doctors really are? The New Yorker, Dec 6 2004.
38. Panel for the Prediction and Prevention of Pressure Ulcers in Adults. Pressure ulcers in adults: prediction and prevention. Clinical practice guideline, Number 3. AHCPR Publication No. 92-0047. Rockville, MD: US Department of Health and Human Services; 1992.
39. Bergstrom N, Bennett MA, Carlson CE, et al. Treatment of Pressure Ulcers. Clinical Practice Guideline, Number 15. AHCPR Publication No. 95-0652. Rockville, MD: US Department of Health and Human Services; 1994.
40. Stechmiller JK, Cowan L, Whitney JD, et al. Guidelines for the prevention of pressure ulcers. Wound Repair Regen. 2008;16:151–86.
41. Bolton L, Girolami S, Slaton S, The association for the advancement of wound care guidelines subcommittee, et al. Assessing the need for developing a comprehensive content-validated pressure ulcer guideline. Ostomy Wound Manage. 2008;54(11):22–30.
42. Bouza C, Saz Z, Munoz A, Amate J. Efficacy of advanced dressings in the treatment of pressure ulcers: a systematic review. J Wound Care. 2005;14:193–9.
43. Leape LL, Berwick DM, Bates DW. What practices will most improve safety? Evidence-based medicine meets patient safety. JAMA. 2002;288:501–7.

44. Redelings MD, Lee NE, Sorvillo F. Pressure ulcers: more lethal than we thought? Adv Skin Wound Care. 2005;18(9):367–72.
45. Coleman EA, Berenson RA. Lost in transition: challenges and opportunities for improving the quality of transitional care. Ann Intern Med. 2004;140:533–6.
46. Coleman EA. Fall through the cracks: challenges and opportunities for improving transitional care for persons with continuous complex care needs. J Am Geriatr Soc. 2003;51:549–55.
47. Brandeis GH, Morris LN, Nash DJ, et al. The epidemiology and natural history of pressure ulcers in elderly nursing home residents. JAMA. 1990;265:2905–9.
48. Bates-Jensen BM. Quality indicators for prevention and management of pressure ulcers in vulnerable elders. Ann Intern Med. 2001;135:744–51.
49. Johnson PW. Why lawyers are still targeting pressure ulcers. Extended Care Product News 2005 Mar 31–35. Malvern, PA: A Journal of HMP Communications.
50. In Conversation with Albert Wu, MD, MPH on Second Victims. http://webmm.ahrq.gov/perspective.aspx?perspectiveID=101. Accessed 21 Aug 2012.

Index

Printed in the United States
By Bookmasters